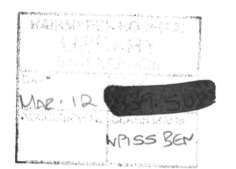

Atlas of
Female Pelvic Medicine and Reconstructive Surgery

Second Edition

Editor

J. Thomas Benson, MD

Clinical Professor
Department of Obstetrics and Gynecology
Associate Director
Female Pelvic Medicine and Reconstructive Surgery Fellowship
Indiana University
Methodist Hospital
Indianapolis, Indiana

With 16 contributors

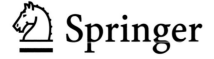

Springer

CURRENT MEDICINE GROUP LLC, PART OF SPRINGER SCIENCE+BUSINESS MEDIA LLC

400 Market Street, Suite 700 • Philadelphia, PA 19106

Senior Developmental Editor	Diana Winters
Developmental Editors	Stephanie Weidel Brown and Colleen Downing
Editorial Assistant	Juleen Deaner
Cover Design	Maureen Looney and Bill MacAdams
Design and Layout	Dan Britt and William Whitman Jr.
Illustrators	Marie Dean, Sara Krause, Wieslawa Langenfeld, Maureen Looney, Annelisa Ochoa, and Giovanna Santori
Production Coordinator	Carolyn Naylor
Indexer	Holly Lukens

Library of Congress Cataloging-in-Publication Data

Atlas of female pelvic medicine and reconstructive surgery / editor, J. Thomas Benson. -- 2nd ed.
   p. ; cm.
 Rev. ed. of: Urogynecology and reconstructive pelvic surgery. c2000.
 Includes bibliographical references and index.
 ISBN 978-1-57340-304-7 (alk. paper)
 1. Urogynecology--Atlases. 2. Generative organs, Female--Surgery--Atlases. 3. Urinary incontinence--Atlases. 4. Fecal incontinence--Atlases. 5. Pelvis--Diseases--Surgery--Atlases. I. Benson, J. Thomas. II. Urogynecology and reconstuctive pelvic surgery.
 [DNLM: 1. Female Urogenital Diseases--Atlases. 2. Fecal Incontinence--Atlases. 3. Prolapse--Atlases. 4. Reconstructive Surgical Procedures--Atlases. WJ 17 A8813 2008]

 RG484.A885 2008
 618.1--dc22

2008019285

ISBN 978-1-57340-304-7
ISBN 1-57340-304-0

www.springer.com

For more information, please call 1 (800) 777-4643
or email us at orders-ny@springer.com

www.currentmedicinegroup.com

10 9 8 7 6 5 4 3 2 1

Printed in China by Hong Kong Graphics and Printing LTD.

This book was printed on acid-free paper

Preface

During the preparation of this atlas, the editor, Dr. J. Thomas Benson, passed away after a 4-year bout with pancreatic cancer. His chapters in this text represent his last work and will serve as a reminder of his many contributions to the field. Dr. Benson was a pioneer in the field of female pelvic medicine and reconstructive surgery who, despite his diagnosis, remained active in patient care and fellow teaching.

Dr. Benson led a full and distinguished career in the field of medicine. He served as chairman and residency program director at Methodist Hospital in Indianapolis for over 20 years. In 1988, Dr. Benson started a fellowship in urogynecology. He, along with the other pioneers in this field, recognized the need for improved care for women with pelvic floor disorders and he dedicated the rest of his life to this mission. In 1996, the American Board of Obstetrics and Gynecology recognized Dr. Benson's program as the first to receive board accreditation in the country. Dr. Benson graduated 18 fellows from this program, the statistic of which he was most proud. He shared his knowledge with others readily and enjoyed helping numerous physicians across the country develop their professional careers.

He served in numerous professional positions including president of American Urogynecologic Society (AUGS) from 1991 to 1992, clinical professor at Indiana University School of Medicine, Advisory Board member for the International Society of Pelvic Neuromodulation, Task Force member of the American Association of Electrodiagnostic Medicine, World Health Organization Committee Member for Definition of Clinical Neurophysiology of the Pelvic Floor, Associate Editor of the International Urogynecology Journal, reviewer for numerous specialty journals, grant reviewer for NIDDK in 2000, American College of Surgeons Advisory Council for Obstetrics and Gynecology member, AUGS Board of Directors and Executive Committee, and United Methodist Children's Home board member, to name but a few. He was sought after as a national and international speaker and enjoyed these opportunities to share his knowledge.

Perhaps what best defined Dr. J. Thomas Benson was his natural curiosity, vision, and passion. Unsatisfied that pelvic floor disorders were the result of simple "defects" in connective tissue, Dr. Benson sought to define the pathophysiology of prolapse and incontinence. He dedicated his later career to the neurodiagnostic evaluation of the pelvis. He progressed from "simple" studies such as pudendal nerve terminal motor latencies to complex pelvic neurophysiologic reflex evaluations and somatosensory-evoked potentials. He became an international expert in needle electromyography of the pelvis and its related pathology. At a time when stress incontinence was thought to be a condition of urethral displacement, Dr. Benson argued the role of the urethral sphincter and its function as the core pathology in stress incontinence.

Likewise, he looked at the levator ani and its dysfunction as the key to women who developed prolapse. He was integral to our understanding of the innervation of the pelvis from both autonomic and somatic views. Although these concepts were initially unpopular, they have become widely accepted in the etiology of prolapse and incontinence. Determined to further his understanding of electrodiagnostic medicine and to legitimize his research, in 1995, at the age of 61, Dr. Benson completed a fellowship in clinical neurophysiology at the Mayo Clinic in Rochester, Minnesota. He became the first and only ob-gyn to become boarded in Electrodiagnostic Medicine.

In addition to his neurophysiologic contributions, early on Dr. Benson discussed issues of fecal incontinence and bowel evacuation problems as an underrecognized component of pelvic floor disorders. At a time when neither patients nor physicians felt comfortable addressing these issues, he was outspoken about the need to discuss these issues with patients.

Of his over 70 peer-reviewed publications, Dr. Benson is perhaps best known for his prospective randomized trial comparing vaginal to abdominal surgery for the treatment of pelvic organ prolapse, the first such study to be completed. A master vaginal surgeon who believed vaginal surgery is what separated gynecologists from general surgeons, Dr. Benson was surprised and somewhat disappointed at the results showing superior outcomes with abdominal surgery. Nonetheless, armed with his results, he informed the medical community of his findings. He won the Society of Gynecologic Surgeons prize paper with this research and often defended his study in lively debates.

Away from medicine, Dr. Benson will be remembered by many in our field for his love of life. He was an avid motorcyclist, owning several Harley Davidsons before their resurgence. His dancing at national and international meetings will be missed as will his challenging of members to different athletic competitions. He was an avid lover of music and played both the guitar and piano. He was an outdoorsman who did not forget the practical lessons learned while being raised on a farm. He was always reading, eager to expose himself and others to new ideas.

Dr. Benson truly believed in the power of teaching and sharing of knowledge as the way to improve patient care. He was disappointed when others with the potential did not dedicate themselves to these same ideals. This text and its contributors represent the ideas and people Dr. Benson believed in. We can best honor Dr. Benson by continuing to push our field forward and challenge current concepts in order to improve patient care.

We all feel a loss with the passing of a person of his stature. We were very fortunate to have him in our field and in our lives. We became better physicians because of him, and our patients received better care through his efforts.

Douglass S. Hale

Contributors

J. Thomas Benson, MD

Clinical Professor
Department of
  Obstetrics and Gynecology
Associate Director
Female Pelvic Medicine and
  Reconstructive Surgery Fellowship
Indiana University
Methodist Hospital
Indianapolis, Indiana

Alfred E. Bent, MD

Professor
Department of Obstetrics
  and Gynecology
Dalhousie University
Head
Division of Gynecology
Department of Obstetrics
  and Gynecology
IWK Health Center
Halifax, Nova Scotia, Canada

**Linda Brubaker, MD, MS,
  FACOG, FACS**

Professor, Departments of
  Ob/Gyn and Urology
Division Director, Female Pelvic
  Medicine and Reconstructive Surgery
Assistant Dean for Clinical and
  Translational Research
Stritch School of Medicine
Loyola University Chicago
Chicago, Illinois

Sarah E. Camp, MD

Resident
Department of Obstetrics
  and Gynecology
George Washington University
Washington, District of Columbia

Renee M. Caputo, MD

Urogynecology and Pelvic
  Floor Associates
Mount Carmel Health Providers, Inc.
Columbus, Ohio

John O. L. DeLancey, MD

Norman F. Miller Professor
  of Gynecology
Director of Pelvic Floor
  Research Group
Director, Fellowship in Female
  Pelvic Medicine/Reconstructive
  Surgery
Department of Obstetrics
  and Gynecology
University of Michigan
Ann Arbor, Michigan

Dee Fenner, MD

Furlong Professor of
  Women's Health
Director of Gynecology
Associate Chair for Surgical Services
University of Michigan
  Health System
Ann Arbor, Michigan

**Douglass S. Hale, MD,
  FACOG, FACS**

Director
Female Pelvic Medicine and
  Reconstructive Surgery Fellowship
Associate Clinical Professor
Department of Obstetrics
  and Gynecology
Indiana University
Director
Urogynecology Research
  Foundation
Department of Urogynecology
Urogynecology Associates
Indianapolis, Indiana

Christina Lewicky-Gaupp, MD

Department of Obstetrics
  and Gynecology
Female Pelvic Medicine and
  Reconstructive Surgery
University of Michigan Hospitals
  and Health Center
Ann Arbor, Michigan

Danielle Markle, MD, MA

Resident Physician
Department of Obstetrics
  and Gynecology
University of California, Irvine
Orange, California

Mary T. McLennan, MD
Associate Professor
Department of Obstetrics,
  Gynecology, and Women's Health
Saint Louis University
Saint Louis, Missouri

Karen L. Noblett, MD
Associate Professor
Department of Obstetrics
  and Gynecology
Director
Division of Female Pelvic Medicine
  and Reconstructive Surgery
University of California Irvine
  Medical Center
Orange, California

Walter S. von Pechmann, MD
Associate Professor of Obstetrics
  and Gynecology
George Washington University
  School of Medicine
National Capitol Consortium
  Fellowship in Female Pelvic Medicine
  and Reconstructive Surgery
Washington, District of Columbia

Laura C. Skoczylas, MD
Resident Physician
Department of Obstetrics
  and Gynecology
University of California, Irvine
Orange, California

**Patrick J. Woodman,
  DO, FACS, FACOOG**
Clinical Associate Professor of
  Obstetrics & Gynecology (Voluntary)
Indiana University School of Medicine
Assistant Director
Female Pelvic Medicine and
  Reconstructive Surgery Fellowship
Indianapolis, Indiana
Assistant Clinical Professor
Department of Osteopathic
  Surgical Specialties
Michigan State University College
  of Osteopathic Medicine
East Lansing, Michigan

Stephen B. Young, MD
Professor
University of Massachusetts
  Medical School
Chief
Division of Urogynecology and
  Reconstructive Pelvic Surgery
Department of Obstetrics
  and Gynecology
University of Massachusetts
  Memorial Medical Center
Worcester, Massachusetts

Contents

Chapter 1
Anatomy. 1
John O. L. DeLancey

Chapter 2
Congenital Anomalies of the Female Genital Tract. 9
Renee M. Caputo

Chapter 3
Neurophysiology of Pelvic Visceral Function. 25
J. Thomas Benson

Chapter 4
Pathophysiology of Pelvic Visceral Dysfunction 53
J. Thomas Benson

Chapter 5
Diagnosis of Urinary Incontinence and Retention 81
Mary T. McLennan and Alfred E. Bent

Chapter 6
Management of Urinary Incontinence and Retention 111
Karen L. Noblett, Danielle Markle, and Laura C. Skoczylas

Chapter 7
Evaluation of Fecal Incontinence and Constipation 149
Dee Fenner and Christina Lewicky-Gaupp

Chapter 8
Treatment of Fecal Incontinence and Constipation 159
Dee Fenner and Christina Lewicky-Gaupp

Chapter 9
Diagnostic Evaluation of Pelvic Organ Prolapse 175
Linda Brubaker

Chapter 10
Nonsurgical Management of Pelvic Organ Prolapse. 187
Stephen B. Young

Chapter 11

Surgical Management of Pelvic Organ Prolapse **203**

Douglass S. Hale

Chapter 12

Urethral Diverticula and Genitourinary Fistulas **229**

Patrick J. Woodman

Chapter 13

Rectovaginal Fistulas **247**

Patrick J. Woodman

Chapter 14

Injuries to the Genitourinary Tract: Prevention, Recognition, and Management **255**

Walter S. von Pechmann and Sarah E. Camp

Index **267**

1

Anatomy

John O. L. DeLancey

Muscles and connective tissues support the pelvic organs by attaching them to the bony pelvis. In women who have pelvic organ prolapse and incontinence, damage to these muscles and fibrous structures results in descent of the vaginal walls and pelvic organs through the urogenital hiatus in the levator ani muscles. Different types of prolapse exist in different women. One woman may have a cystocele, while another may have a cystocele and rectocele. The site at which a muscle or fascia is damaged determines the type of prolapse present. Of course, understanding the nature of these different clinical problems must be based on an accurate understanding of the site and type of defect present. The supportive apparatus that holds the pelvic organs in place was designed to operate in the standing position. This is the orientation in which the pelvic organ supports must be studied and understood. Physicians learn about pelvic anatomy from observing supine cadavers and by examining women in the clinic and operating department who are recumbent. This is somewhat like trying to understand how a parachute works while observing it lying crumpled on the ground. In considering the following anatomy, the reader should keep in mind the anatomic and topographic relationships as they exist under the effects of gravity in the standing individual.

Anatomy is the basic science of reconstructive pelvic surgery. This chapter is intended to provide a view of pelvic anatomy useful to clinicians who wish to understand the nature of pelvic organ prolapse. It is based on illustrative material taken directly from dissections of female cadavers supplemented with macroscopic and microscopic examination of serial sections containing the whole pelvis. Special techniques have been used to minimize embalming artifacts. Careful attention to the illustrations should provide a framework for understanding the clinical topics that follow.

THE BONY PELVIS AND BORDERS OF THE PELVIC FLOOR

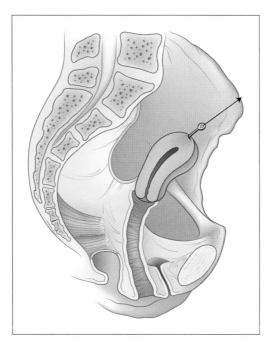

Figure 1-1. Compartments of the pelvis. The pelvis is divided into an anterior and posterior compartment by the vagina and its attachments to the pelvic wall. The walls of the posterior compartment are formed by the sacrum and levator ani muscles. The pubic bones, internal obturator muscles, and the anterior projection of the levator ani muscles form the walls of the anterior compartment. The walls of the vagina are attached to the pelvic walls by the endopelvic fascia and form the separating wall that divides the anterior and posterior compartments.

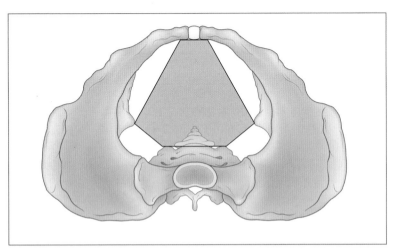

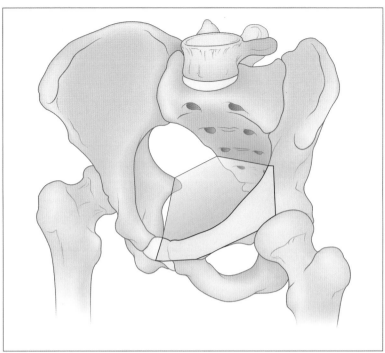

Figure 1-2. Space occupied by the pelvic floor. The boundaries of the pelvic floor are hexagonal. The ventral bounds are the pubic bones anteriorly, the arcus tendinei laterally, and the sacrum and sacrospinous ligaments dorsally. The ischial spines form the lateral points of attachment for both the sacrospinous ligament and the arcus tendinei.

Figure 1-3. Pelvic plane. The plane of the pelvic floor lies oblique to the horizontal plane in the standing position.

LEVATOR ANI MUSCLES AND ENDOPELVIC FASCIA

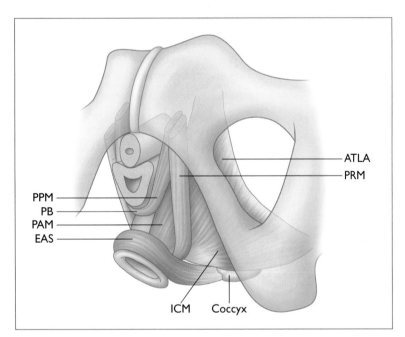

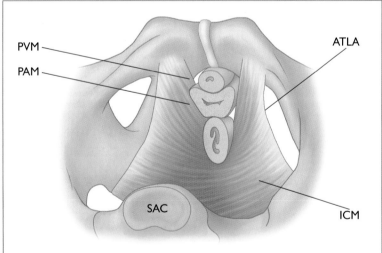

Figure 1-4. Levator ani muscles from below after the vulvar structures and perineal membrane have been removed, showing the arcus tendineus levator ani (ATLA), external anal sphincter (EAS), puboanal muscle (PAM), perineal body (PB) uniting the two ends of the puboperineal muscle (PPM), iliococcygeal muscle (ICM), and puborectal muscle (PRM). Note that the urethra and vagina have been transected just above the hymenal ring.

Figure 1-5. The levator ani muscle seen from above, looking over the sacral promontory (SAC) and showing the pubovaginal muscle (PVM). The urethra, vagina, and rectum have been transected just above the pelvic floor. The internal obturator muscles have been removed to clarify levator muscle origins. PAM—puboanal muscle; ATLA—arcus tendineus levator ani; ICM—iliococcygeal muscle.

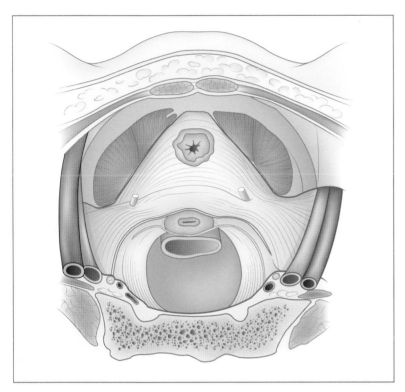

Figure 1-6. Fascial tissues of the pelvis. The fascial tissues that attach the cervix to the pelvic wall are shown from above after the removal of the uterine corpus. Note how the uterosacral ligaments are simply the medial margin of these tissues. Also note the lateral boundary of the pelvic floor formed by the tendinous arch of the pelvic fascia.

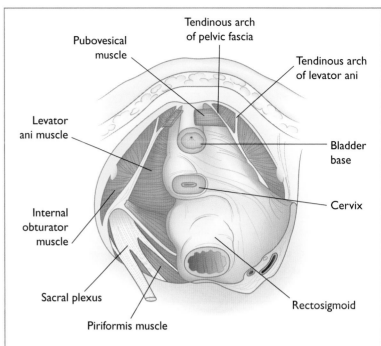

Figure 1-7. The right side of this dissection shows the endopelvic fascia's attachment to the pelvic walls. The other side reveals the position of the levator ani muscles below this level, as well as the nerves of the sacral plexus. Note the proximity of the sacral plexus of nerves to the sacrospinous ligament as they exit the pelvis through the greater sciatic foramen on the inner surface of the piriformis muscle. The boundaries of the pelvic floor, the arcus tendineus, and coccygeus muscle/sacrospinous ligament complex are visible on the cadaver's left side.

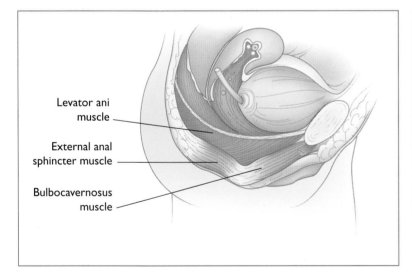

Figure 1-8. Lateral view of the pelvis. The relationship between the pelvic organs and the levator ani muscles is illustrated. A portion of each organ system (urinary, genital, and intestinal) lies above the levator ani muscles. Each system has an orifice below the muscles. As the viscera pass through the pelvic musculature, they are influenced in two ways. First, the sling of the levator ani muscles pulls them toward the pubic bones, constricting their lumens and preventing their downward descent through the attachment of the visceral walls and the muscles. Second, distal sphincters help occlude the lumens of each organ system.

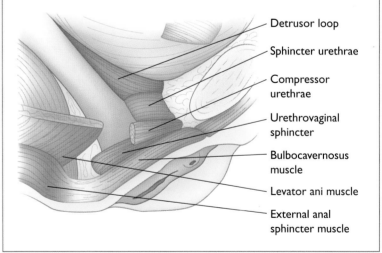

Figure 1-9. In this illustration, the anterior portion of the levator ani muscle has been removed to show the urogenital sphincter muscles. The striated urogenital sphincter muscle has two regions. Just below the vesical neck, the muscle encircles the urethra. Nearer the external meatus, two bands of muscle arch over the dorsal urethral wall. One band, the urethrovaginal sphincter muscle, encircles both the vagina and urethra while the other, the compressor urethra, passes laterally along the ischiopubic rami just cephalad to the perineal membrane (urogenital diaphragm).

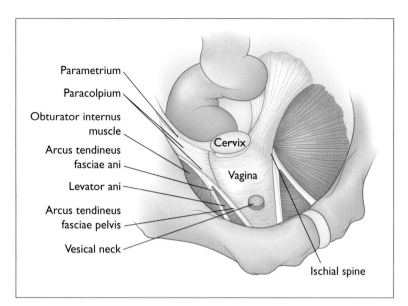

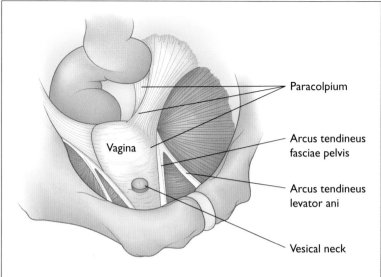

Figure 1-10. Fascial supports of the vaginal apex and anterior vaginal wall. This illustration demonstrates the regional differences in the fascial attachments of the vagina and cervix to the pelvic walls. The bladder and corpus of the uterus have been removed so only the vesical neck and cervix remain. Note that the fascial fibers near the cervix and upper vagina are vertical in orientation, while those attaching to the midvagina are transverse, spanning the space between the fascial arches. It is also possible to see divergence between the two fascial arches. The tendinous arch of the levator ani, from which the levator ani muscle arises, attaches higher on the pubic bone than the tendinous arch of the pelvic fascia, which is the structure to which the endopelvic fascia is attached.

Figure 1-11. Attachments to the pelvic wall after hysterectomy. This figure reveals the situation that is present after hysterectomy. The upper vaginal supports differ from the midvaginal supports.

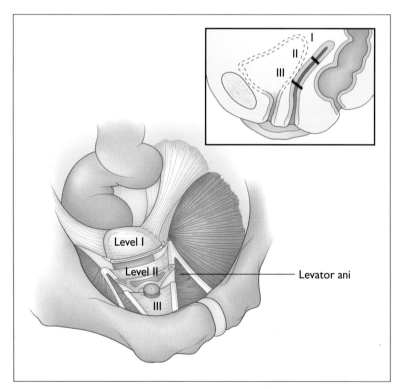

Figure 1-12. The attachments of the vagina to the pelvic walls can be divided into three regions. Note that despite the removal of the cervix, the fibers in level I, the long suspensory fibers of the paracolpium, suspend the upper vagina. In the midvagina, level II, the vagina is attached laterally to the tendinous arch of the pelvic fascia. Level III is characterized by fusion of the vagina to surrounding structures.

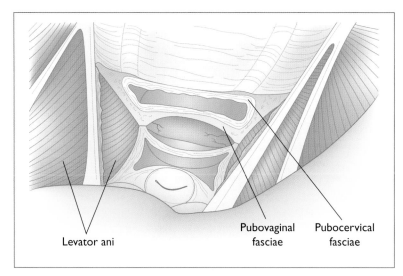

Levator ani   Pubovaginal   Pubocervical
                fasciae   fasciae

Figure 1-13. Nature of level II. This view shows the caudal margin of level II after a triangular wedge of the vaginal wall has been removed, which exposes the distal urethra and the anterior surface of the rectum. The fascial attachment between the anterior vaginal wall and the tendinous arch of the pelvic fascia is visible. The structural layer on which the bladder rests is comprised of the vaginal wall and its connections through the pubocervical fascia to the arcus. At this level of the vagina, there is no separate layer that separates the vagina from the bladder. It is the wall of the vagina itself that is responsible for bladder base support.

ANATOMY OF THE URINARY CONTINENCE MECHANISM

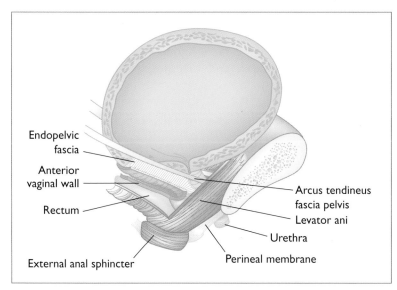

Endopelvic fascia
Anterior vaginal wall
Rectum
External anal sphincter
Arcus tendineus fascia pelvis
Levator ani
Urethra
Perineal membrane

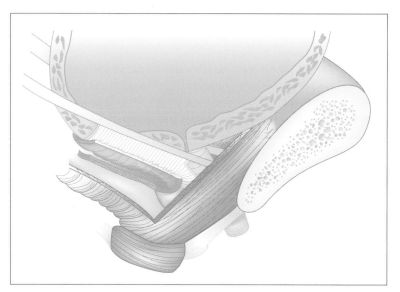

Figure 1-14. The lateral view of the pelvic floor structures related to urethral support is seen from the side in the standing position, cut just lateral to the midline. Note that windows have been cut into the levator ani muscles, vagina, and endopelvic fascia so that the urethra and anterior vaginal walls can be seen. Note that the tendineus arch of the pelvic fascia is stretched from the pubic bone to its eventual attachment to the ischium. The anterior vaginal wall is attached to the arcus by the endopelvic fascia and forms a supportive layer for the bladder and urethra. The levator ani muscle attaches to the endopelvic fascia so that contraction of the levator muscle can elevate the urethra.

Figure 1-15. Closeup view of the urethral support structures shown in Figure 1-14.

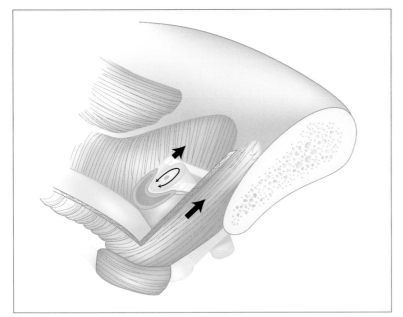

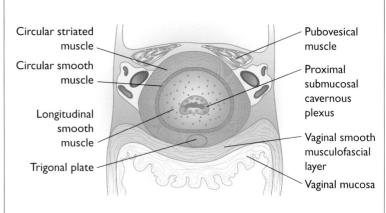

Figure 1-16. There are two ways in which the striated muscles of the pelvic floor can affect urinary continence. The constrictive effects of the striated urogenital sphincter muscle within the wall of the urethra can increase urethral closure pressure during times of increased need and during increases in abdominal pressure. The levator ani muscles can also stiffen the supports of the urethra. As abdominal pressure pushes the urethra downward, this stiffened support system provides a firm and unyielding backboard against which the urethra can be compressed closed.

Figure 1-17. Structures seen in the midurethra. Here the striated muscle of the urethra can be seen to surround the circular and longitudinal smooth muscle layers. The submucosal vaginal musculofascial layer is the layer that provides support for the urethra. Note also the prominent vascular plexus that surrounds the mucosal lining of the urethra. This plexus probably provides a flexible filling between the mucosa and muscular layers. The trigonal plate bridges the gap between the ends of the striated urogenital sphincter muscle. This gap does not impede its ability to constrict the lumen because the trigonal plate spans the separation between the muscles, forming a tendon-like union of the two sides and mechanically connecting them.

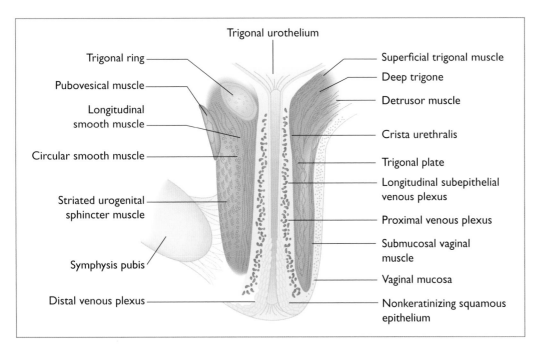

Figure 1-18. The layered structure of the urethral wall can be seen in sagittal section. Just below the internal urinary meatus, the urethral lumen is surrounded by muscle that forms the bladder. The trigonal ring anteriorly marks the most caudal extent of the bladder. Inserting into the vesical neck in the dorsal wall of the urethra are fibers of the detrusor muscle that probably act to help open the vesical neck when the detrusor muscle contracts. The striated urogenital sphincter muscle begins below the vesical neck and extends along the midurethra. The pubovesical muscle is an extension of the detrusor muscle that passes laterally to attach the bladder muscle to the tendinous arch of the pelvic fascia and may also be involved in vesical neck opening at the beginning of micturition.

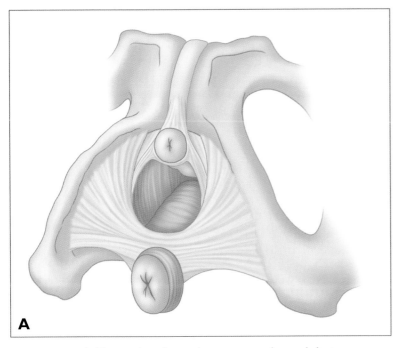

A

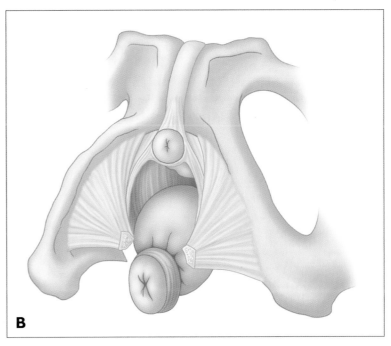

B

Figure 1-19. **A**, The perineal membrane spans the arch between the ischiopubic rami with each side attached to the other through their connection in the perineal body. **B**, Note that separation of the fibers in this area leaves the rectum unsupported and results in a low posterior prolapse.

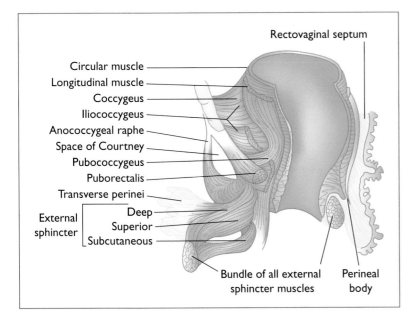

Rectovaginal septum

Circular muscle
Longitudinal muscle
Coccygeus
Iliococcygeus
Anococcygeal raphe
Space of Courtney
Pubococcygeus
Puborectalis
Transverse perinei
External sphincter {
Deep
Superior
Subcutaneous

Bundle of all external sphincter muscles

Perineal body

Figure 1-20. This lateral view of the anal sphincters reveals their important relationships. Note that the internal anal sphincter extends down to overlap the external anal sphincter so that a fourth degree laceration of the perineum during vaginal delivery must transect the internal sphincter as well as the external sphincter. Note also that the puborectalis muscle lies cephalic to the external sphincter behind the anorectum at the anorectal angle. Note that the pubococcygeus muscle lies cephalic to the puborectalis and to the iliococcygeus muscle. The anal sphincter complex is attached to the coccyx by the anococcygeal raphe.

Berglas B, Rubin IC: Histologic study of the pelvic connective tissue. *Surg Gynecol Obstet* 1957, 97:227–289.

Berglas B, Rubin IC: Study of the supportive structures of the uterus by levator myography. *Surg Gynecol Obstet* 1953, 97:677–692.

Campbell RM: The anatomy and histology of the sacrouterine ligaments. *Am J Obstet Gynecol* 1950, 59:1–12.

DeLancey JOL: Anatomic aspects of vaginal eversion after hysterectomy. *Am J Obstet Gynecol* 1992, 166:1717–1728.

DeLancey JOL: Anatomy and biomechanics of genital prolapse. *Clin Obstet Gynecol* 1994, 36:897–909.

DeLancey JOL: Structural anatomy of the posterior pelvic compartment as it relates to rectocele. *Am J Obstet Gynecol* 1999, 180:815–823.

DeLancey JOL: Structural support of the urethra as it relates to stress urinary incontinence: the hammock hypothesis. *Am J Obstet Gynecol* 1994, 170:1713–1720.

Halban J, Tandler J: *Anatomie und Aetiologie der Genitalprolapse beim Weibe.* Vienna and Leipzig: Wilhelm Braumuller; 1907.

Lawson JO: Pelvic anatomy. II. Anal canal and associated sphincters. *Ann R Coll Surg Engl* 1974, 54:288–300.

Lawson JO: Pelvic anatomy. I. Pelvic floor muscles. *Ann R Coll Surg Engl* 1974, 54:244–252.

Oelrich TM: The striated urogenital sphincter muscle in the female. *Anat Rec* 1983, 205:223–232.

Oh C, Kark AE: Anatomy of the perineal body. *Dis Colon Rectum* 1973, 16:444–454.

Paramore RH: The statics of the female pelvic viscera. In *The Uterus as a Floating Organ*, vol 1. London: HK Lewis; 1918:12–15.

Paramore RH: The supports-in-chief of the female pelvic viscera. *J Obstet Gynaecol Br Emp* 1908, 13:391–409.

Range RL, Woodburne RT: The gross and microscopic anatomy of the transverse cervical ligaments. *Am J Obstet Gynecol* 1964, 90:460–467.

Ricci JV, Lisa JR, Thom CH, Kron WL: The relationship of the vagina to adjacent organs in reconstructive surgery. *Am J Surg* 1947, 74:387–410.

2

Congenital Anomalies of the Female Genital Tract

Renee M. Caputo

he urogenital system develops from the intermediate mesoderm, the coelomic epithelium, and the endoderm of the urogenital sinus. It consists of the urinary (excretory) system and the genital (reproductive) system. Although the urinary system develops first, the two systems are closely associated embryologically and, thus, also anatomically. Anomalies of the female external genitalia are diagnosed at birth, while other internal anomalies may not be discovered until puberty, the onset of menstruation, or sexual activity; this puts the gynecologist in a unique position to be the first to recognize these anomalies, which can have devastating physical and psychological consequences. This chapter will review the basic embryology of the female genital tract with references to the urinary tract when appropriate. The more common anomalies of the female genital tract are then presented, along with the diagnostic tools and treatment options that are necessary to manage them.

NORMAL EMBRYOLOGIC DEVELOPMENT OF THE FEMALE GENITAL TRACT

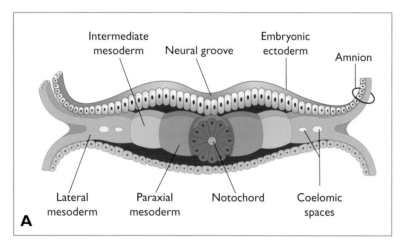

A

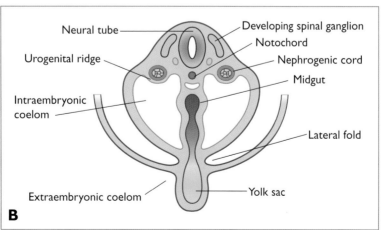

B

Figure 2-1. Urogenital ridges. Dorsal folding of an embryo at approximately 18 days. **A,** The urogenital system develops from the intermediate mesoderm along the dorsum of the embryo. **B,** With transverse folding of the embryo during the 4th week (at approximately 24 days), the intermediate mesoderm migrates ventrally. This bilateral longitudinal mass of mesoderm is called the nephrogenic cord. These cords produce longitudinal bulges, the urogenital ridges, on the dorsal wall of the intraembryonic coelomic cavity. The urogenital ridges become both renal and genital structures. (*Adapted from* Moore and Persaud [1].)

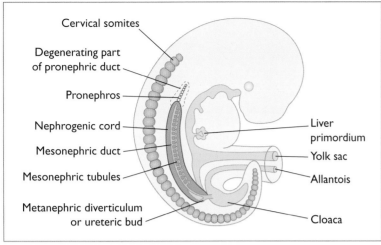

Figure 2-2. Development of the urinary tract. Lateral view of the excretory system in an embryo during the 5th week. Three

sets of kidneys develop in the human embryo, beginning early in the 4th week: the pronephros (the forekidney) and the mesonephros (the midkidney), which are well developed and function as the temporary kidney for approximately 4 weeks until the permanent kidney, the metanephros, begins functioning at approximately 8 weeks' gestation. The metanephros develops from the ureteric bud (metanephric diverticulum), which will give rise to the ureter, the renal pelvis, the calyces, the collecting tubules, and the metanephric mass of mesoderm, which will give rise to the nephrons. The ureteric bud begins dorsally from the mesonephric duct, near its entry into the cloaca. The bud will extend dorsocranially and grows into the metanephric mass of mesoderm. It will open separately into the bladder. Migration of the kidneys from the pelvis to the abdomen occurs due to caudal growth of the embryo; the kidneys reach their adult position by the 9th week. The urinary bladder and urethra develop from the endoderm of the cloaca and the surrounding mesenchyme.

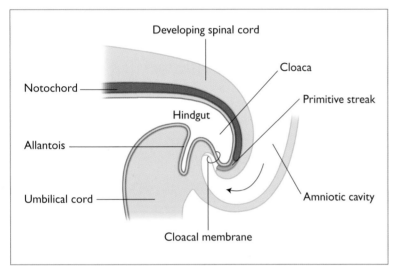

Figure 2-3. Cloaca. Lateral view of a 4-week embryo showing folding of the caudal end. During folding of the caudal end of the embryo in the median plane, part of the endoderm is incorporated into the embryo as the hindgut. The endodermal cloaca, a cavity at the distal part of the hindgut, will become the urinary bladder and rectum. It is in contact with the surface ectoderm at the cloacal membrane. (*From* Moore and Persaud [2]; with permission.)

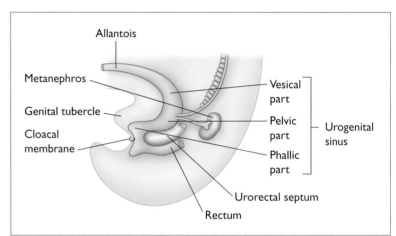

Figure 2-4. Cloaca. Lateral view showing division of the cloaca in 5- to 12-week embryos. The cloaca is divided by the mesenchymal urorectal septum into a ventral urogenital sinus and a dorsal rectum/anal canal. The urogenital sinus is divided into three parts: a cranial vesical part that is continuous with the allantois, an extension of the yolk sac, which will become the bladder; the middle pelvic portion that will become the urethra; and a caudal phallic portion that is closed distally by the urogenital membrane. Distal portions of the mesonephric ducts become the connective tissue of the trigone of the bladder and the remainder degenerates. (*Adapted from* Moore and Persaud [1].)

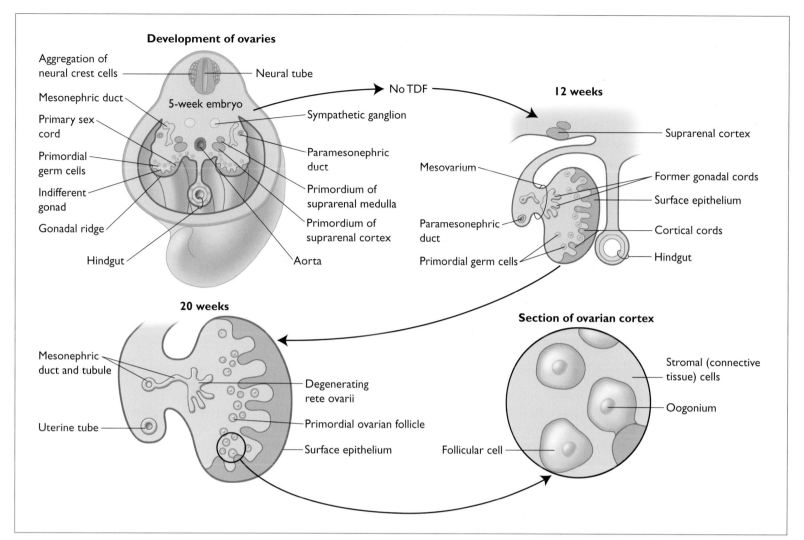

Development of ovaries

Aggregation of neural crest cells

Neural tube

5-week embryo

Mesonephric duct

Primary sex cord

Primordial germ cells

Indifferent gonad

Gonadal ridge

Hindgut

Sympathetic ganglion

Paramesonephric duct

Primordium of suprarenal medulla

Primordium of suprarenal cortex

Aorta

No TDF

12 weeks

Suprarenal cortex

Mesovarium

Former gonadal cords

Surface epithelium

Cortical cords

Hindgut

Paramesonephric duct

Primordial germ cells

20 weeks

Mesonephric duct and tubule

Uterine tube

Degenerating rete ovarii

Primordial ovarian follicle

Surface epithelium

Section of ovarian cortex

Stromal (connective tissue) cells

Oogonium

Follicular cell

Figure 2-5. Development of an ovary from the indifferent gonad of a 5-week embryo. The genetic sex of any embryo is determined at the time of fertilization. However, prior to the 7th week of gestation, the gonads are similar in both sexes. These indifferent gonads are formed from the coelomic epithelium, the underlying mesenchyme, and the primordial germ cells. Development of the indifferent gonads is first noted at about 5 weeks when the germinal epithelium, a thickened area of coelomic epithelium, develops on the medial aspect of the urogenital ridge. Proliferation of cells of the germinal epithelium and underlying mesenchyme produces the gonadal ridge on the medial side of each mesonephros at the urogenital ridge. Epithelial cords, the primary sex cords, grow into the mesenchyme. At about the 6th week, primordial germ cells begin to form in the endodermal cells in the wall of the yolk sac and then migrate along the dorsal mesentery to the gonads, where they are incorporated into the cords that extend from the mesothelial cortex. In the absence of a Y chromosome and testes determining factor (TDF), they differentiate into oogonias, primordial germ cells surrounded by a single layer of follicular cells developed from the surface epithelial cords. The ovary is not histologically identifiable until the 10th week of gestation. At the 12th week of gestation, the ovary descends from the abdominal wall to just inferior to the pelvic brim. Two X chromosomes are required for complete ovarian development. It is the gonad that determines the type of sexual differentiation in the genital ducts and external genitalia. (*Adapted from* Moore and Persaud [1].)

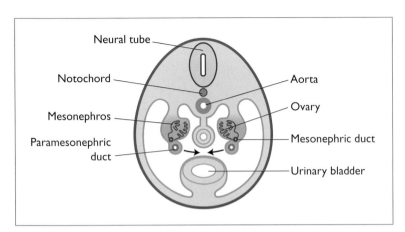

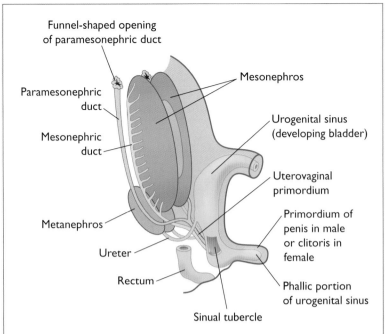

Figure 2-6. Development of the genital ducts. Transverse section of an 8-week embryo showing fusion of the paramesonephric ducts. In the absence of fetal testes and the müllerian-inhibiting substance produced by the Sertoli cells, the paramesonephric ducts develop into the female genital tract. The paramesonephric ducts begin as invaginations of coelomic epithelium at the lateral aspect of the urogenital ridges. The cranial ends open into the coelomic (peritoneal) cavity and become the uterine tubes.

Figure 2-7. Lateral view of the abdomen of a 7- to 10-week embryo showing the relationship of urogenital ducts. Caudally, the paramesonephric ducts cross ventrally to the mesonephric ducts and fuse together in the midline by 10 weeks' gestation to form the uterovaginal primordium or canal, which will become the epithelium and glands of the uterus. The endometrium and myometrium will develop from surrounding mesenchyme. The coelomic epithelium or peritoneal folds in which they are enclosed will give rise to the broad ligaments. By the end of the 10th week, the uterovaginal primordium pushes into the dorsal wall of the urogenital sinus between the two orifices of the mesonephric ducts that are producing the sinus (müllerian) tubercle. (*Adapted from* Moore and Persaud [1].)

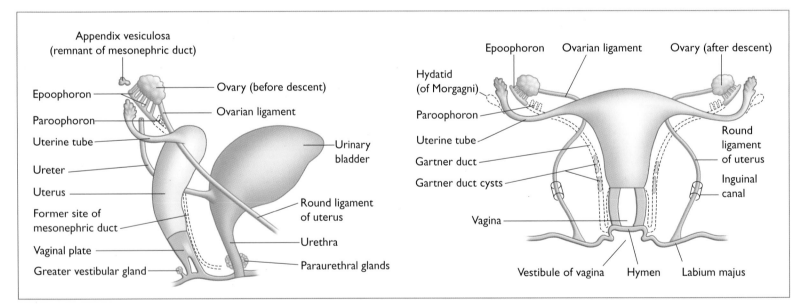

Figure 2-8. Development of the vagina. Formation of the vagina from the uterovaginal primordium and urogenital sinus at 12 weeks' gestation. With the formation of the sinus tubercle, a pair of sinovaginal bulbs develops from the endoderm of the urogenital sinus and grows into the caudal end of the uterovaginal primordium. The sinovaginal bulbs will form a solid structure, the vaginal plate, which eventually breaks down internally to form the lumen of the vagina. The origin of the vaginal epithelium is controversial; some authorities believe that the superior third is derived from the uterovaginal primordium while most believe the entire vaginal epithelium is derived from the vaginal plate. The fibromuscular layer of the vagina develops from the uterovaginal primordium. The caudal end of the vagina descends along the urethra to its separate opening in the vestibule. The lumen of the vagina is separated from the remainder of the urogenital sinus by the hymenal membrane, which usually ruptures during the perinatal period. The hymen is thought to be formed passively by invagination of the posterior wall of the urogenital sinus, which occurs as a result of expansion of the caudal end of the vagina. (*Adapted from* Moore and Persaud [1].)

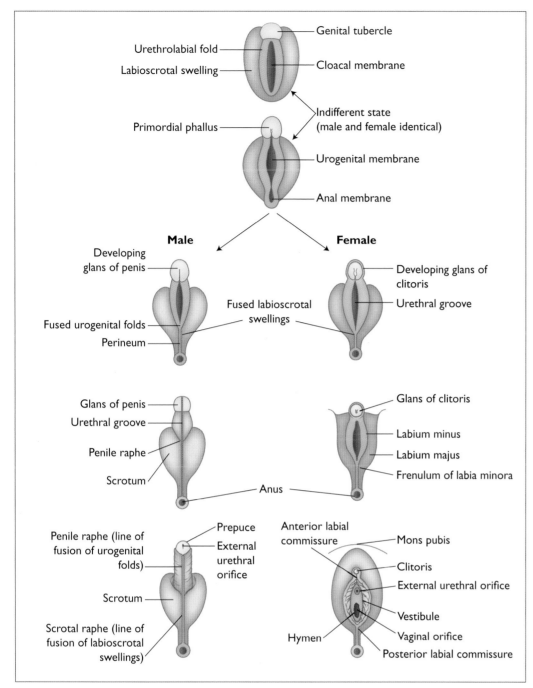

Figure 2-9. Stages in the development of the female external genitalia compared with the male external genitalia. From the beginning of the 4th week until the end of the 9th week, the external genitalia are indifferent. The genital tubercle develops cranial to the cloacal membrane and enlarges to become the phallus. The labioscrotal swellings and urogenital folds then develop lateral to the cloacal membrane. At the end of the 6th week, the urorectal septum fuses with the cloacal membrane and divides the membrane into an anterior urogenital membrane and a posterior anal membrane. Both membranes rupture about 1 week later to create the urogenital opening and anus, respectively. In the absence of androgens, female external genitalia become apparent at the 12th week. The urogenital folds fuse only anteriorly to the anus. The remainder becomes the labia minora. The labioscrotal folds fuse anteriorly to form the mons and posteriorly to become the posterior labial commissure. The unfused portion forms the labia majora. The phallic portion of the urogenital sinus becomes the vestibule into which the urethra and vagina open separately.

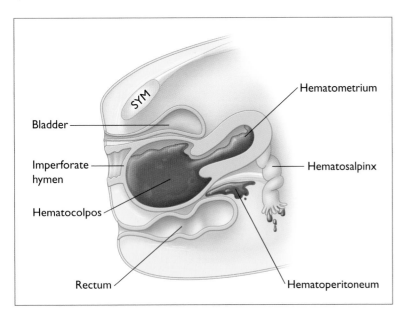

Figure 2-10. Imperforate hymen presenting at menarche. The hymen usually ruptures in the perinatal period, leaving a thin fold of mucus membrane just inside the vaginal opening. An imperforate hymen presents either in infancy as a translucent membrane, distended by mucus, or in adolescence at menarche, distended by blood. SYM—pubic symphysis. (*Adapted from* Mattingly and Thompson [3].)

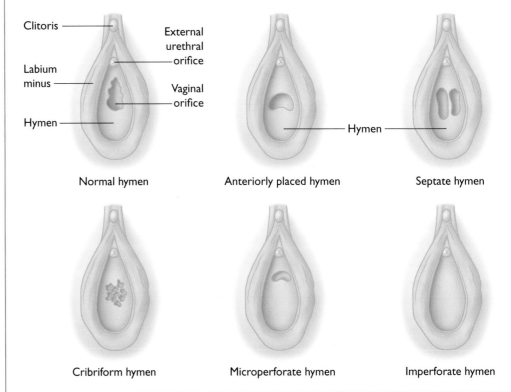

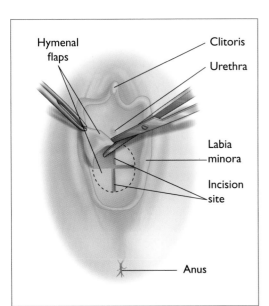

Figure 2-11. Excision of imperforate hymen. A surgical incision and drainage is the first priority in order to evacuate mucus or blood. A cruciate incision is made and the redundant tissue is excised. Because the tissue is avascular, sutures are rarely needed unless excision is carried too far, at which point interrupted sutures of a 3-0 polyglycolic acid suture should be placed. (*Adapted from* Baggish and Karram [4].)

Figure 2-12. Various types of hymenal anomalies. Variations of the imperforate hymen include microperforate, anteriorly placed, hymenal septum, and cribriform hymens. Although not typically responsible for an obstructed genital tract, the developmental anomalies of the hymen pictured here can prevent normal sexual function. In these instances, surgical intervention is required. Surgical excision is best accomplished at times when the tissue is estrogenized, during the newborn period or at puberty. (*Adapted from* Moore and Persaud [1].)

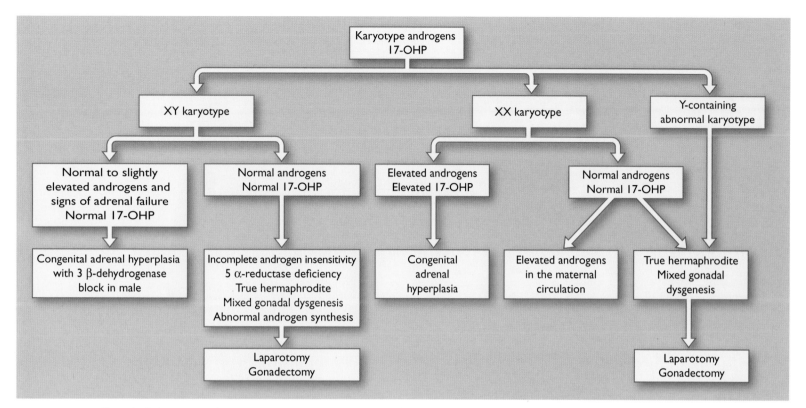

Figure 2-13. Differential diagnosis of ambiguous external genitalia. Hermaphroditism (intersexuality) occurs with errors in sexual determination or differentiation. A hermaphrodite is a person who has a discrepancy between the type of gonads, testes or ovaries, and the appearance of the external genitalia. The varying degrees of intermediate sex seen in hermaphrodites are caused by incomplete (male) or partial (female) virilization of the external genitalia. OHP—17-hydroxyprogesterone. (*Adapted from* Speroff *et al.* [5].)

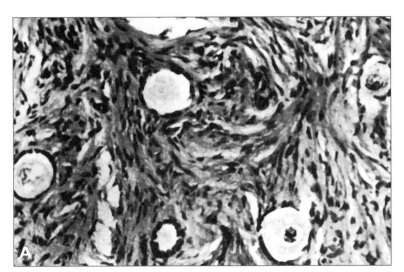

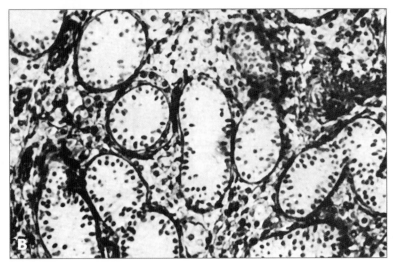

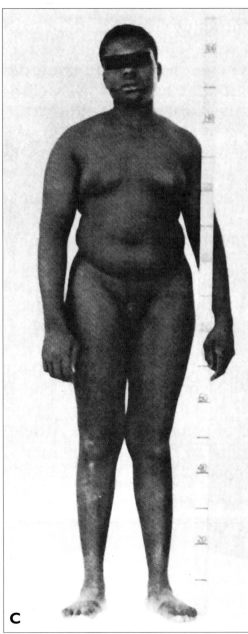

Figure 2-14. A 17-year-old true hermaphrodite with histologic sections of ovotestis. True hermaphroditism is a very rare condition that results from an error in sex determination. True hermaphrodites have ovarian (**A**) and testicular (**B**) tissue, in the same or opposite gonads, on ovaries and testes or an ovotestis. **C,** The phenotype is male or female but the external genitalia are ambiguous. The majority of true hermaphrodites (70%) have a 46,XX chromosome complement; 20% will be 46,XX/46,XY mosaics; and approximately 10% have a 46,XY chromosome complement. Most true hermaphrodites are raised as females. (*From* Copeland [6]; with permission.)

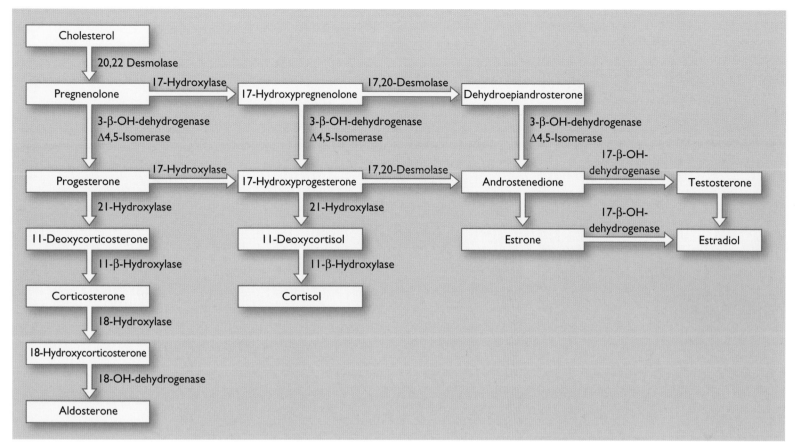

Figure 2-15. Female pseudohermaphrodism. Steroid biosynthesis pathway. A female pseudohermaphrodite is an individual with a 46,XX chromosome complement and normal ovaries but ambiguous genitalia. Female pseudohermaphroditism is caused by exposure of the female fetus to excessive androgens. The most common cause of female pseudohermaphroditism is congenital adrenal hyperplasia (CAH). CAH is caused by a genetic deficiency of one of the enzymes necessary for steroid biosynthesis, which leads to a decline in adrenal cortisol and an increase in adrenocorticotropic hormone, thus an increase in steroid precursors. The excessive production of adrenal androgens virilizes the external genitalia. Although any of the enzymes noted in this figure can be affected, the most common form of CAH (90%) is due to a 21-hydroxylase deficiency. (*From* Speroff *et al.* [5]; with permission.)

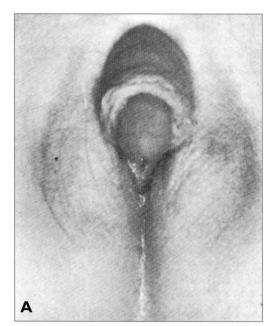
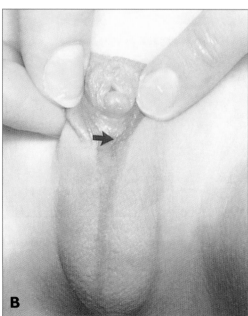
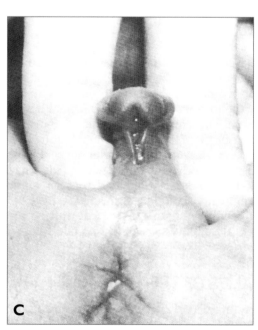

Figure 2-16. Varying degrees of virilization of female external genitalia in congenital adrenal hyperplasia. Virilization can range from (**A**) clitoral enlargement to (**B**) retention of the urogenital sinus (*arrow*) and fusion of the labioscrotal folds to (**C**) almost complete masculinization with a penile/clitoral urethra. The extent of viriliza- tion depends on the timing of exposure during embryogenesis, the length of exposure, and plasma levels of androgens. The earlier the exposure the more extensive the virilization of the external genitalia will be. Exposure after 12 weeks leads only to clitoral hypertrophy. Müllerian and gonadal development is unaffected as neither is androgen dependent. Other causes include virilization by maternal consumption of exogenous androgens (progesterone) in the first trimester and androgen-secreting tumors, either adrenal or ovarian. Treatment for all is surgical correction. (**A** and **C** *from* Copeland [6]; with permission. **B** *from* Moore and Persaud [1]; with permission.)

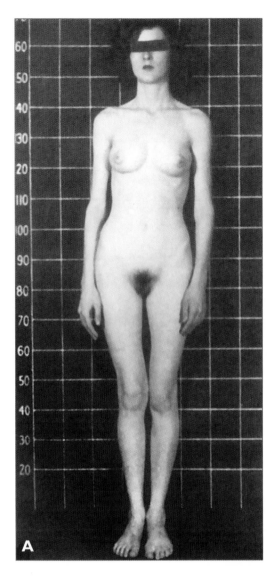

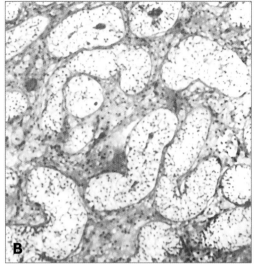

Figure 2-17. Male pseudohermaphroditism. A 17-year-old XY individual with androgen insensitivity syndrome (AIS). **A,** A male pseudohermaphrodite is an individual with a 46,XY chromosome complement whose external genitalia fail to develop as is expected for males. Causes are cytogenetic abnormalities (46,XY gonadal dysgenesis), a central nervous system defect (decreases in luteinizing hormone [LH] and follicle-stimulating hormone), a defect in testosterone biosynthesis, or complete androgen insensitivity. Varying degrees of development of the paramesonephric ducts and external genitalia occur due to the inadequate development of the fetal testes and müllerian inhibiting factor or the production of testosterone. The degree of virilization at birth and the size of the phallus determine the sex of rearing. AIS, also known as testicular feminization, is the result of a defect in the androgen receptor mechanism. These individuals are normal-appearing females with a 46,XY chromosomal complement and height appropriate for males. Testosterone levels are normal and LH levels are elevated. External genitalia are female, but the vagina is typically blind and there are no müllerian derivatives. **B,** Testes are present and can be found anywhere along the pathway of embryonic descent (abdomen, inguinal canal, or in the labia majora). Inguinal hernias are found in approximately 50% of patients with AIS; therefore, all prepubertal females with inguinal hernias need to have cytogenetic testing. Because malignant transformation of the testes is low before 25 to 30 years of age, it is acceptable to leave the testes until after puberty unless herniorrhaphies are performed. (*From* Moore and Persaud [1]; with permission.)

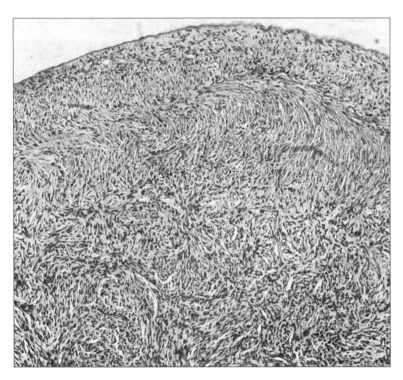

Figure 2-18. Gonadal dysgenesis. Histologic slide of a gonadal ridge from a 15 year old with gonadal dysgenesis. Gonadal dysgenesis refers to a condition in any individual with streak gonads in which interlacing dense fibrous stroma is found at the gonadal ridge with no cortical or medullary elements present. It is a common cause of pubertal failure. Approximately 70% of these individuals have an abnormal karyotype, including 45,XO (most common), an abnormal X chromosome, and mosaicism. Elevated levels of gonadotropins with a low ovarian steroid are typical in patients with dysgenetic gonads. Estrogen-dependent structures are underdeveloped. In 46,XY gonadal dysgenesis, the later the testicular tissue is lost, the less the individual will have of the female phenotype. Gonadal ridges must be removed in these individuals as soon as the diagnosis is made, because up to 30% will develop malignant transformation in the first or second decades of life. (*From* Copeland [6]; with permission.)

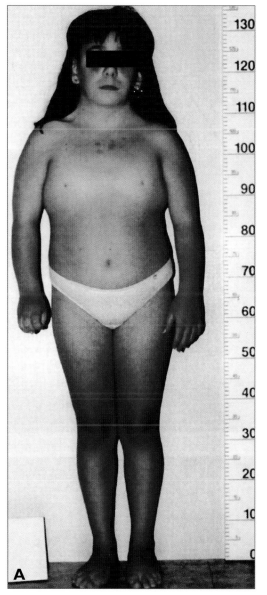

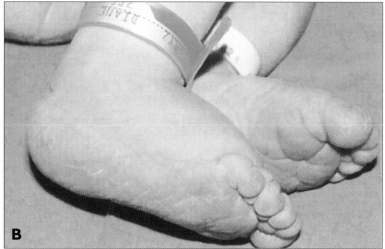

Figure 2-19. Classic physical features of Turner syndrome. **A,** First described by Henry Turner in 1938, Turner syndrome (monosomy X) occurs in one in 8000 live births. It is extremely lethal; only 1% of embryos missing a sex chromosome survive. Turner syndrome is characterized by a female phenotype and short stature, less than 150 cm. It is the most common type of gonadal dysgenesis. Oocytes that are present in children and some adolescents are typically absent in 45,XO adult women, which is caused by increased atresia and failure of germ cell formation. Most individuals with Turner syndrome present during adolescence with delayed puberty, primary amenorrhea, elevated follicle-stimulating hormone and luteinizing hormone levels, and decreased estrogen and androgen levels. External genitalia are well developed, but estrogen-dependent structures such as breast, vagina, and müllerian derivatives are underdeveloped. Hormone replacement is required to increase height and promote the development of secondary sexual characteristics. **B,** Turner syndrome can be diagnosed at birth, with the affected infant demonstrating lymphedema of the feet. (*From* Moore and Persaud [7]; with permission.)

Somatic Features of Turner Syndrome

Decreased adult height (141–146 cm)	Neck webbing
Cognitive defects	Low-set ears
Impaired hearing	Shield chest (widely spaced nipples)
Visual anomalies, usually strabismus	Short 4th or 5th metacarpal
Epicanthal folds	Cubitus valgus
Brachycephaly	Coarctation of the aorta
High arched palate	Ventricular septal defect
Low-set hairline	Horseshoe kidney

Figure 2-20. Individuals with Turner syndrome have a multitude of both physical and internal structural abnormalities. In addition to a karyotype (also to rule out the presence of a Y chromosome, which would require a gonadectomy), screening for internal malformations is necessary, such as an echocardiogram and renal imaging.

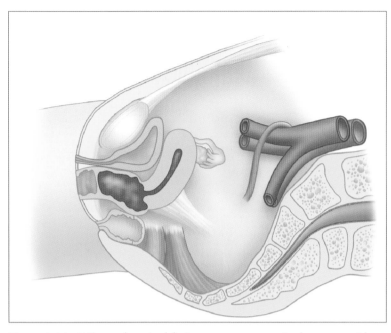

Figure 2-21. Failure of vertical fusion: transverse vaginal septum with hematocolpos. Failure of vertical fusion due to a faulty canalization

results in a transverse septum that can be either complete or incomplete. A complete vaginal septum usually is located midvagina and is diagnosed at menarche, when the patient presents with progressive pain and amenorrhea. Examination reveals a normal perineum, a blind vagina, and a palpable mass representing a hematocolpos during rectal examination. Imaging such as MRI is recommended to determine the thickness of the septum and to confirm the presence of a cervix.

Hematocolpos should be evacuated and vaginal patency established as soon as the diagnosis is made. Under ultrasound guidance, a large bore needle can be guided into the hematocolpos. Repeated saline irrigation may be needed to break up existing clots. The needle placement can also be used to guide surgical dissection into the upper vagina. An abdominal approach with the passage of a probe through the uterine fundus and cervical canal may be necessary to locate the upper vagina. Once open, the septum can be dilated. Revision of the scarred ring can be accomplished when the patient becomes sexually active. Depending on the extent of the vaginal mucosal defect, the upper and lower vaginal margins can be primarily approximated. A split-thickness skin graft may be required to fill the gap if reapproximation is not possible. A vaginal stent is helpful to prevent vaginal narrowing and stenosis. (*Adapted from* Baggish and Karram [4].)

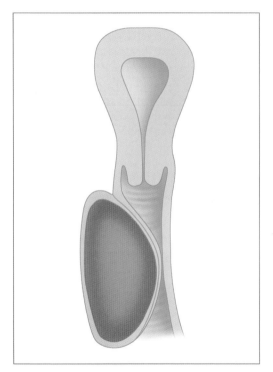

Figure 2-22. Hemivagina: lateral vaginal mass caused by obstructed hemivagina at menarche. When one of the paramesonephric ducts develops abnormally, a lateral vaginal wall cyst with an endometrial lining can occur. An obstructed hemivagina will fill with blood at menarche and form a vaginal mass that bulges into the true vagina. It is almost always associated with ipsilateral renal agenesis and occasionally accompanied by a unicornuate or double uterus. Treatment is excision of the common wall between the vagina and the cyst so that drainage can occur. Removal requires extensive dissection and is not recommended.

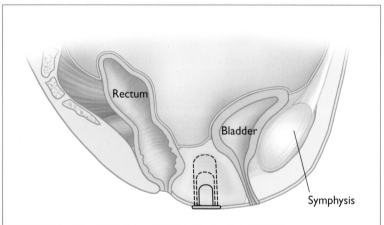

Figure 2-23. Conservative therapy for absence of the vagina: dilation. Müllerian or vaginal agenesis, typically seen in Rokitansky–Kuster–Hauser syndrome, occurs in one in 5000 female births. These genetic females have normal external female genitalia, a very small vaginal pouch, and no uterus. The syndrome is caused by a failure of the müllerian duct to form. Ultrasound may be used to document the absence of the uterus. It is also important that the urinary tract, spine, and hearing apparatus are evaluated due to common coexisting abnormalities in these areas. Vaginal agenesis may also be found in male pseudohermaphroditism; therefore, chromosomal analysis is necessary. Creation of a vagina is the recommended treatment but is delayed until the patient begins contemplating sexual activity. The first and least invasive approach has the patient apply pressure against the vaginal pouch or dimple using dilators graduated in both length and width. This technique requires a motivated patient and can be accomplished in a few weeks to months. (*Adapted from* Baggish and Karram [4].)

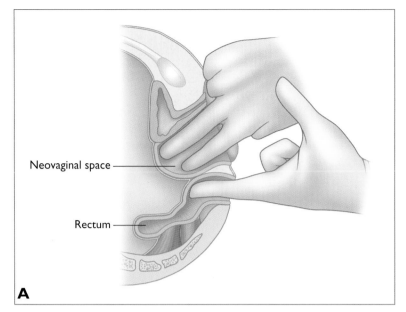

Neovaginal space

Rectum

A

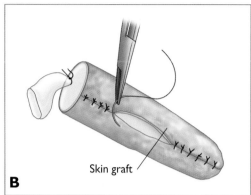

Skin graft

B

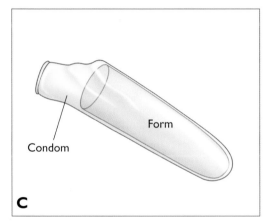

Condom

Form

C

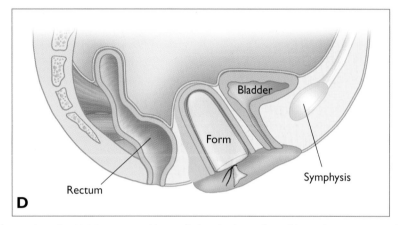

Bladder

Form

Rectum

Symphysis

D

Figure 2-24. Surgical therapy for the absence of a vagina. In 1938, McIndoe and Banister [8] described a vaginoplasty technique that is considered the primary surgical approach for vaginal agenesis today. **A,** Dissection is performed between the urethra and bladder anteriorly and perineal body and rectum posteriorly. **B,** The McIndoe approach utilizes a plastic, foam, or soft silicone mold lined by a split-thickness skin graft that is then placed into the neovaginal canal. **C,** The Wharton technique places a mold that then keeps the vaginal canal patent until it is epithelialized. **D,** Both techniques require that the molds be worn continuously with daily douches and then nightly. Once healing is complete, dilatation is necessary to maintain vaginal patency until sexual activity begins. (*Adapted from* Baggish and Karram [4].)

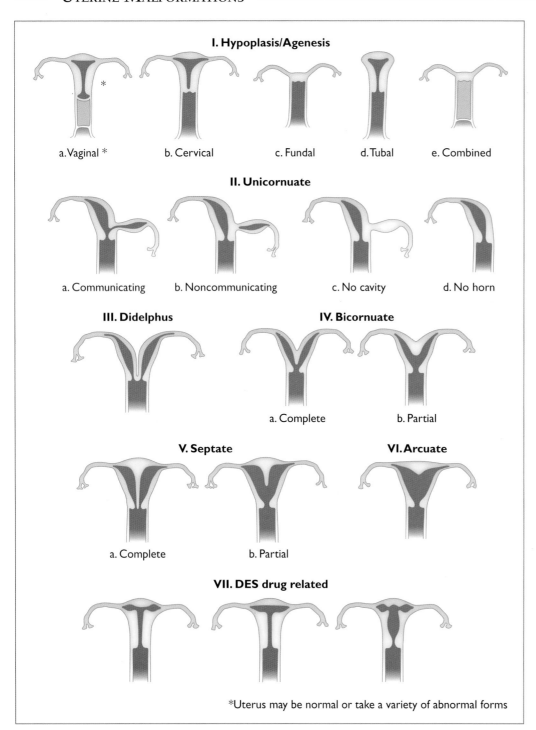

I. Hypoplasis/Agenesis

a. Vaginal *   b. Cervical   c. Fundal   d. Tubal   e. Combined

II. Unicornuate

a. Communicating   b. Noncommunicating   c. No cavity   d. No horn

III. Didelphus   **IV. Bicornuate**

a. Complete   b. Partial

V. Septate   **VI. Arcuate**

a. Complete   b. Partial

VII. DES drug related

*Uterus may be normal or take a variety of abnormal forms

Figure 2-25. Classification and diagnosis of uterine anomalies. Uterine anomalies are caused by defective lateral fusion of the paramesonephric/müllerian ducts. These anomalies include uterine didelphys, bicornuate uterus, septate uterus, and unicornuate uterus with or without obstruction. Although the incidence of spontaneous abortion, premature birth, fetal loss, malpresentation, and cesarean section is increased in the presence of a uterine anomaly, most patients who have them are able to conceive without difficulty and many have perfectly normal pregnancies. In 1988, the American Fertility Society [9] devised a classification system of uterine anomalies based on the degree of failure of normal development. Class I anomalies are incompatible with pregnancy. Uterine anomalies are diagnosed either at menarche or when they interfere with fertility or a successful pregnancy, most often using hysterosalpingography. DES— diethylstilbestrol.

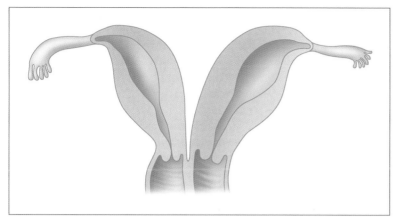

Figure 2-26. Uterine didelphys with longitudinal vaginal septum. Uterine didelphys, a class III anomaly, is defined by separate uterine bodies and is the result of a complete failure of longitudinal fusion

of the inferior parts of the paramesonephric/müllerian ducts. It is easily diagnosed because all patients will have two hemicervices on speculum examination. Most, approximately 75%, will have a longitudinal vaginal septum. True vaginal duplication, when each vagina has its own muscular layer, is rare. Although women with uterine didelphys have reduced fertility and increased pregnancy wastage and premature labor, the didelphic uterus is associated with the best possibility of a successful pregnancy. A unification surgery for the didelphic uterus is technically difficult and few successes have been reported. Because a unification procedure may result in more complications, such as cervical incompetence or stenosis, it is not encouraged. Surgery is indicated when the presence of a longitudinal vaginal septum decreases the caliber of the vagina, causing dyspareunia or obstructing vaginal delivery, or when traumatic lacerations are a concern. Cervical cerclage may be considered in patients whose history suggests an incompetent cervix.

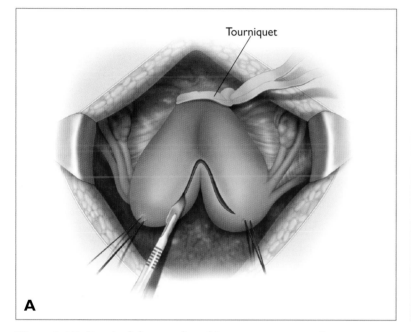

A

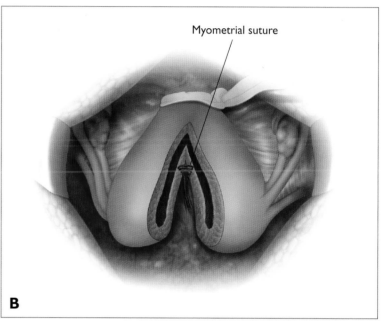

B

Figure 2-27. Surgical therapy for a bicornuate uterus—Strassmann metroplasty. The bicornuate uterus, a class IV anomaly, is the result of failure of the müllerian ducts to fuse at the level of the uterine fundus, with complete fusion inferiorly at the lower uterine segment and cervix. This anomaly is associated with a relatively high rate of spontaneous abortion and premature labor. In patients with a bicornuate uterus and infertility, care must be taken to ensure that all other causes for infertility are ruled out before corrective surgery is considered. For a bicornuate uterus, the corrective procedure

of choice is the Strassmann metroplasty, originally described in 1908. **A,** A transverse incision is made between each fundus and is carried into the uterine cavity. **B,** It is then converted to a sagittal closure using a three-layer technique of interrupted polyglycolic acid sutures starting with the posterior wall. In the medical literature since 1968, live births have been reported in 10 of 11 pregnancies (91%) following this procedure. Because experience with this procedure is limited, careful consideration should be given prior to the performance of a metroplasty in patients with a bicornuate uterus.

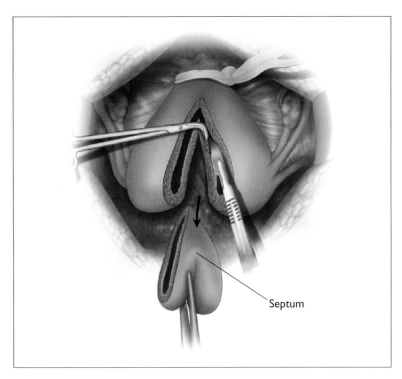

Septum

Figure 2-28. Surgical therapy for septate uterus. The septate uterus, class V, results from either complete or partial failure of resorption of the septum between the müllerian ducts after fusion has occurred. This uterine anomaly is associated with the highest spontaneous abortion rate, up to 89%, which is proportional to the depth of the septum. There also is an increased rate of premature labor in these patients. The Tompkins procedure has been the surgical procedure of choice in patients with a septate uterus and adverse reproductive outcomes. It allows for a septate uterus to be unified without loss of myometrial tissue. A sagittal incision is made in the fundus and is carried through the center of the septum in an anteroposterior direction. The septum is excised and a three-layer closure is performed, which is similar to the Strassmann metroplasty. Although efficacy studies have not been performed, a posttreatment live birth rate of 88% and a spontaneous abortion rate of 5% were reported when data from three reports were combined. Morbidity associated with an abdominal procedure and the need for cesarean section make the Tompkins metroplasty less desirable. A uterine septum can be removed hysteroscopically using sharp dissection, laser, or electrosurgical techniques, and this is currently the procedure of choice. Postoperatively, patients are treated sequentially with conjugated estrogens, 2.5 mg daily for 1 to 2 months, and medroxyprogesterone acetate, 5 mg twice daily for 10 days, to promote healing. A postoperative hysterosalpingogram is recommended to confirm complete resection. Reproductive outcomes from six studies with over 250 patients who have had a hysteroscopic metroplasty showed an 81% conception and live birth rate. Cesarean section is not required for subsequent pregnancies.

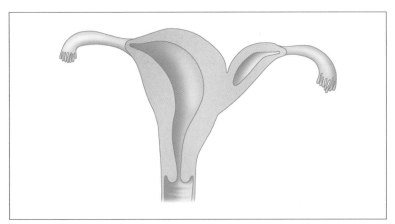

Figure 2-29. Unicornuate uterus with a noncommunicating rudimentary horn. The unicornuate uterus, class II, occurs when one of the paramesonephric/müllerian ducts fails to develop, resulting in a uterus with one fallopian tube. It represents only 1% to 2% of all congenital uterine anomalies, but has the highest rates of spontaneous abortion and premature delivery. A unicornuate uterus may be present alone or in conjunction with a rudimentary horn on the opposite side. Most (90%) of uterine horns are noncommunicating. Patients with a noncommunicating horn are at risk for hematometrium, hematosalpinx, endometriosis, and a rudimentary horn pregnancy. Therefore, the noncommunicating horn should be excised. Urinary tract anomalies are often associated with a unicornuate uterus and are found on the contralateral side. There is no surgical procedure available to increase the size of the uterus, but cervical cerclage has been recommended for patients who have an incompetent cervix.

REFERENCES

1. Moore K, Persaud TVN: Urogenital system. In *The Developing Human: Clinically Oriented Embryology,* edn 7. Philadelphia: WB Saunders; 2003:287–328.

2. Moore K, Persaud TVN: Organogenetic period. In *The Developing Human: Clinically Oriented Embryology,* edn 7. Philadelphia: WB Saunders; 2003:77–99.

3. Mattingly R, Thompson J: Surgery for anomalies of the müllerian ducts. In *Te Linde's Operative Gynecology,* edn 6. Philadelphia: JB Lippincott; 1985:345–380.

4. Baggish M, Karram MM: Unification of bicornuate uterus. In *Atlas of Pelvic Anatomy and Gynecologic Surgery.* Philadelphia: WB Saunders; 2001:94–97.

5. Speroff L, Glass R, Kase N: Normal and abnormal sexual development. In *Clinical Gynecologic Endocrinology and Infertility,* edn 4. Baltimore: Williams and Wilkins; 1989:379–408.

6. Copeland LJ (ed): *Textbook of Gynecology,* vol 1. Philadelphia: WB Saunders; 1993:122–124.

7. Moore K, Persaud TVN: Human birth defects. In *The Developing Human: Clinically Oriented Embryology,* edn 7. Philadelphia: WB Saunders; 2003:157–186.

8. McIndoe AH, Banister JB: An operation for the cure of congenital absence of the vagina. *J Obstet Gynaecol Br Empire* 1938, 45:490.

9. The American Fertility Society classification of adnexal adhesions, distal tubal occlusion, tubal occlusion secondary to tubal ligation, tubal pregnancies, müllerian anomalies and intrauterine adhesions. *Fertil Steril* 1988, 49:944.

3

Neurophysiology of Pelvic Visceral Function

J. Thomas Benson

Urinary and fecal storage and elimination processes are complex and involve the entire nervous system. Processes involving smooth muscle structures (detrusor, urethral sphincters, rectal, internal anal) and skeletal muscle (external anal sphincter, urethral sphincter, pelvic floor muscles) act simultaneously. These activities depend on autonomic (to smooth) and somatic (to skeletal) efferent neural mechanisms that are reflexly stimulated by sensory nerve afferents integrated in the lumbosacral spinal cord, with an element of supraspinal control. The control mechanisms are both excitatory and inhibitory and consist of neural circuits located in the brain, spinal cord, and peripheral ganglia. The neural circuits exhibit phasic, rather than tonic, patterns of activity, which operate to turn "on" or turn "off" patterns of neuronal activity involved in storage and elimination. Such switchlike activity allows voluntary control over urinary and fecal storage and elimination. Some visceral function (eg, the gastrointestinal tract and the cardiovascular system) involves tonic patterns of autonomic pathway activity and maintains an involuntary level of function even after elimination of extrinsic neural input. The urinary and fecal storage and elimination differ from tonic involuntary viscera in their dependence on central nervous control. The neurons of interest, then, include the motor neurons, including the "upper" and "lower" motor neurons, and the interneurons, the sensory neurons, and the autonomic neurons.

The basic unit of the nervous system is the nerve cell. The nerve cell is intended to last the lifetime of the organism and is able to do so by its plasticity—the ability to be dynamic and to constantly reorganize, restructure, and regrow to retain function. The basic function of the nerve cell is transmission of information. The nerve cell is limited in its ability to relay information to a method of conveying electrical signals. These signals, called "action potentials," are transient, all-or-none impulses that are highly stereotyped throughout the nervous system. They have constant form and vary only in frequency. Thus, the signals that convey, for instance, visual information are identical to those that carry information on bladder fullness. The information conveyed by the action potential is determined not by the form of the signal but by the pathway the signal travels. Therefore, circuits, or patterns or pathways, are of utmost importance in the study of organ innervation.

The transmission of the action potential within the nerve cell process is electrical (ionic), using protein channels in the bilayered axon membrane that allow passage of sodium, potassium, and chloride ions. The electrical signals flow in a predictable and consistent direction, and only in that direction, within a nerve cell. The direction runs from the receiving sites of the neuron (usually dendrites and cell body) to the action potential trigger zone at the axon hillock. At the neuroeffector site, or the site of junction with another neural structure, the invading action potential(s) causes release of neurotransmitters from the nerve cell, which act on receptors on the synapsing nerve cell or the effector organ, establishing a chemical method of transmission. Once the "recepted" neurotransmitters reach the postsynaptic target cells, electrical (ionic) processes again occur in the target cell. The communication with postsynaptic target cells is not random, and each cell communicates with certain specific target cells and always at specialized points of synaptic contact. Understanding the neurophysiology leads to possible treatments; neurotransmitters, for example, may be modulated, receptors can be affected, protein channels can be blocked or opened, nerve growth factors and gene therapies may affect neuroplasticity, and electrical stimulation may affect reflex activity.

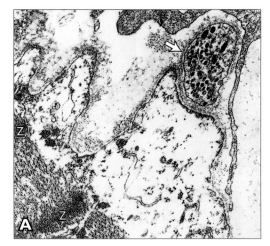 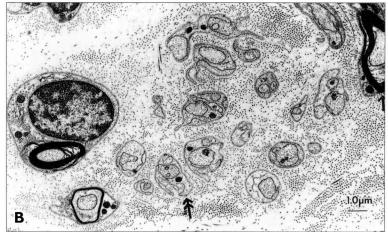

Figure 3-1. Axon terminals. **A**, In this electron microscopic image of a cat urethra, we can see the adrenergic axon terminal (*arrow*) with synaptic vesicles containing neurotransmitter. **B**, In this biopsy of a human female urethra, electron microscopy reveals the axon terminal with vesicles containing neurotransmitter in myelinated (*arrow*) and unmyelinated (*double arrow*) nerves. Z—myofibril. (**A** *from* Elbadawi [1]; with permission. **B** *from* Hale *et al.* [2]; with permission.)

Neurons of the Central and Peripheral Nervous Systems

Upper and Lower Motor Neurons and Interneurons

Many single neurons of the CNS receive thousands of connections from other neurons. The presynaptic nerve terminal contains synaptic vesicles with chemical neurotransmitters and the postsynaptic membrane has specialized receptors for the neurotransmitters. These chemical synapses can be excitatory or inhibitory. Neurotransmitter release is effected by an action potential entering the axon terminal and opening voltage-dependent calcium channels. When the neurotransmitter binds to receptor, ion channels open in the postsynaptic neuron. If excitatory, Na+ channels allow sodium influx and depolarization will generate an action potential. If inhibitory, Cl- channels allow influx, K+ channels allow egress, and hyperpolarization develops, preventing action potential development. Acetylcho-line, the primary neurotransmitter in the body, acts in limited areas of the CNS. The chief excitatory neurotransmitter in the CNS is glutamate, the most plentiful amino acid neurotransmitter in the adult CNS. Sites of action include the cerebral cortex, hippocampus, subthalamic nucleus, and cerebellum. Although excitation of synapses is essential for neuronal function, overstimulation may be toxic to the neuron. Glutamate, acting on N-methyl-D-aspartate (NMDA) receptors, opens calcium channels. If the effect is too prolonged, cell death may occur. Clinical therapies related to blocking NMDA receptors are now available. The chief inhibitory neurotransmitters are γ-aminobutyric acid (GABA) and glycine, and clinical application of agents acting on GABA transmission is being developed.

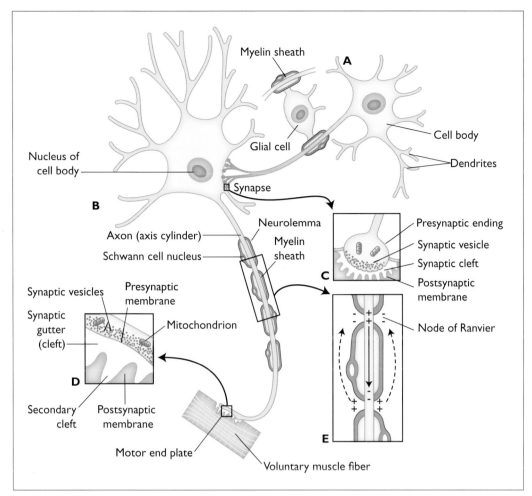

Figure 3-2. Development of the upper and lower motor neurons. The brain and spinal cord develop from the neural tube. Neuron A (**A**) is confined to the central nervous system (CNS), its cell body frequently supraspinal, dendrites communicating with other neurons. Its axon travels in tracts, supported by glial cells, myelinated by oligodendrocytes. It joins neuron B (**B**) at a chemical junction, the synapse (**C**).

Neuron B is a motor neuron, its cell body is within the CNS system, and its axon extends to a peripheral nerve and innervates a striated muscle. The axon is surrounded by myelin, produced by Schwann cells, and interrupted segmentally at the node of Ranvier, an area rich in sodium channels. Action currents flow from node to node ("saltatory" conduction, **E**), a much more effective propagation than is present in unmyelinated nerves. Each functioning skeletal muscle fiber is innervated by an axon (**D**), connecting to the muscle fiber through a neuromuscular junction. (*From* Manter and Gatz [3]; with permission.)

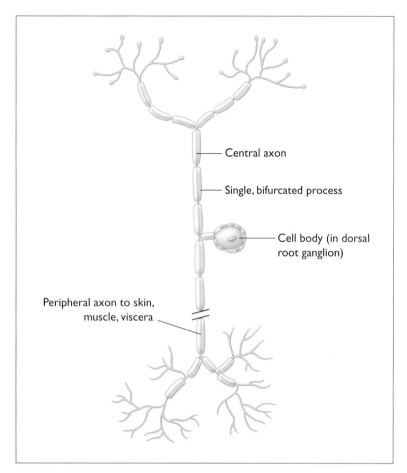

Central axon

Single, bifurcated process

Cell body (in dorsal root ganglion)

Peripheral axon to skin, muscle, viscera

Figure 3-3. Further development of neurons. The sensory neurons develop from a proliferation of the neural crest resulting in cellular aggregations lateral to the neural tube. The nerve cell body has two primary axon processes that fuse into one, dividing like a "T." (*From* Wiesenfeld-Hallin *et al.* [4]; with permission.)

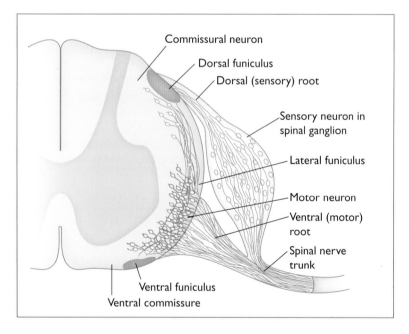

Commissural neuron

Dorsal funiculus

Dorsal (sensory) root

Sensory neuron in spinal ganglion

Lateral funiculus

Motor neuron

Ventral (motor) root

Spinal nerve trunk

Ventral funiculus

Ventral commissure

Figure 3-4. Neuroanatomy of sensory neurons. The cell body is located in the dorsal root ganglion and the peripheral process goes to the peripheral sensory site, and the central process enters the spinal cord through the dorsal root. The action potentials generated at the sensory organ travel to the cord through this single neuron because there are no synapses in the dorsal root ganglion. Sensory small fiber naked terminals may be excited by a variety of substances including histamine, bradykinin, serotonin, acetylcholine, and substance P, whereas various types of touch or pressure sensations are perceived by encapsulated receptors such as muscle spindles, Golgi tendon organs, pacinian corpuscles, Meissner's corpuscles, and others. Neurotransmitters at the central processes include neuropeptides. Unlike neurons that produce acetylcholine and monoamines by alteration of ubiquitous molecules delivered to the cell, peptides are produced de novo in the cell. A number of peptides, many first identified in the gut then later found in neural tissue, are involved in sensory nerve neurotransmission. Peptides so involved include vasointestinal peptide, substance P, cholecystokinin, calcitonin gene–related peptide, and enkephalin. After significant axonal injury, tonic firing of sensory neurons may occur, a process involving nitric oxide neurotransmission [4] in dorsal root ganglion cells. This process is important in chronic pain syndromes and offers a pathway of possible therapy. (*From* Clemente [5]; with permission.)

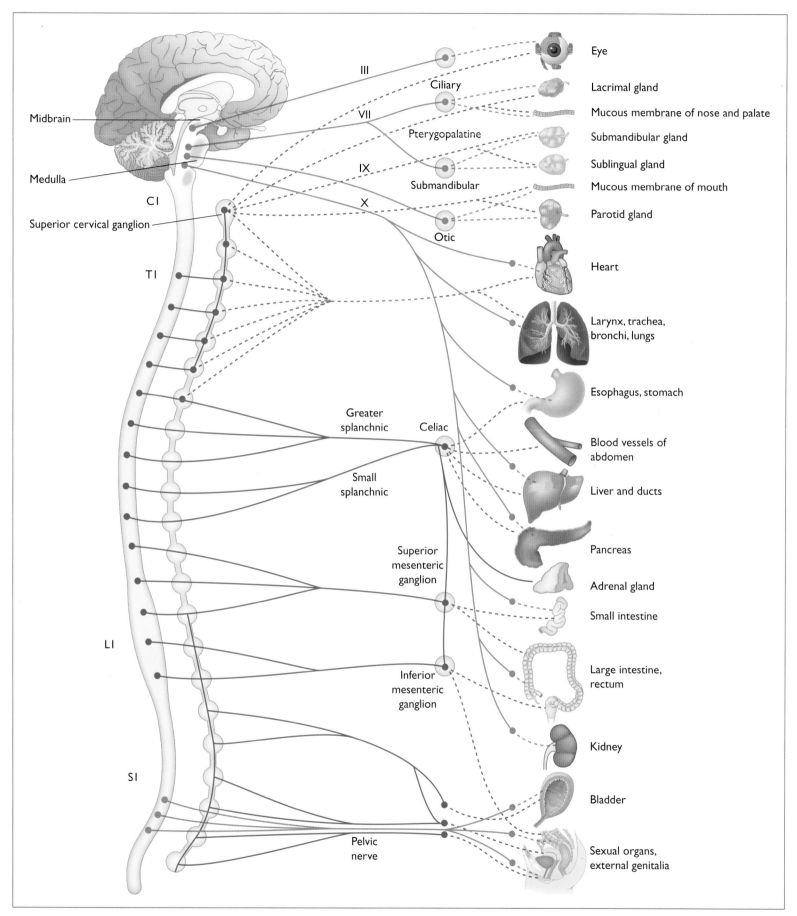

Figure 3-5. The efferent autonomic nervous system. The autonomic system contains the sympathetic (*red*) and parasympathetic (*blue*) divisions. Autonomic nerves are composed of at least two neurons, a preganglionic and a postganglionic neuron. The preganglionic neuron bodies are located in the lateral gray matter of the spinal cord. In the sympathetic division, they are located in a column extending from the first thoracic through the second lumbar segments and the sacral portion of the parasympathetic system in a similar column in the second, third, and fourth sacral segments.

Continued on the next page.

Neurophysiology of Pelvic Visceral Function 29

Figure 3-5. *(Continued)* The cranial portion of the parasympathetic division's preganglionic neurons arises in the visceral efferent nuclei of the brainstem. The postganglionic neurons of the sympathetic and sacral parasympathetic system arise, like the sensory neurons, from the neural crest. The sympathetic ganglia neurons form paravertebral chains and outlying collateral ganglia located adjacent to branches of the abdominal aorta. The sacral parasympathetic ganglionic neurons are located adjacent to the organ innervated. Sympathetic preganglionic axons exit the cord through the ventral root and course to the sympathetic chain via white rami communicantes. Some synapse in the chain and the postganglion axon joins the spinal nerves via gray rami communicantes (the paravertebral sympathetic system), whereas others course through the chain to synapse with ganglion cells in the outlying collateral ganglia (prevertebral sympathetic system). Sacral preganglionic axons exit the cord via the ventral roots to the pelvic splanchnic nerves (nerve erigens) and traverse the pelvic plexus to synapse with the ganglion cell at the organ. *(From Clemente [5]; with permission.)*

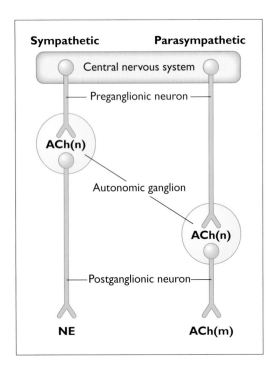

Figure 3-6. Preganglionic autonomic neurons. The preganglionic autonomic neurons use acetylcholine as a primary neurotransmitter and synthesize nitric oxide; some sympathetic preganglionic neurons release enkephalin or neurotensin. Acetylcholine acts on nicotinic receptors—ACh(n)—for excitation and on muscarinic receptors—ACh(m)—for excitation and inhibition. The autonomic ganglion neurons are not just relay stations but are the site of complex interactions. At the neuroeffector junctions, sympathetic terminals release norepinephrine (NE), neuropeptide Y, and ATP except at sweat glands where acetylcholine is used. NE acts on different types of adrenergic receptors. NE is mainly inactivated by reuptake by prejunctional terminals. The limiting of NE activity by its reuptake is a process that can be clinically modulated by the use of NE reuptake inhibitors. Parasympathetic terminals release acetylcholine, vasointestinal protein, ATP, and nitric oxide. Acetylcholine acts on different subtypes of muscarinic receptors. Cotransmitters such as purine (ATP, adenosine), local factors (histamine, serotonin, prostaglandins), and circulating influences (epinephrine, steroids, cytokines) modulate autonomic neurotransmission. The previously unrecognized bladder neurotransmitter substance simply called "nonadrenergic, noncholinergic neurotransmitter" is now recognized to be ATP [6]. There are now five recognized muscarinic receptor subtypes corresponding to five distinct genes (*m1-m5*) for muscarinic receptors. The detrusor and salivary glands possess subtype *m3* and the detrusor also possesses *m2*. Subtype-specific antimuscarinic drugs may not necessarily be effective, however, as the receptor expression is variable [7].

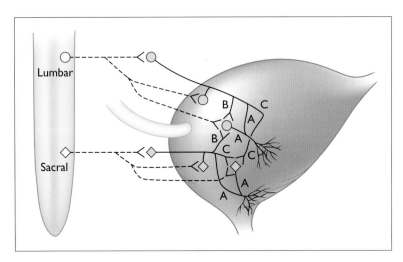

Figure 3-7. The pathways of postganglionic synapses in vesicourethral peripheral neural systems. Visceral effectors are characterized by automatic activity, the ability to sustain rhythmic contractions in the absence of innervation, intramural conduction, transmission of electric inputs between syncytial fibers, and denervation supersensitivity. Whereas the main consequence of denervation in striated muscle is paralysis and atrophy, most autonomic effectors develop no atrophy and an exaggerated response to the specific neurotransmitter, secondary to upregulation of postjunctional receptors. This property allows clinical testing for postganglionic bladder denervation by measuring the bladder response to bethanechol injection, which is a rarely used clinical test. Sympathetic pathway (*top*) and parasympathetic pathway (*bottom*).The *open circle* is preganglionic and the *solid circles* are postganglionic. The *open diamond* is preganglionic and the *solid diamonds* are postganglionic with synapses as shown (**A–C**). (*From* Elbadawi and Schenk [8].)

FORMATION

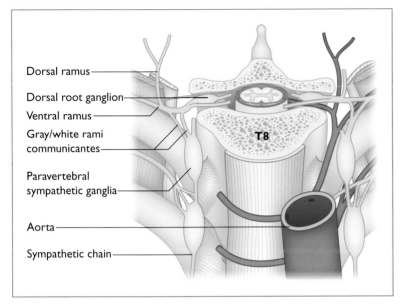

Dorsal ramus

Dorsal root ganglion

Ventral ramus

Gray/white rami
communicantes

Paravertebral
sympathetic ganglia

Aorta

Sympathetic chain

T8

Figure 3-8. Formation of a peripheral nerve. The motor neurons from the anterior horn cells, the sensory neurons with cell bodies in the dorsal root ganglia, and the preganglionic parasympathetic (in cranial and sacral cord levels) and postganglionic sympathetic neurons (from paravertebral sympathetic ganglia at all spinal cord levels) constitute a peripheral nerve. In this section from the T8-9 cord level, the white rami communicantes (so-called because they are myelinated) convey preganglionic sympathetic neurons to the sympathetic chain and the gray rami communicantes convey some of the postganglionic neurons back to the peripheral nerve. (*From* Low [9]; with permission.)

ANATOMY

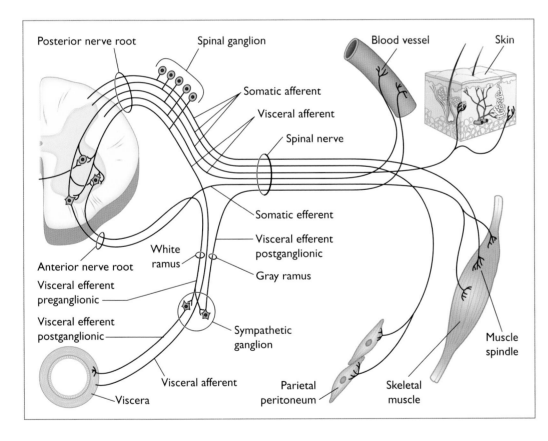

Posterior nerve root

Spinal ganglion

Blood vessel

Skin

Somatic afferent

Visceral afferent

Spinal nerve

Somatic efferent

Visceral efferent
postganglionic

White
ramus

Gray ramus

Anterior nerve root

Visceral efferent
preganglionic

Visceral efferent
postganglionic

Sympathetic
ganglion

Visceral afferent

Viscera

Parietal
peritoneum

Skeletal
muscle

Muscle
spindle

Figure 3-9. Structure of a typical spinal nerve. The peripheral nerve thus contains the sensory, motor, and autonomic nerves necessary for visceral innervation. (*From* Clemente [5]; with permission.)

Classification of Nerve Fibers

Sensory and Motor Fibers	Sensory Fibers	Largest Fiber Diameter	Fastest Conduction Velocity, *m/s*	Comments
A–α	Ia	22	120	Motor: The large alpha motor neurons of lamina IX, innervating extrafusal muscle fibers
				Sensory: The primary afferents of muscle spindles
A–α	Ib	22	120	Sensory: Golgi tendon organs, touch and pressure receptors
A–β	II	13	70	Motor: The motor neurons innervating both extrafusal and intrafusal (muscle spindle) muscle fibers
				Sensory: The secondary afferents of muscle spindles, touch and pressure receptors, and pacinian corpuscles (vibratory sensors)
A–γ		8	40	Motor: The small gamma motor neurons of lamina IX, innervating intrafusal fibers (muscle spindles)
A–δ	III	5	15	Sensory: Small, lightly myelinated fibers; touch, pressure, pain, and temperature
B		3	14	Motor: Small, lightly myelinated preganglionic autonomic fibers
C	IV	1	2	Motor: All postganglionic autonomic fibers (all are unmyelinated)
				Sensory: Unmyelinated pain and temperature fibers

Figure 3-10. Classification of nerve fibers. (*From* Erlanger and Gasser [10]; with permission.)

SPINAL PATHWAYS

EFFERENT SPINAL NEURONS

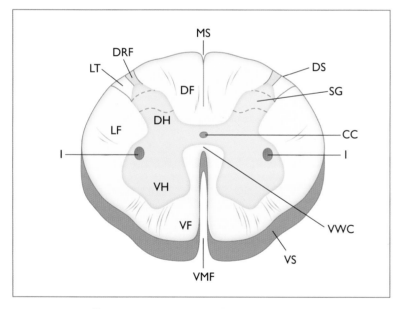

Figure 3-11. Efferent autonomic spinal neurons. 1) Parasympathetic: The preganglionic neurons are in the sacral cord segments. Dendrites of these neurons go to the lateral and dorsolateral funiculus, receiving glutaminergic neurons from the pontine micturition center, the "M" region of the pons. These terminals are excitatory and responsible for bladder contraction during micturition. Other dendrites go to the lateral edge of the dorsal horn, dorsal gray commissure, which also has excitatory connection to the pons "M" region, and to the ventral gray matter. The sacral parasympathetic outflow is critical for defecation, micturition, and erection, mediated chiefly by muscarinic cholinergic receptors.

2) Sympathetic: The preganglionic neurons are in the lumbar intermediolateral gray matter (T11-L2). Lumbar sympathetic neurons mediate inhibitory viscerosympathetic reflexes, activated by low bladder pressure afferent activation, which ascends to the lumbar cord to reflexly activate the sympathetic continence reflex. This reflex pathway is facilitated by norepinephrine and serotonin. The efferent limb of this reflex has an inhibitory effect on parasympathetic ganglionic transmission, increases outlet resistance by α-adrenergic receptors in the bladder neck, and may cause bladder contractility decrease by β-adrenergic receptors in the body of the bladder. CC—central canal; DF—dorsal funiculus; DH—dorsal horn; DRF—dorsal root fibers; DS—dorsolateral sulcus; LF—lateral funiculus; LT—Lissauer's tract; MS—dorsal median sulcus; SG—substancia gelatinosa; VF—ventral funiculus; VH—ventral horn; VMF—ventral median fissure; VS—ventrolateral sulcus; VWC—ventral white commissure; 1—intermediolateral gray matter.

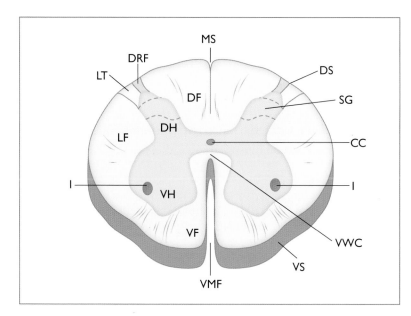

Figure 3-12. Sphincter motoneurons (Onuf's nucleus). In the sacral cord, these anterior horn cells differ from other somatic anterior horn cells in many respects; they are structurally smaller, have resistance to anterior horn cell disease (amyotrophic lateral sclerosis, polio), and have supraspinal connection similar to autonomic preganglionic neurons. The dendritic projections are similar to the distribution of the sacral preganglionic neurons. Onuf's nucleus activity is controlled by another group of neurons in the pons, the "L" region. The terminals from the pons micturition center are excitatory to the dorsal commissural gray, where they make contact with inhibitory γ-aminobutyric acid neurons that, in turn, inhibit the Onuf motor neurons. During storage, this inhibition is not present, allowing the sphincter to contract. Again, norepinephrine and serotonin input to the Onuf's nucleus motor neurons tends to facilitate storage. CC—central canal; DF—dorsal funiculus; DH—dorsal horn; DRF—dorsal root fibers; DS—dorsolateral sulcus; LF—lateral funiculus; LT—Lissauer's tract; MS—dorsal median sulcus; SG—substancia gelatinosa; VF—ventral funiculus; VH—ventral horn; VMF—ventral median fissure; VS—ventrolateral sulcus; VWC—ventral white commissure; 1—intermediolateral gray matter.

AFFERENT PROJECTIONS TO SPINAL CORD

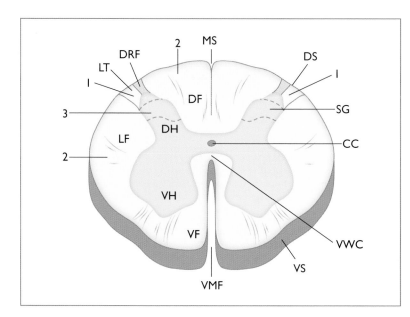

Figure 3-13. Afferent spinal cord projections from the lower urinary tract. Afferent activity in the bladder is transmitted to the central nervous system over both sets of autonomic nerves, the ones initiating micturition passing through pelvic nerves to the sacral cord. The majority of the afferents are alpha-delta neurons, although C fibers can be activated by chemical irritation or cold temperature. The C-fiber pathway bladder overactivity induced by noxious stimuli can be blocked by capsaicin, a neurotoxin that desensitizes C-fiber afferents. The C-fiber reflex pathway is weak in animals with an intact nervous system but emerges in chronic spinal animals (see Fig. 3-38). Pelvic nerve afferent pathways (1) from the lower urinary tract project into Lissauer's tract and pass rostrocaudally, giving off collaterals passing to the base of the dorsal horn. The synaptic connections in the dorsal horn involving alpha-delta and C-fiber transmission use substance P, which has an excitatory effect of long duration. Vasointestinal peptide is the most common peptide involved with sensory afferent activity from the pelvis and is only released from myelinated neurons. Other involved peptides are calcitonin gene–related peptide, enkephalin, and cholecystokinin. Terminations are made in the region of the sacral parasympathetic nucleus and dorsal commissure. Pudendal afferents from the urethra follow a similar pattern.

Some interneurons, synapsing with the afferent projections to the cord, send long projections to supraspinal areas, whereas others make local connections to participate in segmental spinal reflexes. Ascending pathways are in the lateral and dorsal funiculus (2). Neurons in the lateral dorsal horn (3) project via ascending pathways to the periaqueductal gray, where they are relayed to the pontine micturition center where they initiate the micturition reflex. Interneurons located near the parasympathetic nucleus have both excitatory glutamatergic and inhibitory γ-aminobutyric acid (GABAergic) actions on the preganglionic neurons. Descending serotonergic pathways tonically suppress afferent activity at the spinal level, inhibiting the micturition reflex. With increased stretching of the smooth muscle of the bladder, proprioceptive information (bladder "fullness") is carried to pontine and sacral reflex centers, the former resulting in excitation of parasympathetic sacral neurons and inhibition of sacral motor neurons to produce coordinated bladder contraction and urethral relaxation. Interruption of the pontine and sacral connections leads to incoordinated activity (detrusorsphincter dyssynergia). CC—central canal; DF—dorsal funiculus; DH—dorsal horn; DRF—dorsal root fibers; DS—dorsolateral sulcus; LF—lateral funiculus; LT—Lissauer's tract; MS—dorsal median sulcus; SG—substancia gelatinosa; VF—ventral funiculus; VH—ventral horn; VMF—ventral median fissure; VS—ventrolateral sulcus; VWC—ventral white commissure.

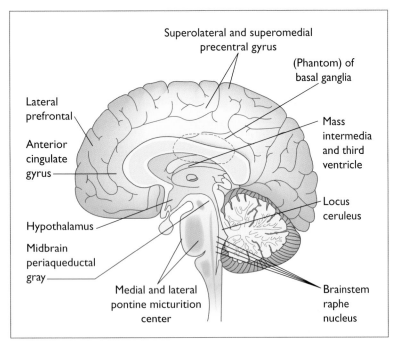

Figure 3-14. Areas of the brain known to be associated with pelvic organ (especially bladder) activity. Newer methods for mapping pathways include 1) positron emission tomography scans, which demonstrate increased activity in the central nervous system (CNS) associated with a given activity such as micturition; 2) transneuronal virus tracing (pseudorabies viruses pass by retrograde axonal transport from a target organ to the CNS where they infect second- and third-order neurons across synapses) [11]; and 3) measurements of gene expression (irritation of target organ increases level of immediate early gene, c-*fos*, in spinal neurons involved in processing afferent input. Areas of involvement for lower urinary tract activity include precentral gyrus, lateral prefrontal cortex, and anterior cingulate gyrus of the cortex, basal ganglia, brainstem raphe nuclei, locus ceruleus, hypothalamus, the midbrain periaqueductal gray, and medial and lateral pons.

Anterior cingulated gyrus and lateral prefrontal cortex are activated during attempted micturition whether micturition is achieved or not. Pelvic floor muscular contraction is associated with activation of the superomedial part of the precentral gyrus. These cortical areas maintain bladder capacity by tonic inhibition, which can be eliminated by N-methyl-D-aspartate glutaminergic receptor antagonist. Basal ganglia are associated with dopaminergic bladder inhibition. Raphe nuclei are cell bodies of origin for serotonin, which suppresses afferent bladder information, thus inhibiting the micturition reflex. The locus ceruleus has norepinephrine cell bodies. Norepinephrine facilitates continence-related reflexes. The anterior hypothalamus induces bladder contraction by neurons, which stimulate medial pontine center parasympathetic pathways, and the posterior portion of the hypothalamus inhibits bladder activity by sympathetic pathways. Lumbosacral cord interneurons project to the periaqueductal gray, which in turn projects to the pons micturition center, or "M" region. The periaqueductal gray and the hypothalamus are activated during micturition. The coordination between sacral cord parasympathetic motor neurons and the nucleus of Onuf motor neurons to the sphincters does not occur in the spinal cord, but in the "M" ("medial") region of the pons, known as the pontine micturition center (PMC) or Barrington's nucleus. A group of neurons in the lateral pons, the "L" region, is associated with contraction of pelvic floor musculature. The PMC, glutaminergic excitatory to sacral parasympathetics and to inhibitory sacral dorsal commissural gray neurons to Onuf's nucleus, is activated during micturition, whereas normal subjects who could not urinate on command had activation of the "L" region [12]. (*From* Manter and Gatz [3]; with permission.)

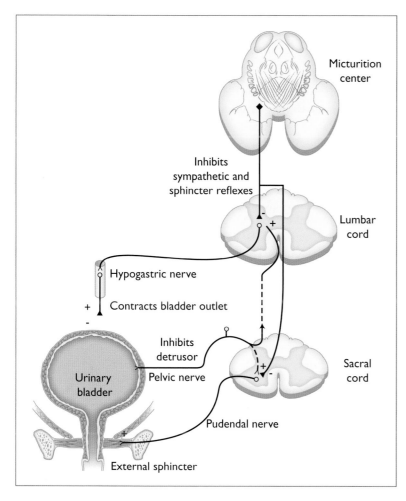

Figure 3-15. Urethral sphincter storage reflexes. The urethral skeletal sphincter muscles have a tonic discharge that increases with bladder filling. This reflex pathway is probably direct spinal, responding to low-level bladder afferent input from sensory neurons (*see* Fig. 3-3) that activate Onuf's nucleus (*see* Fig. 3-12).

During storage, bladder distention produces low-level afferent firing with sacrolumbar intersegmental reflex activation of lumbar sympathetic preganglionic neurons (*see* Fig. 3-11). The efferent pathway is via prevertebral hypogastric ganglionic sympathetic nerves that cause bladder outlet contraction and parasympathetic ganglionic inhibition by α-receptor activity and detrusor relaxation by β-receptor activity. Surgical or pharmacologic sympathetic blockade can reduce urethral resistance, bladder capacity, and compliance and increase bladder contractions. (*From* DeGroat and Booth [13]; with permission.)

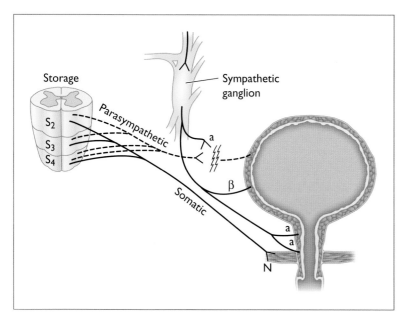

Figure 3-16. Additional storage mechanisms. Through spinal reflex pathways, somatic facilitation of the external sphincter, sympathetic contraction of the bladder neck, and sympathetic inhibition of detrusor and parasympathetic ganglia bladder storage are promoted.

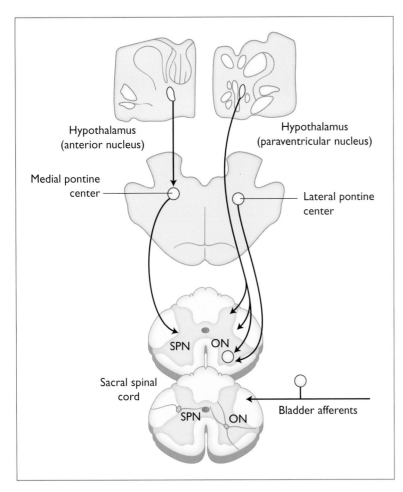

Hypothalamus
(anterior nucleus)

Hypothalamus
(paraventricular nucleus)

Medial pontine
center

Lateral pontine
center

SPN   ON

Sacral spinal
cord

SPN   ON

Bladder afferents

Figure 3-17. Micturition reflexes. The afferent pathways for micturition reflexes are high-level afferent activity via pelvic nerve and, except for the spinal direct reflex activating the sacral parasympathetic preganglionic neurons (*see* Fig. 3-11), involve supraspinal pathways. For inhibition of external sphincter activity, a "set-point" in the pontine micturition center has tonic inhibitory γ-aminobutyric acid modulation and when it is adequately stimulated, urethral sphincter electromyographic activity is inhibited, the first step in micturition, and the sacral preganglionic neurons increase firing, with resultant bladder contraction. The parasympathetic efferent outflow to the bladder is activated via the medial pontine center using glutamic acid as neurotransmitter using both *N*-methyl-D-aspartate (NMDA) and non-NMDA glutaminergic receptors. Inhibition of sympathetic outflow during micturition is probably a function effected through the same pontine center.

Suprapontine controls over the reflexes are largely inhibitory. Frontal cortical areas inhibit the anterior hypothalamus to prevent activation of medial pontine stimulation of parasympathetic sacral neurons. Paracentral cortical connections with the brainstem and cord activate tonic activity in Onuf's nucleus and can reflexly and voluntarily stop the tonic sphincter activity. This activity may be interrelated with the posterior hypothalamic region, including the paraventricular nucleus, which sends direct sacral projections to the parasympathetic nucleus (SPN) and Onuf's nucleus (ON). (*From* DeGroat and Booth [13]; with permission.)

Function of the Abdominal Sympathetic, the Pelvic Parasympathetic, and Somatic Nerves in the LUT and LBT

	Sympathetic	Parasympathetic	Somatic
Bowel and detrusor	–	+	
Internal AS and bladder neck	+	–	
External AS and external US			+
Pelvic floor			+

Figure 3-18. Embryologic origin and related innervation. The lower urinary tract (LUT) and the lower bowel tract (LBT) are embryologically interrelated, both coming from the cloaca and sharing muscular structures of the pelvic floor. The innervation of both depends on autonomic and somatic nerves, with similar functions as depicted here. AS—anal sphincter; US—urethral sphincter.

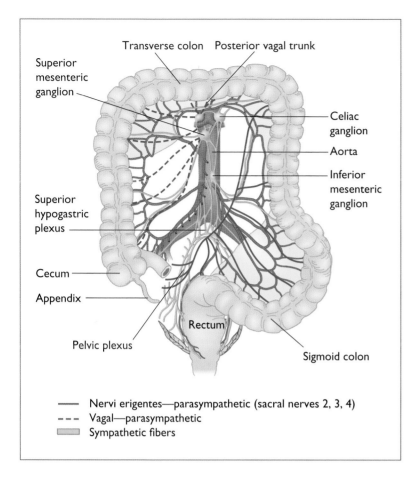

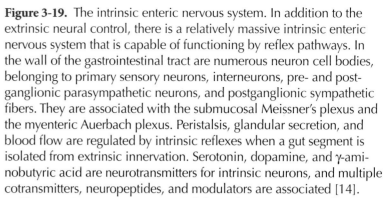

Figure 3-19. The intrinsic enteric nervous system. In addition to the extrinsic neural control, there is a relatively massive intrinsic enteric nervous system that is capable of functioning by reflex pathways. In the wall of the gastrointestinal tract are numerous neuron cell bodies, belonging to primary sensory neurons, interneurons, pre- and postganglionic parasympathetic neurons, and postganglionic sympathetic fibers. They are associated with the submucosal Meissner's plexus and the myenteric Auerbach plexus. Peristalsis, glandular secretion, and blood flow are regulated by intrinsic reflexes when a gut segment is isolated from extrinsic innervation. Serotonin, dopamine, and γ-aminobutyric acid are neurotransmitters for intrinsic neurons, and multiple cotransmitters, neuropeptides, and modulators are associated [14].

The enteric nervous system modulates the continuous influence of the parasympathetic and sympathetic systems. Parasympathetic preganglionic fibers reach the gut via vagus nerves to celiac plexus and superior mesenteric plexus to over half way in transverse colon. Pelvic splanchnic nerves via nervi erigentes from sacral nerves 2, 3, and 4 supply the rest of the tract, going through the pelvic plexus. Postganglionic parasympathetic nerurons use acetylcholine to increase peristalsis, increase secretions, and dilate blood vessels. The sympathetic postganglionic cell bodies in the prevertebral sympathetic ganglia follow blood vessels for the noradrenergic innervation promotion of vasoconstriction, smooth muscle sphincter contraction, and inhibition of peristalsis. The visceral afferents have cell bodies in the dorsal root ganglia and their reflex afferent arcs retrace parasympathetic or sympathetic nerves. The pain pathway from the rectum and upper anal canal follows parasympathetic pathways to sacral cord (hence, it is unaffected by sympathectomy).

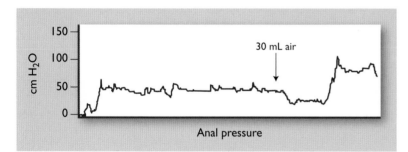

Figure 3-20. Sensorimotor reflexes are important in the regulation of continence. The somewhat debatable concept of "anal sampling," by which the individual chooses whether to discharge or retain rectal contents, depends on the measurable rectoanal inhibitory reflex (RAIR). The balloon distention of the rectum (at "30 mL air" notation) is followed by relaxation of the internal anal sphincter (IAS) (and prior or subsequent contraction of the external anal sphincter), which may allow rectal content to enter the anal canal where rich sensory appreciation evaluates the nature of the

"sampled" content. The smooth muscle of the IAS, unlike the rest of the intestinal smooth muscle, may be contracted (this is debated) by sympathetically mediated α-adrenergic activity; some studies have shown relaxation of the IAS with stimulation of presacral sympathetic nerves [11]. The RAIR is not abolished by spinal anesthesia, indicating an intramural reflex demonstrating the integrative ability of prevertebral ganglion neurons. Absence of the RAIR is suggestive of Hirschsprung's disease.

It is taught that during defecation the external anal sphincter relaxes and that this reflex activity can be diagnosed by electromyographic recording during attempted defecation. Testing in asymptomatic subjects has not consistently demonstrated this, however.

Rectal sensory activities are important for cognitive decisions of voluntary control and for sensorimotor activities regulating contraction in the rectum. The pelvic nerves convey visceral afferent activity that influences the efferent parasympathetic activity of the nervi erigentes, affecting rectal accommodation and defecation. Resection of the nervi erigentes can abolish both rectal sensation and the ability to defecate.

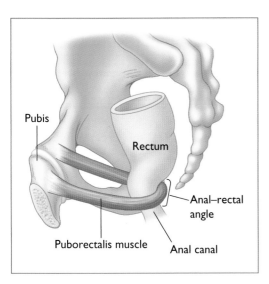

Figure 3-21. Innervation of the skeletal anal sphincter. The function of the skeletal (external) anal sphincter (EAS) is complemented in its continence maintainence by the levator musculature, particularly the puborectalis portion. Continence was believed to be due to a flap valve mechanism dependent on the puborectalis muscle [15]. However, the finding that continence after successful sphincter repair was related to higher sphincter pressures and not to altered anal–rectal angle negated this theory. The nerve supply to the EAS is the pudendal nerve. The nerve supply to the puborectalis muscle is variably the direct sacral branches from S3 and S4 and/or the pudendal nerve. The smooth muscle internal anal sphincter contributes about 80% of the resting anal pressure and is therefore chiefly responsible for anal continence at rest. The EAS, which is slow-twitch, fatigue resistant, with constant tonic activity, contributes some to the resting anal pressure but is more active in responding to sudden demands for resistance.

VAGINA

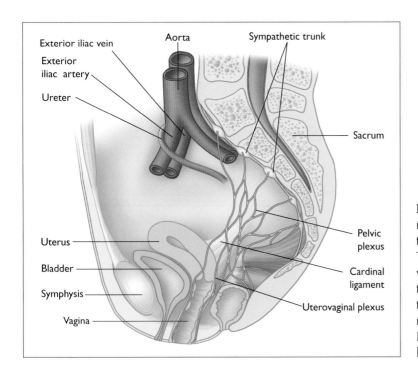

Figure 3-22. Innervation of the vagina. The nerve supply of the vaginal walls originates mostly in the uterovaginal plexus, derived from the pelvic plexus and located strongly in the cardinal ligament [16]. Thus, sympathetic postganglionics, parasympathetic preganglionics, visceral afferents, and somatic nerves all are available. Branches go to the vaginal muscularis and the lamina propria and the erectile tissue of the vestibule and clitoris. Ganglion cells are in the perivaginal fascia, especially laterally and anteriorly, beneath the bladder. No sensory corpuscles are in the vaginal wall, coinciding with the lack of light touch or pain sensation [17].

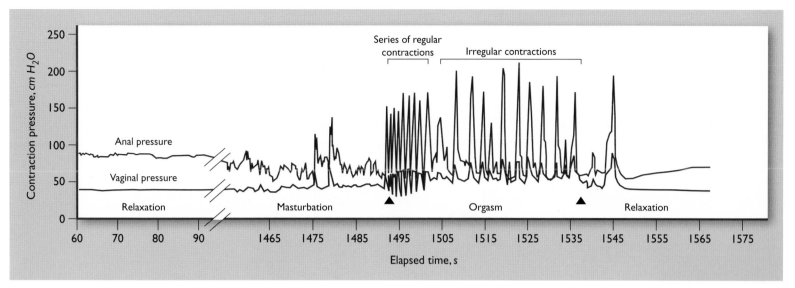

Figure 3-23. Vaginal innervation and sexual function. Vaginal sexual physiology involves marked physical changes in response to somatogenic or psychogenic erotic stimuli, classified by Masters and Johnson into a four-phase sexual response model; excitement, plateau, orgasmic, and resolution phases. During excitation, the vagina is lubricated by a transudative "sweating" phenomenon, and the vaginal walls assume a purplish color. The transudate is a result of fluid from plasma, as indicated by increases in pH, electrolytes, lipid constituents, and organic compounds. In the excitation phase, the inner two thirds of the vagina lengthen and the transcervical diameter widens. In the plateau phase, the orgasmic platform develops. Outer vaginal constriction occurs secondary to muscle contractions and vasocongestion of erectile genital tissue. Clitoral venous congestion and a fivefold increase in vaginal blood flow occur. The orgasmic phase is characterized by the orgasmic platform undergoing a series of regular, involuntary contractions, varying somewhat in duration, frequency, and amplitude [18].

The resolution phase sees resolution of these changes, a process taking a period of 10 to 30 minutes after orgasm. Differentiation of vaginal and clitoral orgasm, proposed by Freud [19], who qualified the former as being more "mature," is now discounted, with mul-

tiple studies indicating that all orgasmic responses are from direct or indirect clitoral stimulation.

The vaginal function in infertility is likely limited to its role as seminal receptacle and reservoir. Sperm capacitation probably does not commence until sperm enter cervical mucus. Age-related vaginal changes vary with hormonal status, vasculature status, and continuation or lack of sexual activity. Estrogen is trophic for the vagina and much of the lower urinary tract, with estrogen receptors found in the vagina, vestibule, distal urethra, bladder trigone, and pelvic muscles. Postmenopausal decrease in estrogen causes many physiologic changes in these tissues; however, hormone replacement may not reverse changes or reduce symptoms. Data are equivocal on whether and how estrogen receptors decrease in number, density, or function [20]. Following menopause, the vaginal epithelium loses the majority of its superficial and intermediate layers, and mucosal pH changes from acidic to neutral or basic. Loss of normal adherent flora (*Lactobacillus*) takes place and colonization with pathologic organisms may occur, leading to urinary tract infections. Few randomized trials of estrogen for urogenital atrophy including women older than 75 years are available, but expert opinion suggests that if estrogen therapy is elected, it should be limited to topical formulations.

The history is necessary to identify neurologic disease in patients who are referred for pelvic floor disorders, to characterize pelvic organ function in patients with known neurologic disease and to determine the prognosis and treatment options by understanding underlying neuropathology. Symptoms frequently correlate poorly with objective evaluations such as urodynamics in patients with neurologic disorders, especially with conditions that fluctuate, such as multiple sclerosis. Objective evaluations are of utmost importance to improve pelvic organ function and to eliminate factors that promote infection, which can themselves negatively influence the course of the neurologic disease. Standard examination forms are found helpful by many, as in the example here.

Name _____ Age _____ Sex _____ Number _____

Referral _____ Date _____

Chief complaint and present illness

Past history—medications

Urinalysis	Culture		Radiology
			Endoscopy

Spinal cord injury

Date	Level		Complete	Incomplete	Dysreflexia

Muscle stretch reflexes

R	KJ	AJ	Babinski	Clonus	Vibration	Toe position
L						

Sensation

R	52	53	54	Lower limb
L				

Cutaneous reflexes

R	Abdominal	Anal	Clitoral–anal	
L				

Muscle contraction

R	Pubococcygeus	Anal sphincter	
L			

Standing stress test   Noninstrumental uroflow

	Volume
	Peak flow
	Average flow
	Residual urine

Cystometrogram   Medium   Position   Filling rate

First sensation   Urge   Capacity   Compliance

			Voluntary	Coordinated
Detrusor contraction	Volume	Amplitude	inhibit	EMG

Instrumental voids   Detrusor   Abdominal   EMG   UPP   AMP   Length

External anal sphincter needle EMG

		MUP recruitment/
Insertional	Spontaneous activity	MUP morphology

Sacral (clitoral–anal) reflex

Sensory threshold   Latency

Impression

Figure 3-24. The pelvic floor disorders neurological examination. The examination begins with observing the patient ambulating to evaluate gait and talking with the patient to evaluate mental status. Skin examination for lesions associated with neurologic disease such as neurofibromata and café-au-lait spots is performed. Excessive hair at spinal base, skin dimples, and fat deposits may suggest spina bifida. Feet abnormalities such as high arch or pes cavas may be associated with spinal deformities or with congenital neuropathies. Examination then proceeds to evaluate cranial nerves, motor function, reflexes, and sensory function [21].

Cranial nerve function indicates status of midbrain, pons, and medulla. The most important cranial nerve evaluation is the extraocular eye movement examination. The medial longitudinal fasciculus is near pontine structures related to micturition, and lesions here are not infrequent in multiple sclerosis. The finding is impairment of conjugate gaze to one or both sides with failure of the adducting eye to cross the midline and nystagmus in the abducting eye.

Motor function examination is to detect changes in tone, strength, atrophy as a sign of denervation, and presence of abnormal movements. Paresis is incomplete loss of strength and plegia is complete loss. Tone is important to evaluate as well as strength. Decrease in tone is seen in peripheral nerve lesions, loss of proprioception, or various myopathies. Tone increase is seen in suprasegmental disorders (upper motor neuron disorder). Spasticity is seen when the muscle stretch reflexes are overactive and may be seen as a response to passive limb movement. If increase in tone is equal in limb flexors and extensors, resistance to passive movement characterized as rigidity may be present. Rigidity is a feature of basal ganglia disease (Parkinson's). AMP—amplitude; EMG—electromyogram; MUP—motor unit potential; UPP—urethral pressure profile.

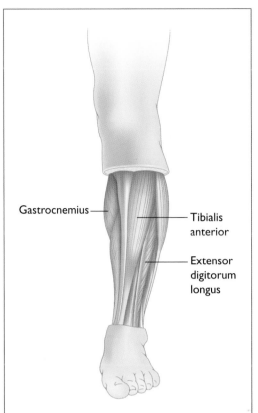

Figure 3-25. Myotomes of importance for pelvic floor disorder evaluation. Certain muscle myotomes have more importance in pelvic floor disorders such as when lumbosacral radiculopathies are associated with pelvic organ dysfunction. Then evaluation is helpful. These include the tibialis anterior (L4-5, peroneal nerve; dorsiflexes foot), the gastrocnemius (S1, S2, tibial nerve; plantar flexes foot), and the extensor digitorum longus (L5, S1, peroneal nerve; extends lateral four toes).

Sacral assessment is made by examination of the levator and anal sphincter muscle. Presence of voluntary contraction implies that the sacral and suprasacral innervation is intact. Careful examination for muscle tone is important. Presence of anal sphincter tone with absence of voluntary contraction may imply intact sympathetic (hypogastric) innervation or suprasegmental somatic neural dysfunction. Atrophy of levators and of external anal sphincter may be detected in denervation states.

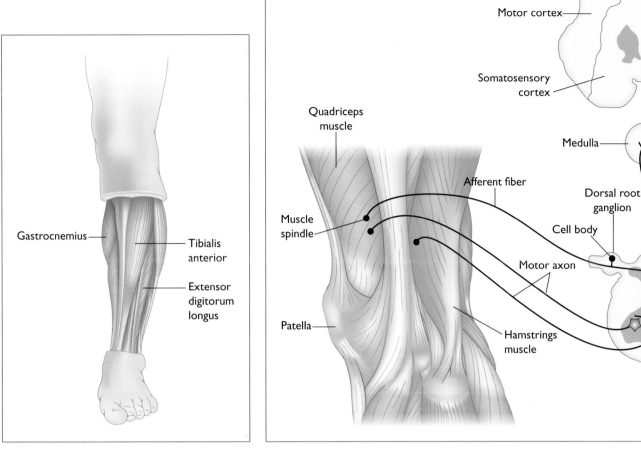

Figure 3-26. Reflexes of importance for pelvic floor disorder evaluation: The types of reflexes are muscle stretch reflex, cutaneous reflex, and pathologic reflexes. The muscle stretch reflex is created by stimulation of the large afferent nerves in the muscle spindle when the muscle tendon is struck. In the spinal cord, the sensory neurons act directly on motor neurons, which contract the muscle. In addition, the sensory neurons act on inhibitory interneurons to inhibit the motor neurons that would contract the opposing muscle. The muscle stretch reflexes of greatest importance to the pelvic floor specialist are the knee reflexes (L2, L3, and L4), and the ankle reflex (S1 and S2). The muscle stretch reflexes reflect segmental and suprasegmental cord function. Segmental lesions diminish the reflexes, and suprasegmental lesions, especially pyramidal tract lesions, are associated with hyperactive reflexes. Other muscle stretch reflexes to test include biceps (C5 and C6) and triceps (C7).

Cutaneous reflexes are segmental and suprasegmental motor responses to cutaneous stimuli. The abdominal reflexes (T6 to L2) are obtained by stroking the abdominal skin toward the umbilicus with a response of the umbilicus moving toward the stimulus. It is absent with obesity and tension and presence of scars. The cremasteric reflex (L1 and L2) is stroking the inner thigh with resultant elevation of ipsolateral testicle. The anal reflex (S2-5) is elicited by stroking para-anal skin with resultant anal contraction. The sacral reflexes directly assess sacral segments. The clitoral–anal reflex is with stroke of clitoris and resultant anal sphincter contraction, also referred to as bulbocavernosus reflex (S2-5). Absence of cutaneous reflexes may indicate peripheral nerve lesions. The abdominal cutaneous reflex is absent in pyramidal tract disease, especially if associated with increased muscle stretch reflexes. Absence of sacral reflexes may indicate segmental or peripheral nerve lesions and may be associated with urodynamic abnormalities, *eg*, detrusor areflexia. They are preserved or even exaggerated in suprasegmental lesions.

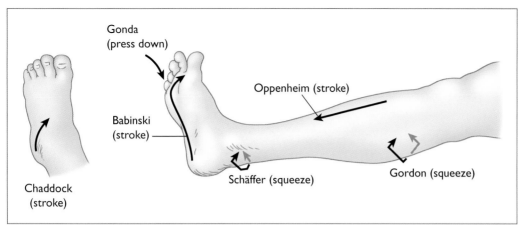

Figure 3-27. Pathologic reflexes of importance for pelvic floor disorders. Pathologic reflexes are sensitive for neurologic lesions. In the upper limbs, pyramidal tract disease (upper motor neuron disorder) may be detected by a pathologic reflex, the Hoffmann reflex. The Hoffmann reflex occurs when the flexed distal phalanx of digit 2, 3, or 4 is suddenly released (or "flicked" with the examiner's thumbnail), leading to flexion of the terminal phalanx of the thumb. In lower limb examination, the toe extensor response observed with the Babinski response is a sign of pyramidal tract disease. It may be elicited by varying maneuvers. It is important for the specialist in pelvic floor disorders to realize that bilateral positive Babinski responses are closely associated with detrusor-sphincter dyssynergia in patients with multiple sclerosis. Cutaneous stimulation of the lower limbs with resultant ipsilateral hip and knee flexion and ankle dorsiflexion with Babinski is seen in patients with spinal cord injury and is called the flexion spinal defense reflex. If there is contralateral lower limb extension, it is the crossed extensor reflex.

Sensory function: Sensory testing evaluates for touch, pressure, pain, temperature, toe position, and vibratory sensation. Touch may be light, tested with a brush, or more firm and tested with a needle. Pressure is tested with manual compression. Pain may be tested with a needle and temperature with hot or cold objects. Loss of position sense deserves special mention for the testing. The big toe should be grasped by the examiner's index finger and thumb on the lateral aspects, without touching adjacent toe or anterior or posterior aspects of the big toe, so that pressure sensation perceived by the patient does not give a false-negative finding. Moving the toe only 10° is adequate to see if the patient can (without observing) tell whether the toe is positioned anteriorly or posteriorly. Vibration may be tested with a tuning fork at the malleoli and compared with the upper limb.

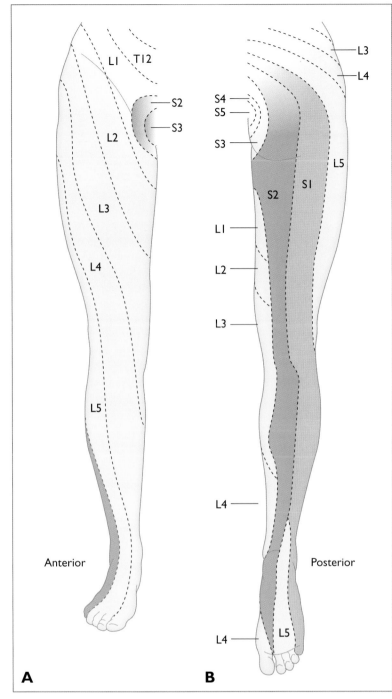

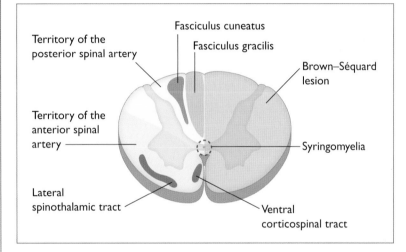

Figure 3-28. Dermatomes of importance for pelvic floor disorders. Upper body dermatomes to remember are C7 (middle finger), C8 and T1 (little finger), T5 (nipples), and T10 (umbilicus). The dermatomes of most importance to the pelvic floor specialist are in the lower limbs and perineum (**A** and **B**). L3 is at the front of the knee, L5 in the lateral leg and dorsum of foot, S1 in the lateral foot, S2 in the back of the leg and thigh, and S3–5 is at the perineum and the para-anal skin, including the posterior labia majora. The anteriormost part of the labia majora is supplied by thoraco–upper lumbar nerves.

Symmetric losses of all types of sensory function (pain, thermal, touch, vibration, and position sense), especially in the distal lower limbs, are seen in polyneuropathies, most commonly diabetes and alcoholism. Absence of toe position and vibration sense is seen in posterior column disease. If sensory loss follows a dermatome, nerve root disorder (radiculopathy) is suspected. Patients with pelvic floor disorders may have multiple lumbosacral radiculopathies associated with their pelvic organ dysfunction, as seen in spinal stenosis.

Figure 3-29. Spinal cord lesions produce sensory loss dependent on the cord area affected. Figure shows a cross-section of the C8/T1 cord. Transverse myelitis or complete spinal cord transection produces complete sensory loss (pain, touch, vibration) below the lesion. Disorder of posterior columns produces loss of vibration and toe position below the lesion, the lower limb afferents traversing the fasciculus gracilis. If the anterior spinal area is affected (eg, anterior spinal artery syndrome), there is loss of pain (conveyed by the spinothalamic tract, which crosses within one or two segments) and touch (conveyed by the anterolateral system of fibers located near the anterior and lateral funicular cord junction) but preservation of vibratory sensation. In hemisection of the spinal cord (Brown–Séquard syndrome), there is loss of pain and temperature on the contralateral side and loss of vibration on the ipsilateral side. In syringomyelia, there is cavitation near the central canal, most commonly in the cervical region. Sensory dissociation occurs with loss of pain and temperature (decussating fibers lost) and sparing of position, vibration, and touch.

It is interesting to note that the visceral pain pathway is not limited to the crossed spinothalamic tract, but visceral pain information ascends both ipsilaterally and contralaterally. The visceral tracts are located adjacent to, but deep to, the spinothalamic tracts, close to the cord gray matter [22].

Electrodiagnostic Tests

	Technical Performance	Diagnostic Performance	Therapeutic Performance
Kinesiologic EMG	Good	Fair	Good, grade C
Concentric needle EMG	Fair	Good	Grade C
Single-fiber EMG	Fair	Fair	Poor, grade C
Pudendal nerve terminal motor latency	Good	Poor	Controversial, grade D
Anterior sacral root stimulation	Unknown	Unknown	Research only
Motor evoked potential	Unknown	Unknown	Poor, grade C
Quantitative sensory testing	Variable (different techniques)	Unknown	Research only
Pudendal cerebral SEP	Good	Fair	Poor, grade B
Pelvic visceral SEP	Unknown	Unknown	Research only
Sacral reflex test	Good	Good	Grade B
Viscerosomatic reflex	Unknown	Unknown	Research only
Autonomic testing	Variable (different techniques)	Fair	Research only

Figure 3-30. Evidence-based recommendations for neurophysiologic testing. The clinical recommendations given here are based on the report by the Committee on Clinical Neurophysiology at the 3rd International Consultation on Incontinence (June 26–29, 2004, Monaco) [23], based on available published data and classified by type of research or clinical publication.

Neurophysiologic tests may enhance information from clinical examination and urodynamic testing. The tests should be performed by trained and certified staff with formal quality control. Organization of interdisciplinary teams with urogynecology, urology, proctology, and neurology would be the ideal. EMG—electromyography; SEP—somatosensory evoked potential.

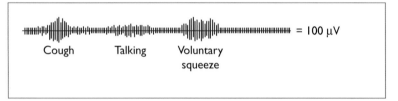

Figure 3-31. Kinesiologic electromyography (EMG). Kinesiologic EMG measures dynamic skeletal muscle activity during a given activity. The skeletal muscle activity is a function of "motor units," a motor unit being an anterior horn cell, its axon and axonal branches, and all the muscle fibers innervated by the anterior horn cell axon branches. The kinesiologic EMG measures the aggregate of activated motor units in the recording territory of the electrode. This type of EMG examination is used widely in urodynamic studies. Usually surface electrodes are applied para-anally, but needle electrodes in the external anal sphincter or urethral sphincter are preferable in patients with spasticity as they will record more localized and specific muscle activity. Outlet skeletal muscle activity as coordinated with bladder activity may be evaluated. Normally, there is quieting of EMG activity prior to detrusor contraction with voiding, a coordination secondary to activity in the pons. Disruption of the pontine–sacral pathway leads to loss of this coordination, a condition known as detrusor-sphincter dyssynergia. Similar studies of the external anal sphincter or puborectalis to demonstrate "paradoxical" contraction during defecation have met with varying results.

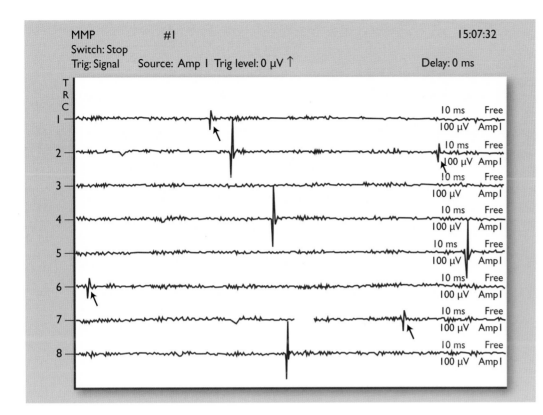

MMP   #1   15:07:32
Switch: Stop
Trig: Signal   Source: Amp 1 Trig level: 0 µV ↑   Delay: 0 ms

Figure 3-32. Concentric needle electromyogram (EMG). Concentric needle EMG evaluation may be applied to the external anal sphincter, urethral sphincter, or pubococcygeus and puborectalis muscle. The study assists in diagnosing myopathic or neuropathic conditions, evaluating states of denervation or reinnervation, and ability to "recruit" motor units to increase strength, and the needle electrode may also be used for recording in sacral reflex studies. Amp—amplifier; MMP—multimotor unit potential; TRC—recording channel; Trig—trigger.

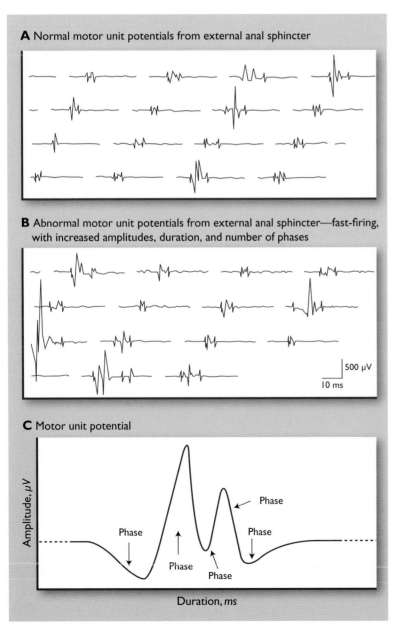

A Normal motor unit potentials from external anal sphincter

B Abnormal motor unit potentials from external anal sphincter—fast-firing, with increased amplitudes, duration, and number of phases

500 µV

10 ms

C Motor unit potential

Amplitude, µV

Phase

Phase

Phase

Phase

Phase

Phase

Duration, ms

Figure 3-33. Electromyogram (EMG) interpretation. Typically in needle EMG studies, the examiner will look for insertional activity (defines presence of muscle or absence as in fibrous replacement), spontaneous activity (which acts as a hallmark of denervation states or states of abnormal neuromuscular activity), recruitment (an activation of motor units that occurs with attempt to increase strength of a muscle's contraction; recruitment is decreased in neuropathic states and is "increased" in myopathic conditions), and motor unit potential morphology and stability (morphology is altered in reinnervation, and stability denotes active versus static neural activity states). Advanced EMG systems now offer computer-assisted programs so that motor unit activity may be analyzed by examining individual motor unit potentials, examining multiple motor units simultaneously, or by analyzing intermingled motor units during muscle contraction. Normative data are now available for these advanced types of needle EMG analysis of anal sphincter muscle, but careful attention to the EMG instrument make, filter parameters, and method of data collection is necessary. The study is then objective and clinically useful, and the normative data are not significantly affected by age, gender, vaginal deliveries, and the part of the external anal sphincter examined.

Needle EMG of sphincter muscles has suggested that pelvic floor denervation is a component of pelvic floor disorders. Patients with sacral radiculopathies or cauda equina or conus medullaris disorders are helped in the diagnosis by sphincter needle EMG. Anal sphincter needle EMG is helpful in distinguishing multiple system atrophy (or Shy–Drager syndrome) from Parkinson's disease [24]. In this condition, urinary incontinence frequently precedes the neurologic features. Urethral needle EMG has revealed complex repetitive discharges or "pseudomyotonia" in a group of young women with urinary retention and features of polycystic ovary syndrome. The syndrome has gained the term *Fowler's syndrome* [25]. The abnormal EMG activity has also been seen in asymptomatic subjects.

Single-fiber needle EMG was used in original research demonstrating relationships of neuropathy to pelvic floor disorders. It now is used very little clinically, mainly because the information gained is not as great as with concentric needle EMG and the cost of the needles is considerable.

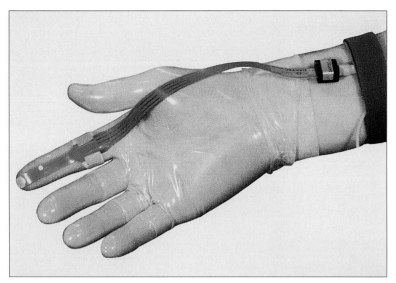

Figure 3-34. Pudendal nerve conduction tests. Motor nerve conduction velocities are routinely used in limb studies, the test requiring measurement of at least two points where the nerve is stimulated to calculate velocities. Such measurement is not possible in the pelvis. A single stimulation of a nerve to a muscle with recording of the response over the muscle is another way to evaluate the nerve and is termed a *distal* or *terminal motor latency*. The response over the muscle is called the compound muscle action potential (CMAP). Such a study of the pudendal nerve is most commonly performed with the "St. Mark's pudendal electrode" [26]. The stimulating cathode and anode and the two recording electrodes are on a disposable adhesive sheet that can be applied to an examining glove. The stimulating electrodes are located at the finger tip and the recording electrodes at the base of the examiner's index finger. It is used rectally so the examiner may stimulate the pudendal nerve at the ischial spine and the recording electrodes at the base of the examiner's finger records the CMAP at the external anal sphincter.

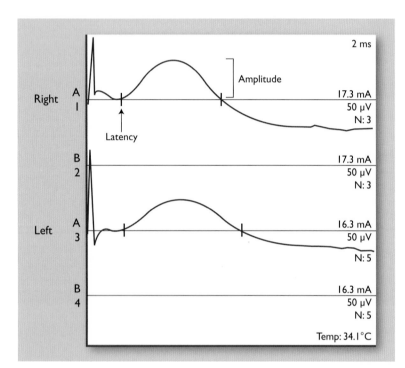

Figure 3-35. Interpretation of pudental nerve conduction tests. The resulting pudendal compound muscle action potential (CMAP) has measurable latency and amplitude. However, there are varying opinions on the validity of the test because reproducibility, sensitivity, and specificity are uncertain. The test was thought to predict response to anal sphincter surgery but more recent studies have not shown this [27]. The American Gastroenterological Association has stated that the pudendal terminal motor latency test cannot be recommended for evaluation of patients with fecal incontinence. Any utility in urinary incontinence is doubtful.

Anterior sacral root stimulation: Transcutaneous stimulation of the deeply situated sacral roots has become possible with the development of special electrical and magnetic stimulators, and recorded responses can be made in the pelvic floor muscles. Stimulation over the sacrum allows anterior root stimulation. Needle electrode recording is preferable in the sphincter because the stimuli are nonselective and activate several muscles innervated by lumbosacral segments. The most important clinical use of anterior sacral root stimulation is with the treatment of sacral neuromodulation. In this, patients with lower urinary tract or colorectal dysfunction have invasive percutaneous stimulation of the sacral roots, chiefly S3. Before implanting a permanent stimulator, a temporary external stimulator is used to test response as judged by patients' urinary (or colorectal) diaries. Observable muscle contractions in the foot and the perineum occur with proper stimulation when placing the anterior sacral stimulating lead, and CMAP responses may be obtained with appropriate recording electrodes placed over a muscle supplied by the respective sacral root. The latencies of the response differentiate CMAP (muscle response to stimulation of its supplying nerve or nerve root) from reflex response (muscle response from stimulating the sensory nerve in the segmental reflex arc). Clinical value of the test is yet to be established.

Motor evoked potentials: The muscle response to stimulation of its neural supply in the central nervous system is termed motor evoked potentials (MEP), and pelvic floor muscle MEPs from stimulation over the motor cortex or the spine are possible. The cortical stimulation is now mainly done with magnetic stimulation, as this type of stimulation is much less painful than electrical. Normative data for the urethral sphincter and the puborectalis muscle in adult women for transcranial magnetic stimulation have been reported [28]. Again, it is preferable to use concentric needle electrodes for recording. Clinical use for MEPs has not been well established.

Quantitative sensory testing (QST): Sensory testing is used commonly as in dermatomal skin testing, sensations during bladder fill on cystometric study, and anorectal sensations with anal manometry. More objective sensory testing can be performed with QST. QST of the urogenitoanal system may be performed with stimulation by vibration, temperature, or electrical methods. There is no commonly accepted, detailed, standardized test, and thus no established utility for incontinence evaluation.

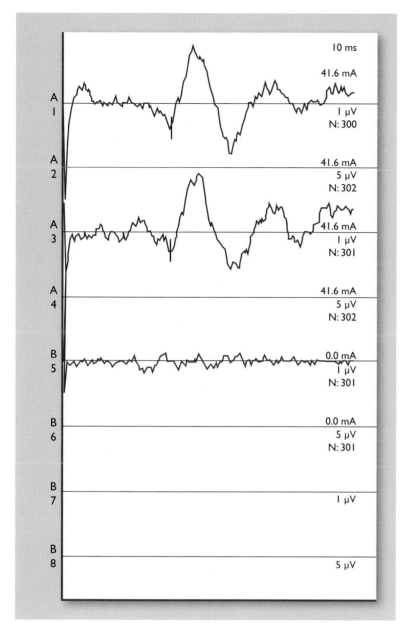

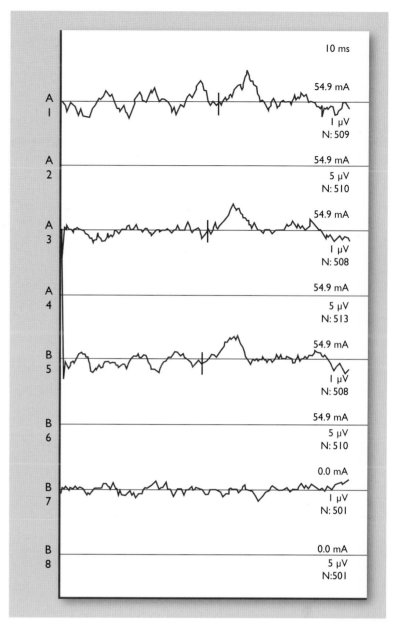

Figure 3-36. Somatosensory evoked potentials (SEPs) relevant to the evaluation of pelvic floor disorders. Pudendal SEPs are waveforms recorded over the central nervous system (spinal cord or cortex) that are elicited by stimulation of a sensory nerve or sensory innervated area (dermatome). Cerebral SEPs from stimulation in the leg or pelvic area are best recorded at the scalp site designated Cz-2cm and Fz for recording electrodes G1 and G2. These sites are part of the international 10–20 electroencephalography (EEG) system for scalp electrode placement. Cz-2 is in the sagittal midline, 2 cm posterior to the coronal plane realized by an imaginary line over the scalp, connecting the ears. The stimulus is applied adjacent to the clitoris with a 3-cm bar electrode, anode medial. Multiple stimuli are given, at a rate not to be divisible into 60 (50 in Europe) Hz so that interference is less likely to be problematic (usually 2.9 Hz). The stimulus intensity is three times sensory threshold and averaging of a few to many hundreds of stimuli is performed. The test is replicated and controlled by repeating without stimuli. The response latency at the cortex is about 40 ms for the first positive peak. This is similar to the latency of the cortical response to stimulation of the posterior tibial nerve at the ankle. The conduction time from the stimulus to the cord is, of course, longer with tibial stimulation, meaning that the cord conduction time for the tibial is shorter than for the pudendal nerve, leading to interesting theories of why this should be. The test may be done in conjunction with tibial SEP, wherein an abnormal pudendal SEP with normal tibial SEP suggests conus (sacral) involvement. Following spinal cord injury, tibial and pudendal SEPs are of prognostic value for bladder control [29].

Figure 3-37. Interpretation of somatosensory evoked potentials (SEPs). Stimulation of the urethra or bladder or anorectum can be done to obtain cerebral SEPs. This gives information about pelvic visceral pathways, which traverse the pelvic plexus. The response is very small and technically difficult to obtain. The latency (varying from 50 to 100 ms) is greater than pudendal SEPs, as would be expected with the afferent nerves being small, slowly conducting visceral afferents.

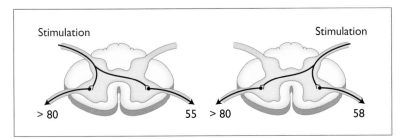

Figure 3-38. Sacral reflexes: The Third International Consultation on Incontinence Committee on Clinical Neurophysiology has graded the sacral reflex test as "good" for technical and diagnostic performance and a grade of "B" for clinical performance. Only kinesiologic electromyography (EMG) and needle EMG have such positive recommendation [23]. The sacral reflex study has been given the term *bulbocavernosus reflex* but, as performed in women, it is better termed *clitoral–anal* reflex. The stimulation may be performed with right and left paraclitoral stimulation and with right and left anal recording. The recording is more specific if needle electrodes are used. As a practical matter, the clinical neuro-physiologic examination of the pelvic floor patient usually consists of initial concentric needle electromyography of the external anal sphincter (EAS) and the respective needles for the right and left EAS examination are left in place to record the responses in the clitoral–anal reflex. The stimulation is done at about three times sensory threshold and the stimulus is double, with an interstimulus interval of 5 ms, as double stimuli are more effective in obtaining response in polysynaptic reflex pathways. Measured parameters include sensory threshold and latency of response. With this study, efferent and afferent as well as side-to-side localization of dysfunction are possible.

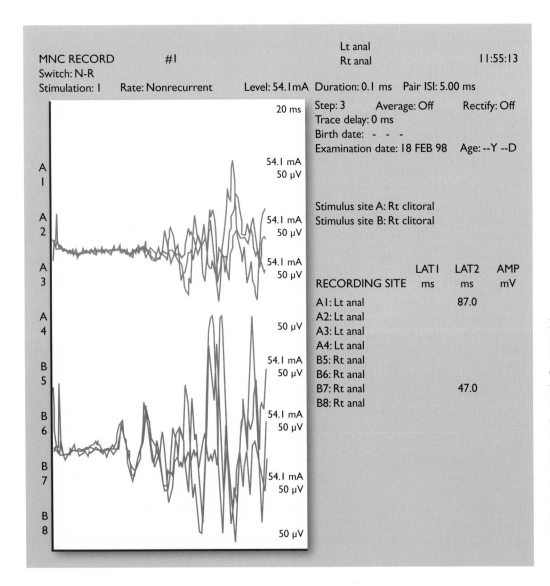

Figure 3-39. Interpretation of sacral reflexes. In cases of unilateral or asymmetric lesions, a healthy reflex arc may obscure a pathologic one if both clitoral–anal reflex arcs are not tested. The reflex may be absent or delayed in incontinent patients or patients with voiding dysfunction who have conus/cauda equina lesions. Abnormality may be seen with pudendal neuropathies. The reflex is abolished during micturition (just as sphincter electromyography quiets) if suprasegmental tracts are intact. Sacral reflex recording is suggested as a supplementary test to concentric needle electromyography of pelvic floor muscles in patients with suspected peripheral nervous lesions [30].

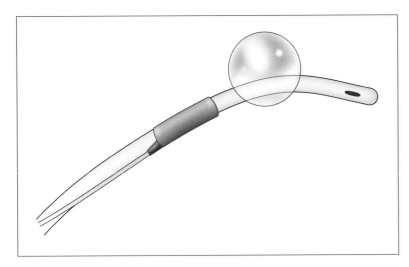

Figure 3-40. Viscerosomatic reflexes: anal. Anal responses may be recorded, in the manner described, with stimulation at the urethra or in the bladder. The stimulation may be applied, as with evoked responses from the bladder base, with catheter-mounted ring electrodes. These consist of two lengths of platinum wire wound into a thin cylinder and coated with plastic.

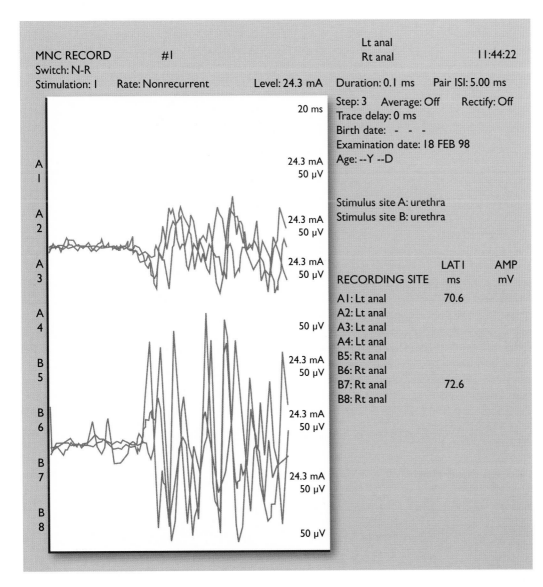

Figure 3-41. Viscerosomatic reflexes: urethral. The urethra is stimulated with the ring electrode located 1 cm distal to the urethrovesical junction. The stimulus is paired as with other sacral reflexes. The stimulus is three to four times sensory threshold and a series (usually four) of responses is collected. Averaging is not done as there is some variability in the latencies as is seen in polysynaptic reflexes. Stimulation, with the same electrodes, may be done in the bladder to obtain a bladder–anal reflex. To ensure electrode contact with the bladder, the bladder is emptied, the Foley balloon is deflated, the catheter is advanced into the bladder, and the catheter-mounted electrodes are connected to the preamplifier to do impedance testing. The catheter is manipulated until impedance is under 10 kΩ, ensuring electrode contact with the bladder wall. The electrodes are then reconnected to the stimulator to do the test. Measured parameters include sensory threshold and latency of response. The response latency is longer than the clitoral–anal reflex because slowly conducting, smaller sensory afferents constitute the afferent side of the reflex.

As indicated by the Clinical Neurophysiology Committee, clinical data are not sufficient to recommend the clinical use of the viscerosomatic reflexes at this time, but the potential is significant [23].

Localizing Disorders

Clinical Condition	Clitoral–anal reflex	Urethroanal reflex	Bladder–anal reflex
Pudendal neuropathy	Abnormal	Abnormal	Abnormal
Cauda equina disorder	Abnormal	Abnormal	Abnormal
Conus medullaris disorder	Abnormal	Abnormal	Abnormal
Pelvic plexopathy (radical surgery, radiation, etc.)	Normal	Abnormal	Abnormal
Intrinsic bladder afferent disorder (overdistention, bladder neuropathy)	Normal	Normal	Abnormal
Urethral denervation (multiple periurethral dissections)	Normal	Abnormal	Normal

Figure 3-42. Neurophysiologic testing for voiding dysfunction. Because the afferent arms of the reflexes have different origin and pathways [31], localizing dysfunction is possible and can be of value especially in patients with voiding disorders.

Bethanechol supersensitivity test: As mentioned in Figure 3-7, when smooth muscle is denervated, it assumes hypersensitivity to its neurotransmitter. A neurologically intact bladder should have a pressure increase less than 15 cm of H_2O after subcutaneous injection of 5 mg of bethanechol. The increase in pressure is noted 10 to 20 minutes after the injection (simultaneously with sweating and salivation as drug effects). One method is to completely empty the bladder and instill 100 mL of CO_2 at 5-minute intervals. A positive test (> 15-cm H_2O pressure increase) indicates bladder denervation, specifically of postganglionic parasympathetic nerves or their reflex pathway. The test value is debated. The committee on Neurologic Urinary and Fecal Incontinence at the Third International Consultation on Incontinence recommends that the test should be optional for differentiation between neurologic and nonneurologic detrusor areflexia and should be interpreted in conjunction with other diagnostic results. When patients with detrusor areflexia were studied in conjunction with sphincter needle electromyography and clitoral–anal reflex, the combined accuracy approached 100% [32].

OTHER TESTING

Autonomic testing: Most electrophysiologic testing evaluates large-fiber nerves (see Fig. 3-10 for nerve fiber size) and not small, lightly myelinated or "unmyelinated" nerves such as the autonomic nerves. Methods for evaluating the autonomic nerves to the pelvis, with the exception of the bethanechol supersensitivity test, are not available, although cystometry indirectly evaluates the parasympathetic innervation. Small, visceral sensory fibers are tested by stimulating the proximal urethra or bladder and recording the sacral visceroanal reflex or cerebral somatosensory evoked potentials as described, and this is an indirect way to evaluate the autonomic fibers because the pathways are similar. Generalized autonomic dysfunction may be studied by cardiovascular autonomic function tests, and these may be helpful in patients with bladder or gastrointestinal motility disturbances. Smooth muscle electromyography has been limited by technical problems.

The sympathetic skin response (SSR): The sweat gland activity in the skin is sympathetically mediated, and noxious stimulation (electrical shock, sudden noise, etc.) will cause a recordable potential. The recording is done with surface electrodes on the palms and soles and can also be recorded from the perineum. The SSR, when produced by an electrical stimulus, is a reflex with large, myelinated sensory fibers, a complex central integrative function, and a sympathetic efferent limb with postganglionic, nonmyelinated C fibers. The test is not sensitive for partial lesions as only its absence can be considered pathologic. Its utility in evaluating bladder dysfunction is not established.

REFERENCES

1. Elbadawi A: Comparative neuromorphology in animals. In *The Physiology of the Lower Urinary Tract*. Edited by Torrens M. Berlin: Springer-Verlag; 1987.

2. Hale D, Benson JT, Brubaker L, et al.: Histologic analysis of needle biopsy of urethral sphincter from normal and stress incontinent women with comparison of electromyographic findings. *Am J Obstet Gynecol* 1999, 180:342–348.

3. Manter JT, Gatz AJ: In *Essentials of Clinical Neuroanatomy and Neurophysiology*, edn 8. Edited by Gilman S, Newman SW. Philadelphia: FA Davis; 1992.

4. Wiesenfeld-Hallin Z, Hao JX, Xu XJ, Hokfelt T: Nitric oxide mediates ongoing discharges in dorsal root ganglion cells after peripheral nerve injury. *J Neurophysiol* 1993, 70:2350–2353.

5. Clemente CD: *Gray's Anatomy*, edn 30. Philadelphia: Lea & Febiger; 1985:940, 1192, 1248.

6. Andersson K-E: Pharmacology of lower urinary tract smooth muscles and penile erectile tissues. *Pharmacol Rev* 1993, 45:253.

7. Alexander SPH, Mathie A, Peters JA: Acetylcholine receptors (muscarinic). *Trends Pharmacol Sci (Nomenclature Suppl)* 2001:15–18.

8. Elbadawi A, Schenk EA: A new theory of the innervation of bladder musculature. Part 3. Postganglionic synapse in uretero-vesical-urethral autonomic pathways. *J Urol* 1971, 105:373.

9. Low PA: *Clinical Autonomic Disorders*. Boston: Little, Brown; 1993.

10. Erlanger J, Gasser HS: *Electrical Signs of Nervous Activity*. Philadelphia: University of Pennsylvania Press; 1937.

11. Shepherd JJ, Wright PG: The response of the internal anal sphincter in man to stimulation of the presacral nerve. *Am J Dig Dis* 1968, 13:421–427.

12. Blok BF, Sturms LM, Holstege G: Brain activation during micturition in women. *Brain* 1998, 121(Pt 11):2033.

13. DeGroat WC, Booth AM: Autonomic systems to the urinary bladder and sexual organs. In *Peripheral Neuropathy*. Edited by Dyck PJ, Thomas PK, Lambert EH, et al. Philadelphia: WB Saunders; 1984:285–299.

14. Furness JB, Llewellyn-Smith IJ, Bornstein JC, Costa M: Chemical neuroanatomy and the analysis of neural circuitry in the enteric nervous system. In *The Peripheral Nervous System: Handbook of Chemical Neuroanatomy*, vol 6. Edited by Bjorklund A, Hokfelt T, Owman C. New York: Elsevier Biomedical Publishers; 1988:161–218.

15. Parks AG: Anorectal incontinence. *Proc R Soc Med* 1975, 68:681–690.

16. Platzer W, Poisel S, Hafez ESE: Functional anatomy of the human vagina. In *The Human Vagina*. Edited by Hafez ESE, Evans TN. New York: Elsevier/North Holland Biomedical Press; 1978.

17. Maclin VM: Anatomy and physiology of the vagina. In *Female Pelvic Floor Disorders*. Edited by Benson JT. New York: Norton Medical Books; 1992.

18. Bohlen JG, Held JP, Sanderson MO, Ahlgren A: The female orgasm: pelvic contractions. *Arch Sex Behav* 1982, 11:367.

19. Freud S: *Obras Completas.* Madrid: Biblioteca Nueva; 1967.

20. Forsberg JG: A morphologist's approach to the vagina: age related changes and estrogen sensitivity. *Maturitas* 1995, 22:S7.

21. Siroky MB, Krane RJ: The history and examination in neuro-urology. In *Clinical Uroneurology*. Edited by Krane RJ, Siroky MB. Boston, Toronto, London: Little, Brown; 1991.

22. Gilman S, Newman SW, eds: *Manter and Gatz's Essentials of Clinical Neuroanatomy and Neurophysiology*, edn 8. Philadelphia: FA Davis; 1992:61.

23. Abrams P, Cardozo L, Khoury S, Wein A, eds: *Incontinence.* Paris: Editions 21; 2002.

24. Palace J, Chandiramani VA, Fowler CJ: Value of sphincter electromyography in the diagnosis of multiple system atrophy. *Muscle Nerve* 1997, 20:1396–403.

25. Fowler CJ, Christmas TJ, Chapple CR, *et al.*: Abnormal electromyographic activity of the urethral voiding dysfunction, and polycystic ovaries: a new syndrome? *BMJ* 1988, 297:1436–1438.

26. Kiff ES, Swash M: Normal proximal and delayed distal conduction in the pudendal nerves of patients with idiopathic (neurogenic) fecal incontinence. *J Neurol Neurosurg Psychiatry* 1984, 47:820–823.

27. Malouf AJ, Norton CS, Engel AF, *et al.*: Long term results of overlapping anterior anal sphincter repair for obstetric trauma. *Lancet* 2000, 355:260–265.

28. Brostrom S, Jennum P, Lose G: Motor evoked potentials from the striated urethral sphincter and puborectal muscle: normative values. *Neurourol Urodyn* 2003, 22: 620–637.

29. Curt A, Rodic B, Schurch B, *et al.*: Recovery of bladder function in patients with acute spinal cord injury: significance of ASIA scores and somatosensory evoked potentials. *Spinal Cord* 1997, 35:368–373.

30. Podnar S, Vodusek DB: Protocol for clinical neurophysiologic examination of the pelvic floor. *Neurourol Urodyn* 2001, 20:669–682.

31. Maiden C, Fuller E, Brizendine E, Benson JT: The bladder-anal reflex. *Neurourol Urodyn* 2003, 22:683–686.

32. Sidi AA, Dykstra DD, Peng W: Bethanechol supersensitivity test, rhabdosphincter electromyography, and bulbocavernosus reflex latency in the diagnosis of neurologic detrusor areflexia. *J Urol* 1988, 140:335.

4

Pathophysiology of Pelvic Visceral Dysfunction

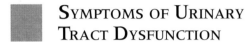
SYMPTOMS OF URINARY TRACT DYSFUNCTION

PATHOPHYSIOLOGY

Dysfunction of the lower urinary tract such as incontinence or voiding dysfunction may decrease a patient's quality of life.

Symptoms of overactive bladder (OAB) (urgency, with or without incontinence, usually with frequency and nocturia) may be related to urodynamically demonstrable involuntary detrusor contractions during filling cystometry. When there is a relevant neurologic condition that is known to affect urinary function, detrusor overactivity may be characterized as "neurogenic detrusor overactivity."

OAB is associated with female stress urinary incontinence. The hypothesis in this situation involves the loss of pelvic floor afferent inhibition of detrusor contraction. Although yet unproven, this is an exciting example of an anatomic defect leading to a functional consequence. In nonneurogenic OAB, the mechanisms listed in this section may contribute to its pathophysiology (see Fig. 4-4). Nonneurogenic causes of OAB are nearly always idiopathic. Neurophysiologic mechanisms in animal experiments provide some potential mechanisms for detrusor overactivity.

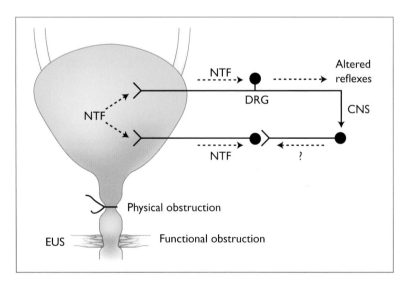

Figure 4-1. Neuroplasticity in bladder neural pathways following partial urethral obstruction. In paraplegic cats that develop reflex voiding, the voiding is inefficient secondary to detrusor–sphincter dyssynergia. The bladder becomes enlarged and the afferent neurons increase in size markedly (by 50%). In animals with urinary diversion after spinal transection, the bladder distention and hypertrophy were avoided and the afferent neuron hypertrophy was prevented, suggesting that factors released in the hypertrophied bladder are responsible for the neural changes. Outlet obstruction produced by urethral ligation in cats with intact spinal cords induces hypertrophy of bladder afferent and efferent neurons, which is accompanied by increased levels of nerve growth factor (NGF). Changes in afferent neuron pathways can also be elicited by other agents (eg, bradykinin, histamine, nitric oxide) that can be released in the urinary bladder by afferent neurons.

Continued on the next page

Figure 4-1. *(Continued)* Hence, disorders of the central nervous system (CNS) can increase bladder activity by altering central neural mechanisms; however, these mechanisms may also be altered by local bladder conditions, such as obstruction, inflammation, or injury, and may lead to overactive bladder (OAB). With these conditions, a C fiber–mediated spinal reflex develops, which can be tested with the ice-water test. An increase in NGF occurs with each of these conditions and, if blockage is present, the urinary frequency following obstruction or inflammation does not occur [1]. Manipulating the NGF production or blocking its receptors may influence an OAB. DRG—dorsal root ganglia; EUS—external urethral sphincter; NTF—neurotrophic factor. *(From DeGroat [2].)*

Aging is clinically associated with OAB in both men and women. Elderly patients with OAB have a characteristic ultrastructural pattern of abundant protrusion junctions between bladder muscle cells, which allows ion transfer and may promote electrical coupling and generate myogenic contractions. Superimposed degeneration of bladder muscle was associated with clinical poor emptying, the detrusor hyperactivity with impaired contractility syndrome [3].

Age-related changes in cholinergic and purinergic ATP neurotransmission result in a decrease of the former and an increase of the latter during electrical stimulation in humans, which may contribute to changes in bladder function in the elderly.

Idiopathic detrusor overactivity has distinct mechanisms that are considered to be involved in the pathophysiology of the disorder. A primary mechanism is sensory afferent activation. Normally, lightly myelinated A delta nerve fibers, with endings located in the detrusor smooth muscle, serve as bladder afferents in the pathways involved with storage or elimination. Smaller unmyelinated C fibers also exist; most are "silent" and not actively involved in bladder reflex activity. However, a group of C fibers that are neuropeptide containing and sensitive to capsaicin (the chemical producing the "hot" sensations when eating hot peppers) may become active. These may be referred to as capsaicin-sensitive sensory afferents. Local release of tachykinins (substance P, calcitonin G–related peptide, neurokinin) in the bladder wall from these sensory nerves produces detrusor muscle contraction and increased vascular permeability.

Figure 4-2. The bladder urothelium has a vital role in afferent activation. While many bodily afferent activities begin with the afferent nerve (eg, the somatic sensations carried from the skin begin with cutaneous afferent nerves), other places, such as the hearing organ and auditory nerves, the gustatory afferent epithelium, and afferent nerve, have afferent impulse initiation in combined structures involving epithelium and nerve. Such appears to be the case with the bladder, in which the urothelium is actively involved with the afferent nerves. The C fibers generally end in the suburothelial layer of the bladder wall, but they can penetrate the urothelium. The urothelium is involved in transduction, the release of mediators/transmitters, and the intermediate layer of transitional epithelium in the bladder has cells that contain cytoplasmic vesicles filled with such mediators. NGF—nerve growth factor; NO—nitric oxide.

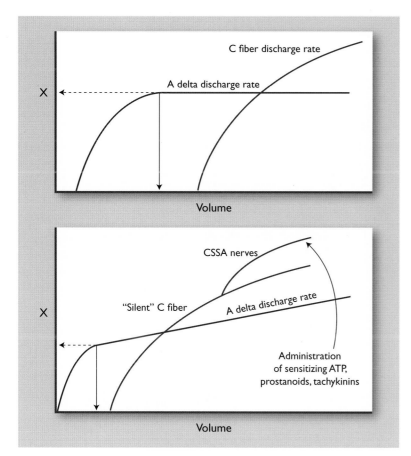

Figure 4-3. Correlation of afferent discharge with a cystometrogram. ATP is released by bladder distention and ATP receptors (P2X3) are expressed on sensory afferent nerves. Thus, bladder distention can evoke neural discharges. In humans, this P2X3 immunoreactivity is found near myofibroblasts in close apposition to C fiber endings. Prostanoids and nitric oxide (NO) are also synthesized in mucosa and muscle, and it is likely that stimulatory ATP, prostanoids, tachykinins, and inhibitory NO mediators are involved in transduction underlying the activation of sensory afferents. Upregulation of urothelial afferent transduction can induce overactive bladder (OAB). The density of capsaicin-sensitive sensory afferent (CSSA) nerves is increased in idiopathic OAB [4].

Muscle, nerve cells, and urothelial cells produce nerve growth factor (NGF), which is retrogradely transported to the nerve nucleus and causes responses that include altered gene expression. This allows neurons to prevent atrophy and maintain important gene products including ion channels. Mediators from different cell types including urothelium, myofibroblasts, nerve endings, smooth muscle cells, mast cells, and others influence the sensitivity (the action potential firing rate) of afferent neurons. NGF is included with the abovementioned stimulatory mediators. The increase in CSSA nerves is not seen if NGF is inhibited and the NGF influencing the increase in C fiber afferentation is produced in the bladder.

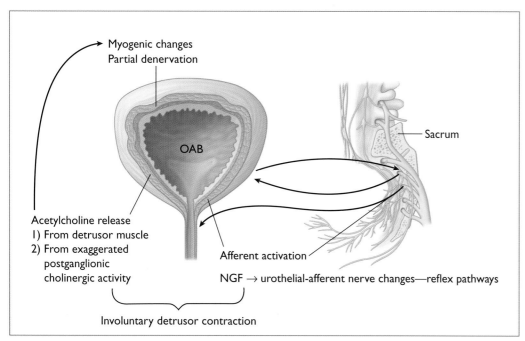

Figure 4-4. Myogenic changes may contribute to the pathophysiology of overactive bladder (OAB). It is hypothesized that partial denervation of the detrusor increases cell coupling. The proposed increased coupling between muscle cells in OAB has been refuted by findings of the reduction of gap junctions (intercellular connections allowing the passage of electrical or ionic activity), but changes in muscle cell properties are consistently found in bladders with involuntary contractions [5].

Acetylcholine release. There is a basal release of acetylcholine, of a nonneuronal origin, in the human detrusor associated with stretch. The production is in the urothelium or possibly occurs by increased postganglionic cholinergic neurons activated by increased afferent activity in patients with OAB [6].

Stress urinary incontinence (SUI) has been dichotomized to urethral hypermobility versus intrinsic urethral sphincter deficiency. Fifty years ago, the posterior urethrovesical angle was implicated and a correlation of loss of the angle with SUI has been documented. Many cases were not associated, however, and the idea that primary urethral weakness could cause SUI became evident. Originally called type III incontinence (types I and II having mobility of the urethra and changes in the urethrovesical angle), the name of the condition has become intrinsic sphincter deficiency (ISD). Important elements in ISD include pudendal innervation; striated sphincter mass and function; and urethral smooth muscle, mucosa, and submucosal cushions. The dichotomy of hypermobility versus ISD has given way to a continuum, in part due to the development of the concept of Valsalva leak point pressure (VLPP) [7]. The amount of pressure that is required to produce leakage in the absence of detrusor contraction (VLPP) has emerged as correlating well with incontinence symptoms.

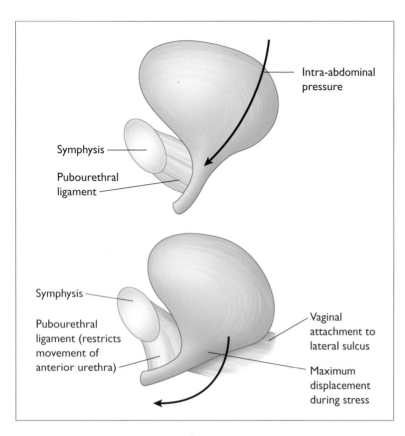

Intra-abdominal pressure

Symphysis

Pubourethral ligament

Symphysis

Pubourethral ligament (restricts movement of anterior urethra)

Vaginal attachment to lateral sulcus

Maximum displacement during stress

Figure 4-5. Effects of intra-abdominal pressure. Real-time ultrasonography suggests that the anterior and posterior walls of the proximal urethra move differently during increases in intra-abdominal pressure [8]. The anterior urethra becomes arrested in its rotational descent by the pubourethral ligaments and the posterior urethra continues to descend with the vaginal wall, supported by the vagina and its lateral attachments that form the lateral sulcus. With intra-abdominal pressure increases, the proximal urethra first has a "funneling" or shearing force produced by the unequal separation of the urethral walls, then an expulsive force produced by pressure transmission of abdominal forces to the bladder and urethra. The urethra resists this by closure of the pudendally innervated sphincter. The relative contributions of vaginal mobility and urethral function are part of a continuum, not a dichotomy.

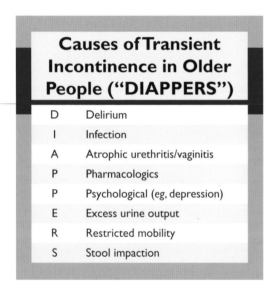

Causes of Transient Incontinence in Older People ("DIAPPERS")

D	Delirium
I	Infection
A	Atrophic urethritis/vaginitis
P	Pharmacologics
P	Psychological (eg, depression)
E	Excess urine output
R	Restricted mobility
S	Stool impaction

Figure 4-6. Transient incontinence. Thanks to our colleagues in geriatric medicine, we have the useful mnemonic "DIAPPERS" to assist in the recall of transient factors that lead to incontinence. Delirium (D) is a fluctuating, confused state, its onset and duration measured in hours rather than years as with dementia, and incontinent episodes of essentially normal voiding occur during the confusion. Infection (I) may cause incontinence as the chief symptom in the elderly, who frequently lack irritative symptoms with urinary tract infection. Atrophy (A), based on more recent epidemiologic studies, may not be causative of incontinence and more research is needed. Medications (P, pharmacologics) are one of the most common causes of incontinence in older people and include sedatives, diuretics, anticholinergics, antihistamines, antispasmotics, opiates, α-adrenergic blockers, and calcium channel blockers. Psychologic factors (the second P), eg, depression, are states in which vegetative signs may include a loss of regard for continence. Excess (E) urine

output, including that seen with diabetes, alcoholism, congestive states, and edema, can cause incontinence. Restricted mobility is often overlooked. Fecal impaction usually involves both urinary and fecal incontinence, fecal incontinence being the seepage of liquid stool (S) around the impaction, which maintains a constant rectoanal inhibitory reflex and keeps the internal anal sphincter relaxed. Reflexes involving the lower urinary tract are probably also involved with the urinary incontinence, but data on this are inadequate.

Neurogenic overactive bladder. Because not all patients with a given neurologic condition develop typical urinary symptoms or urodynamic findings, a specific understanding of each individual's dysfunction is absolutely necessary. The understanding must include a description of the function of the bladder, urethra, and pelvic floor; their coordination during filling and voiding; and their influence on other conditions, eg, autonomic dysreflexia or renal function. Generally, urodynamic investigation is necessary to provide the specific understanding required for therapy. When observed in urodynamic study, involuntary detrusor activity may lead to incontinence, which is called neurogenic detrusor overactivity incontinence. If accompanied by a sensation of the desire to void, it may be termed urge incontinence. If a sensation is absent, the term reflex incontinence was used in the past but is no longer recommended.

If the urethra contracts when the detrusor contracts, detrusor–sphincter dyssynergia is diagnosed. Functional obstruction may be produced. If a high-pressure situation develops, renal impairment may occur.

Urodynamic findings of little phasic detrusor activity with poor compliance and urinary loss when intravesical pressures elevate, the so-called detrusor leak point pressure, represent a condition formerly termed overflow incontinence. Again, elevated pressures may be associated with endangered renal function. The level of pressure that is considered to be too elevated is about 40 cm H_2O, but the evidence for this is not completely clear.

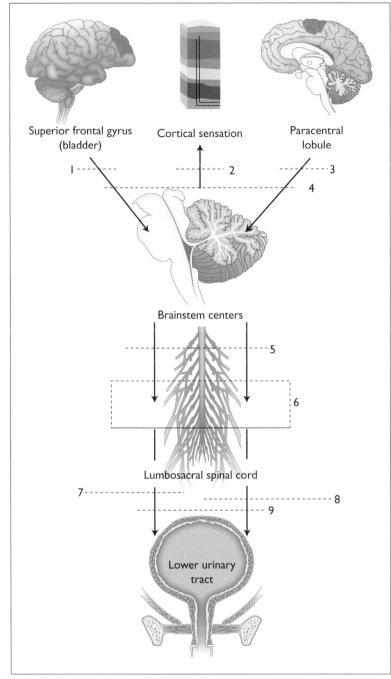

Figure 4-7. Clinical stigmata of lesions relating to function of the lower urinary tract. A simplified scheme shows the interaction of various levels of the nervous system in micturition. The locations of certain possible nervous lesions are denoted by numbers and explained as follows. 1) Lesions isolating the superior frontal gyrus prevent the voluntary postponement of voiding. If sensation is intact, this produces urge incontinence. If the lesion is larger, there is an additional loss of social concern about incontinence. 2) Lesions

isolating the paracentral lobule, sometimes associated with a hemiparesis, cause spasticity of the urethral sphincter and retention. This will be painless if sensation is abolished. Minor degrees of this syndrome may cause difficulty in the initiation of micturition. 3) Pathways of sensation are not known accurately. In theory, an isolated lesion of sensation above the brainstem would lead to unconscious incontinence. Defective central conduction of sensory information would explain nocturnal enuresis. 4) Lesions above the brainstem centers lead to involuntary voiding that is coordinated with sphincter relaxation. 5) Lesions below brainstem centers but above the lumbosacral spinal cord, after a period of bladder paralysis associated with spinal shock, lead to involuntary reflex voiding that is not coordinated with sphincter relaxation (detrusor–sphincter dyssynergia). 6) Lesions destroying the lumbosacral cord of the complete nervous connections between the central and peripheral nervous system result in a paralyzed bladder that contracts only weakly in an autonomous fashion due to its remaining ganglionic innervation. However, if the lumbar sympathetic outflow is preserved in the presence of conus or cauda equina destruction, there may be residual sympathetic tone in the bladder neck and urethra that may be sufficient to be obstructive. 7) A lesion of the efferent fibers alone leads to a bladder of decreased capacity and decreased compliance that is associated experimentally with an increased number of adrenergic nerves. 8) A lesion confined to the afferent fibers produces a bladder that is areflexic with increased compliance and capacity. 9) Because there are ganglion cells in the bladder wall, it is technically impossible to decentralize the bladder completely, but congenital absence of bladder ganglia may exist, producing megacystitis.

Work by DeGroat [2] and others has led to a new era in the understanding of neural activity relating to urogynecologic disorders. Together, clinicians and scientists, working in conjunction with manufacturers and the interested public, can use this knowledge to dramatically improve patient care.

In humans, the medial frontal lobes of the cerebral cortex and the basal ganglia suppress the micturition reflex. Suprapontine lesions affect the glutaminergic excitatory and inhibitory regulation of micturition from the cortex and the central dopaminergic dual excitatory and inhibitory influences on reflex bladder activity. Cerebral infarction and Parkinson's disease alter the excitatory/inhibitory balance.

Spinal cord injury invokes the bladder effects seen in idiopathic detrusor overactivity. Capsaicin-sensitive C fiber afferentation develops, which does respond to intravesical administration of capsaicin or its ultrapotent analogue resiniferatoxin.

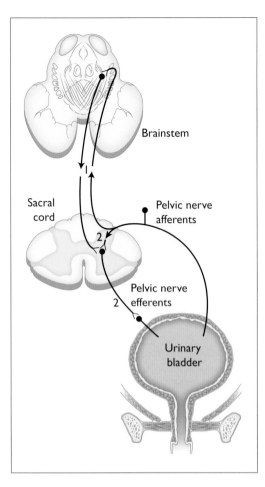

Figure 4-8. Micturition reflex. DeGroat's [2] theories have evolved. The micturition reflex in normal animals (pathway 1) with the stimulation of myelinated (alpha–delta) afferents from the bladder and recording from postganglionic nerves on the bladder surface had latencies of 100 ms with a demonstrated central delay of 60 to 75 ms, suggesting a supraspinal reflex mechanism. This reflex remained present in decerebrate animals but was lost in acute and chronic spinal injury animals. Sixty percent of animals with an intact spinal cord had a second reflex (pathway 2) with a latency of 180 to 200 ms with a demonstrated central delay of 15 to 40 ms, occurring only at stimulus intensities sufficient to activate unmyelinated afferent fibers (C fibers). This reflex was abolished with spinal cord transection, but 3 to 7 days later it returned and increased in magnitude in conjunction with development of reflex micturition. Capsaicin, a neurotoxin that disrupts C fiber function, blocks the bladder contractions induced by bladder distention in cats with chronic spinal injury, but not in normal cats. Thus, chronic spinal injury animals have the facilitation of C fiber–evoked reflex and lose alpha–delta-evoked reflexes, indicating two distinct central pathways (supraspinal and spinal) using different afferent limbs (alpha–delta and C fiber, respectively). Clinically, this C fiber–mediated reflex may be tested by instillation of cold water into the bladder, activating C fibers. There is no resulting voiding reflex in normal patients, but reflex voiding in response to cold water appears in patients with upper motor neuron lesions (multiple sclerosis, cerebrovascular disease, Parkinson's disease, the elderly with a loss of sensation, normal infants), suggesting that C fiber afferents are involved in several pathologic conditions associated with bladder overactivity. There are many possible mechanisms for the emergence of C fiber reflexes in paraplegic cats—eg, cord changes, loss of supraspinal inhibition, and changes in neurotransmitters—but there is considerable evidence that one important factor is changes in the afferent neurons.

The C fiber plasticity seen with a spinal cord injury involves an increase in size and excitability due to a shift in sodium channels from high-sensory (tetrodotoxin-resistant) to low-sensory (tetrodotoxin-sensitive) thresholds [9]. The capsaicin first stimulates, then depletes, the C fiber activity, resulting in increasing bladder capacity, reducing micturition contraction pressure, decreasing autonomic dysreflexia, and reducing incontinence frequency.

In a chronic spinal cord injury, the bladder afferent nerves increase in size, a change prevented by urinary diversion, suggesting that a factor released by the bladder—nerve growth factor (NGF)—is responsible for the afferent nerve changes. The release of NGF may be related to obstruction, produced in the chronic spinal cord–injured animal by the detrusor–sphincter dyssynergia. Spinal cord transection has recently been shown to alter the urothelial barrier function by producing ultrastructural changes with increased permeability, allowing irritating urinary constituents to change the properties of sensory pathways [10]. (*From* Krane and Siroky [11].)

URETERAL OBSTRUCTION AND REFLUX

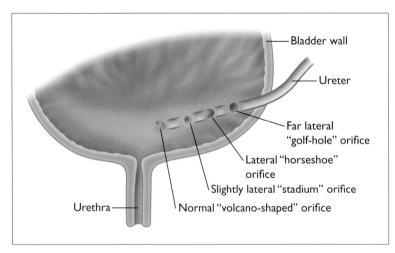

Figure 4-9. Surgical obstruction of the ureter is every pelvic surgeon's nightmare. Ureteral obstruction can occur with procidentia or vaginal vault prolapse. Ureteral reflux may be congenital or acquired. Congenital vesicoureteral reflux is a disorder of ureteral termination in which the orifice is too high and lateral. In total ureteral duplication, reflux is common and most frequently involves the lower pole ureter. Acquired reflux may be secondary to detrusor overactivity and not a primary anatomic abnormality at the ureterovesical junction. Thus, treating the overactivity may be helpful for reflux resolution.

Lyon classification. A ureterovesical dysfunction is frequently present and the degree of reflux varies directly with the length of the intravesical ureter. The 8- to 15-cm water pressure that is normally present in the bladder passively compresses the ureter. The ureteral orifice's appearance is affected by the intrinsic longitudinal muscular coat of the submucosal ureter. The orifice normally resembles a cone but can assume the appearance of a stadium, horseshoe, or golf hole with shortening of the muscular coat and with an increasing tendency toward laterality and reflux.

Prognostic factors for reflux resolution include the degree of hydronephrosis, laterality of orifice, morphology of orifice, length of intravesical ureter, age, and lower urinary tract dysfunction. One of the most sensitive studies for diagnosing reflux is retrograde cystography; a voiding cystogram is almost as reliable.

Continued on the next page

Figure 4-9. *(Continued)* Anatomic outlet obstructions may be associated with reflux, as can physiologic dysfunction. Detrusor–sphincter dyssynergia is associated with neurogenic detrusor overactivity and functional outlet obstruction with high intravesical pressures, which may result in reflux and renal dilatation. Bladder overactivity and noncompliance may be associated with hydronephrosis also.

Urinary tract infection is associated with reflux. Surgical intervention is suggested for children whose reflux persists beyond puberty, especially for girls, as reflux is a risk factor that predisposes to pyelonephritis during pregnancy. In adults, surgery for reflux is indicated in patients with severe derangement of ureterovesical junction or intractable recurrent urinary tract infection [12].

UPPER TRACT PROTECTION

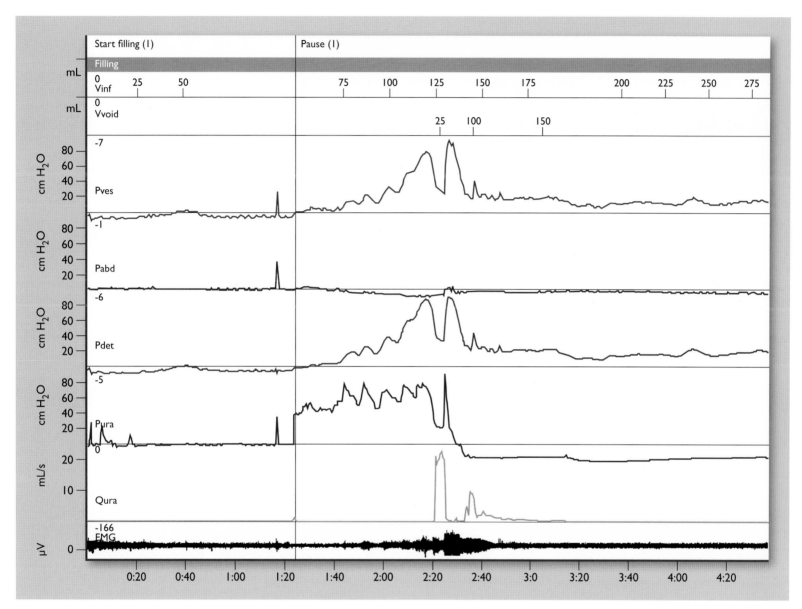

Figure 4-10. Cystometric study showing detrusor–sphincter dyssynergia. The *blue line* is intravesical pressure (Pves); the *red line* is abdominal pressure (Pabd); the *purple line* is "detrusor" pressure (Pdet), which is intravesical pressure minus abdominal pressure; the *green line* is intraurethral pressure (Pura); the *pink line* is urine flow; and the *black line* is anal electromyogram (EMG), measured with EMG needles in the right and left external anal sphincter muscle.

An involuntary detrusor contraction occurs without urethral relaxation and with a simultaneous increase in sphincter EMG activity and urinary loss occurs near the end of the involuntary contraction.

The "neurogenic bladder" may be classified in varying ways, but the most practical involves urodynamic pattern recognition. International Continence Society classification of overactive detrusor, underactive detrusor, overactive sphincter, and underactive sphincter is helpful. Four major patterns are usual in describing detrusor–sphincter dysfunction: 1) detrusor overactivity with sphincter overactivity (mostly dyssynergia), 2) detrusor overactivity and sphincter underactivity, 3) detrusor underactivity with sphincter overactivity, and 4) detrusor underactivity with sphincter underactivity. Patients with dysfunction of the lower urinary tract frequently need measures to protect the upper urinary tract. These measures include catheterization, pharmacologic management, and surgical management of contracted bladder states.

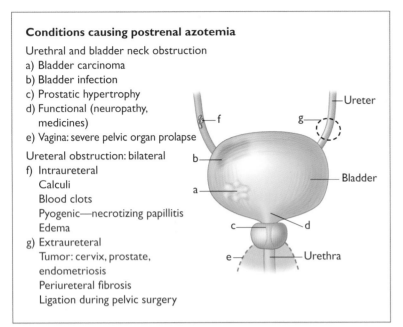

Conditions causing postrenal azotemia

Urethral and bladder neck obstruction
a) Bladder carcinoma
b) Bladder infection
c) Prostatic hypertrophy
d) Functional (neuropathy, medicines)
e) Vagina: severe pelvic organ prolapse

Ureteral obstruction: bilateral
f) Intraureteral
   Calculi
   Blood clots
   Pyogenic—necrotizing papillitis
   Edema
g) Extraureteral
   Tumor: cervix, prostate, endometriosis
   Periureteral fibrosis
   Ligation during pelvic surgery

Figure 4-11. The pelvic floor relationship to acute renal failure is in the postrenal category. The diagnosis is clinically suggested by findings such as palpable bladder or hydronephrotic kidneys and abnormal pelvic examination findings, particularly with findings that may be obstructive to the urinary tract, large residual urine volumes, and a history of calculi. Renal failure may be predicted based on urodynamic patterns of altered bladder function: detrusor overactivity, poor compliance, obstructive sphincter dyssynergia, and myogenic failure with increased residual urine are the most likely causes.

SEQUELAE OF PELVIC FLOOR DISORDERS

Skin breakdown. Urine is toxic to skin. This realization has led to marked improvements in padding and bedding for patients with urinary incontinence who are unable to attend to their own perineal hygiene. Frequently, it is incontinence that leads to nursing home placement and deterioration of the patient's relationships. Careful management of this factor is a primary focus of good patient care. Studies of skin-cleansing or moisturizing/barrier products have been limited because they have been uncontrolled, small, and lacking power. Perineal dermatitis is common among users of absorbent products, and skin wetness is the main cause. Fecal incontinence is more irritating than urinary incontinence and the combined effects are even more damaging. Skin cleansers may be better than soap and water for skin health. Less frequent pad changing is associated with pressure ulcers. Barrier creams may be recommended in buttock, sacral, and pad areas.

Sexual dysfunction and reconstructive surgery. It remains paradoxical that sexual function is addressed so infrequently by health care providers in the field of female pelvic medicine. The effects of pelvic floor disorders on sexual function are ubiquitous. No area of medical specialty is more closely related to sexual dysfunction and it is imperative that research and clinical management become a requirement of the subspecialty of female pelvic medicine and reconstructive surgery.

Unstructured, rather than structured, interviews are preferred by many clinicians. However, questionnaires may allow more effective evaluations in many situations. The quality of existing questionnaires was studied by the Committee on Symptom and Quality of Life Assessment at the Third International Consultation on Incontinence, held in Monaco in June 2004. The highest recommended questionnaire was the Golombok–Rust Inventory of Sexual Satisfaction. Designed for men and women in a current heterosexual relationship, it takes about 15 minutes to complete. The five female-specific domains are anorgasmia, vaginismus, avoidance, nonsexuality, and dissatisfaction.

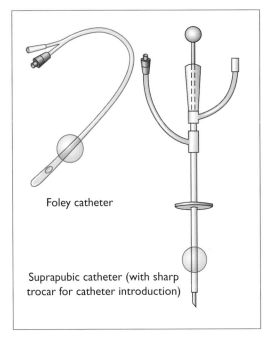

Foley catheter

Suprapubic catheter (with sharp trocar for catheter introduction)

Figure 4-12. Indwelling catheters are inserted urethrally or suprapubically through an abdominal wall incision. Urinary catheters are effective in bladder drainage, both in short- and long-term situations, by intermittent or indwelling catheterization. They may have some advantage over Valsalva and Credé bladder expression, which may be unsafe in certain situations, as high pressures may be generated. Therefore, the lower urinary tract function must be shown to be urodynamically safe before recommending these methods of bladder expression. In general, bladder expression should be replaced by clean, intermittent catheterization in patients with neurologic bladder–sphincter dysfunction. Catheters, however, are rarely trouble-free.

Catheter Material

Preferred	Short-Term Use Only
Silicone	Polytetrafluoroethylene-coated latex
Silicone elastomer-coated latex	Plastic
Hydrophilic polymer-coated latex	Silver-alloy coated material

Figure 4-13. Catheter material. The catheter material is important because bacteriuria increases 5% to 8% per day of indwelling catheterization and a strongly adherent biofilm of bacteria and host proteins rapidly colonizes the catheter. Bacteria in a biofilm are less susceptible to antibiotics than are free-living organisms [13]. Catheter coatings with silver, antiseptics, or antibiotics are undergoing development. Encrustation that leads to catheter blockage occurs in 50% of long-term (> 14 day) users, most commonly under alkaline conditions caused by urea-splitting bacteria, eg, *Proteus mirabilis*. No current long-term catheter materials are resistant to biofilm formation and encrustation. The 12 to 16 Ch sizes are usually adequate for adults; there is a preference for smaller balloon sizes (10 mL for adults) and a 25-cm length is adequate for women. In addition to biofilm formation and encrustation, other complications of long-term indwelling urethral catheterization include urethral trauma, fistula, stone formation, bladder neck incompetence, metal erosion, and bladder carcinoma, which are found with an incidence of 0.11% in patients with a spinal cord injury [14].

In summary, transurethral long-term indwelling catheter use is not safe for neurologic patients. Its use may be required in debilitated patients when intermittent catheterization is not feasible. As a short-term solution, it may be used in patients with low-pressure vesicoureteral reflux, severe bilateral hydronephrosis, and acute pyelonephritis with reflux, and in women with total incontinence for whom other procedures are not feasible. Siliconized catheters with frequent changes are encouraged, with sterile techniques and aseptic, closed drainage systems advisable. As a routine, bladder irrigation and antibiotic prophylaxis are not recommended. Urodynamic testing, renal function testing, and bladder screening are performed at least yearly.

At times, suprapubic tubes are preferable to urethral catheters. The incidence of bacteriuria is less than with urethral catheterization, because there is less urethral damage and fewer urethral spasms. One key disadvantage is that it requires a surgical procedure that can have complications (especially bowel perforations), and all the other complications of long-term urethral catheterization continue to exist with suprapubic catheters, except for urethral damage. Both suprapubic and urethral catheterization are inferior to intermittent catheterization.

Types of Catheterization

	Intermittent	Indwelling (Urethral/Suprapubic)
Purpose	Resume bladder storage and regularly empty	Empty the bladder
Safety	Safe for the treatment of neurologic bladder	Unsafe for the treatment of urologic bladder
Complications	Infection	Infection
	Urethral trauma	Urethral trauma
	Bladder stones with long-term use	Fistulae
	More problematic in patients who are difficult to catheterize	Stones
		Cancer
		Bladder neck incompetence
		Loss of bladder compliance

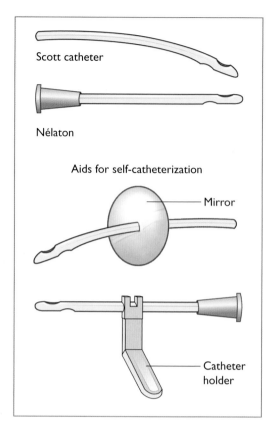

Figure 4-14. Intermittent catheterization (IC) and self-catheterization have been in use for the past 40 years. These types of catheterization have revolutionized the care of spinal cord–injured patients, replacing long-term indwelling catheterization, as well as the management of neurogenic bladder in children. Initially in these children, long-term renal preservation was the only goal of therapy and early diversion was employed with ileal conduits and cutaneous urostomies. The introduction of IC made conservative management a successful treatment option and made the surgical creation of continent reservoirs an alternative. The rationale for IC differs from continuous drainage, as bladder storage function is preserved and may be helped.

Figure 4-15. Catheters for intermittent catheterization. Self-catheterization may be taught to patients of all ages and assisting devices are available. Sufficient dexterity is required, but if the patient can write and feed herself, dexterity is adequate. Obesity, with large panniculus, may prevent self-catheterization. Catheters are managed by two methods, aseptic and clean; the latter is simpler.

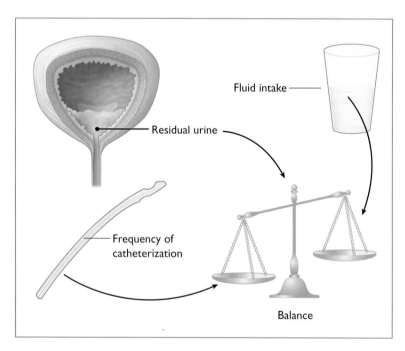

Figure 4-16. The effectiveness of intermittent catheterization (IC) and intermittent self-catheterization (ISC) is improved when there is adequate bladder capacity; bladder pressure is low; urethral resistance is adequate; and there is balance among fluid intake, frequency of catheterization, and residual urine. The amount of residual urine that indicates a need for IC may vary, but a residual amount greater than 150 mL is an independent risk factor for urinary tract infection [15]. The chief goal of IC is to empty the bladder and prevent its overdistention to improve urologic conditions. Complications such as urinary tract infection are regularly seen with IC and ISC and increase in the long term. Key factors for success include an adequate frequency of catheterization, a nontraumatizing technique, and suitable materials. Catheterization should be used as a first choice therapy for patients who are unable to effectively empty their bladders and is valuable for achieving continence in neurologic voiding dysfunction.

The principal causes of urinary incontinence in patients with neurologic conditions associated with incontinence are neurologic detrusor overactivity or incompetence of sphincter function. The clinical situation is often clouded by detrusor–sphincter dyssynergia. Therapies are aimed at decreasing detrusor activity, increasing bladder capacity, and changing outlet resistance.

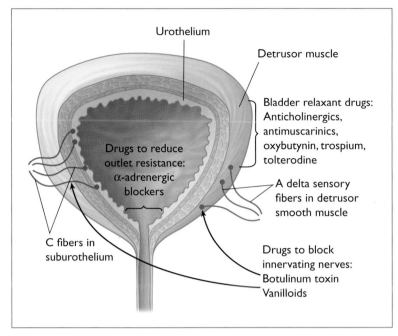

Figure 4-17. Drugs for neurologic bladder/urethral dysfunction. The most widely used drugs are the antimuscarinic agents, which may be given orally, transvesically, transdermally, and intrarectally. They may alleviate incontinence symptoms but are also important for lowering urinary tract pressures and protecting upper tracts. They are often used effectively in conjunction with intermittent catheterization (IC). Side effects (dry mouth, constipation, and urinary retention) are common but appear to be less with tolterodine, propiverine, trospium, and controlled-release oxybutynin compared with immediate-release oxybutynin.

Vanilloids. Capsaicin and resiniferatoxin are used for their anti–C fiber afferentation effects. They act by first stimulating the responsive C fibers (a painful experience akin to eating red peppers) and then eventually depleting C fiber activity. Resiniferatoxin is more comfortable to use as it has less excitatory effect than capsaicin, while exerting 1000 times more potency in vanilloid receptor (TRPV1) agonist action. TRPV1 is a cation channel protein expressed by nociceptive-afferent neurons and regulated by nerve growth factor. Studies are needed to determine the therapeutic role of resiniferatoxin. Intravesical instillation has improved "spinal reflex" incontinence for several months. Vanilloid intravesical therapy is experimental and should be used within clinical trials.

Botulinum toxin A is a powerful toxin known to inhibit acetylcholine release at the presynaptic portion of the neuromuscular junction. The resulting chemical "denervation" leads to decreased skeletal muscle contractility that lasts for 3 to 6 months. The toxin's effects on smooth muscle and afferent neuronal activity are not adequately studied at this time. Its current use is as an injection into the sphincter of patients with functionally obstructive detrusor–sphincter dyssynergia and in injecting the bladder wall in patients with overactive bladder (OAB). Decreasing outlet resistance with sphincter injection in patients with neurologic detrusor–sphincter dyssynergia, and improving incontinence and increasing bladder capacity in spinal cord–injured patients, have been reported, which may make it an alternative to sphincterotomy.

There currently are no controlled studies of drugs that are used to increase urethral outlet resistance. α-Blockers have been shown to reduce urethral resistance whereas cholinergics are of limited benefit for detrusor areflexia and are not appropriate in detrusor–sphincter dyssynergia as detrusor pressure could be increased. IC remains the gold standard for detrusor areflexia.

Neuromodulation. Electrical stimulation to improve lower urinary tract function has been tried over the past decades. Direct bladder stimulation has produced poor results. Intravesical stimulation is an option to induce/improve bladder sensation and to enhance the micturition reflex, but the selection of patients is crucial. Intravesical stimulation may be applied to patients with neurologic hyposensitive and hypocontractile bladders, in whom intact sensory fibers between the bladder and the cortex are demonstrable. Such demonstration is possible by viscerosensory cortical evoked potentials.

Splanchnic nerve stimulation has been abandoned because these nerves include fibers that are sympathetic to the bladder neck. Conus medullaris stimulation is unsound due to the multiplicity of neuronal functions confined to this small space. Sacral anterior root stimulation with posterior rhizotomy has been used in selected spinal cord–injured patients. The posterior rhizotomy is done to affect detrusor areflexia and to improve compliance. However, the rhizotomy also abolishes reflex bowel emptying and sexual function.

Sacral neuromodulation, stimulating the sacral nerve (which is usually the third nerve) in the sacral canal, where the anterior and posterior roots join to form the peripheral nerve, has been confirmed to be a valuable treatment option in patients with OAB and emptying disorders and may be beneficial in neurogenic bladder/urethral dysfunction. It is recommended for use if pharmacotherapy fails.

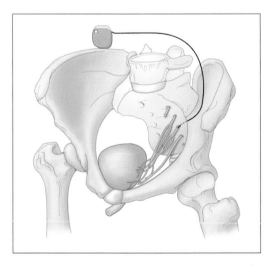

Figure 4-18. Implant therapy. Sacral neuromodulation has been shown to be clinically effective in bladder overactivity and voiding dysfunctions. The mechanisms of action are complex and may involve counteracting the development of new pathologic micturition reflexes. Rat studies using cystometric and electrophysiologic recording and measurements of C fiber–stored neuropeptides (calcitonin gene–related peptide, substance P, neurokinin A) revealed that the elevation of C fiber neuropeptides found in the dorsal root ganglia after spinal cord transection returned to control values with sacral neuromodulation.

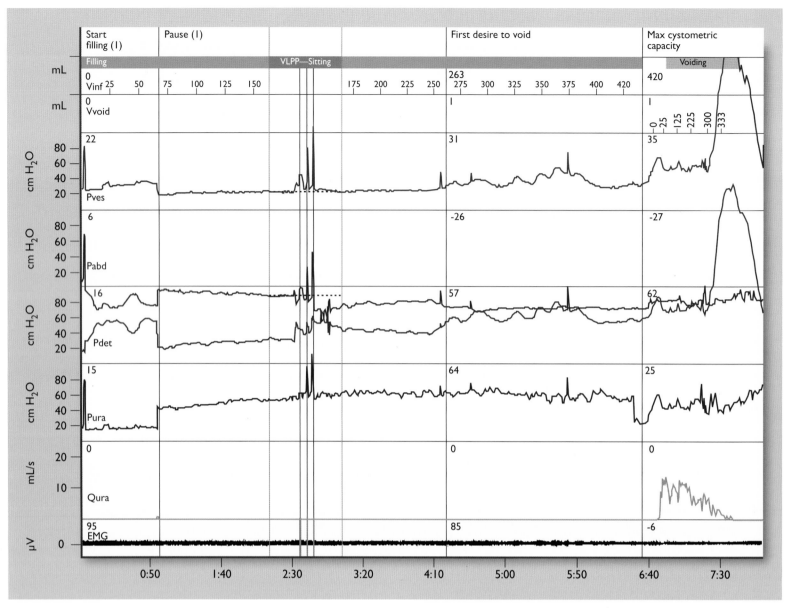

Figure 4-19. Urodynamic evaluation. The bladder may become contracted from many diverse causes. Problems with voiding, incontinence, and upper tract deterioration frequently led to supravesical diversion until advances in urodynamic evaluation and the wider acceptance of intermittent catheterization made reconstruction preferable to diversion.

The *blue line* is intravesical pressure (Pves); the *red line* is intraabdominal pressure (Pabd); the *purple line* is "detrusor" pressure (Pdet), which is intravesical pressure minus abdominal pressure; the *green line* is intraurethral pressure (Pura); the *pink line* is urine flow; and the *black line* is para-anal electromyogram (EMG) activity. At a 150-mL volume, the patient does Valsalva and coughs without urinary loss. At a 255-mL volume, the patient has involuntary detrusor contraction without a fall in urethral pressure (noncoordinated detrusor contraction) and an increase in EMG activity (detrusor–sphincter dyssynergia). Beyond the 200-mL volume fill, the bladder accommodation is decreased (decreased compliance). Bladder capacity is 420 mL and the patient voids with failure of urethral relaxation and without diminished EMG activity, generating very high intravesical pressure that could be artifactual from bladder wall contact with the intravesical pressure transducer. Nevertheless, upper urinary tract evaluation is advisable.

Etiologies affect surgical decision-making. Congenital causes vary remarkably but some are well managed with cystoplasty. Inflammatory causes require that true bladder contracture be present to benefit from cystoplasty. Radiation therapy may cause bladder contracture but major healing problems make cystoplasty a difficult therapy. A defunctionalized bladder becomes physiologically small, but it may achieve satisfactory capacity after urinary flow is restored, so a period of bladder cycling to evaluate expansibility is important before planning augmentation. Neurogenic bladder dysfunction and idiopathic instability may cause a functional small-capacity bladder. If there is intractable hypertonicity, and especially if there is upper tract dilatation, augmentation cystoplasty may be indicated. Conservative treatment alternatives should be exhausted before resorting to surgical intervention.

The various methods of bladder augmentation suggest that no single method has gained universal acceptance as the "best." The goal is to have a low-pressure reservoir to store urine; achieve continence with convenient, voluntary urine expulsion; protect the upper tracts from reflux; and avoid the shift of water and electrolytes.

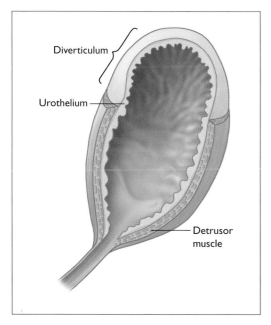

Figure 4-20. Autoaugmentation has been proposed as having advantages such as being simpler to perform, having an absence of urine salt resorption, having less mucus production, and perhaps having less carcinogenic potential. The detrusor muscle is removed with the urothelium intact, creating a large diverticulum to increase bladder capacity with low pressure. However, most authors are unable to reproduce the initial success rates and long-term results are disappointing. It is sometimes considered to be a step that can be taken prior to enteroplasty (bladder augmentation with bowel).

Simple bladder augmentation with bowel can create a low-pressure reservoir. There needs to be bladder tissue, a competent sphincter or bladder neck, and a catheterizable urethra. Augmentation with additional bladder-outlet procedures is necessary when both the bladder and outlet are deficient. Augmentation with surgical closure of the bladder neck will then require a continent stoma. It may be wiser to leave the bladder neck patent as a safety precaution. Augmentation with continent stoma may be used following failed bladder outlet surgery and when the inability to catheterize the urethra is anticipated.

Controversy exists regarding the choice of bowel segment, shape of bowel segment reconstruction, and removal of diseased bladder. Using the minimal amount of bowel possible is a guiding principle. To create a large-capacity reservoir, detubularization of any intestinal segment is necessary. The jejunum is contraindicated because of metabolic consequences. Achieving an antireflux ureteral anastomosis into the reservoir is desired. A continent urinary outlet must be ensured. Because there is a risk of stone formation, only resorbable sutures and staples should be used.

Supratrigonal cystoplasty preserves the basic essentials to control micturition; if the sphincter mechanism is intact, a sensation of bladder fullness is present and ureteral function may be preserved. Most authorities believe the bladder wall should be excised down to the trigone in the structurally contracted bladder, but in the functionally poorly compliant bladder without contracture, the wall may be preserved.

The choice of bowel segment is debated; the small intestine is able to form a more docile storage area than the large bowel (motility is mainly peristaltic in the small bowel whereas the large bowel has more mass contraction) and the cecum is more docile than the sigmoid. The ileocecal segment is preferred by many because it is easily mobilized, the shape requires no refashioning, the ureter can anastomose to the ileum, and it can be reversed to a conduit. The stomach produces less mucus, is less likely to be colonized with bacteria, and is not prone to hyperchloremia. However, there are drawbacks, which include more dysuria and pain due to stomach acids.

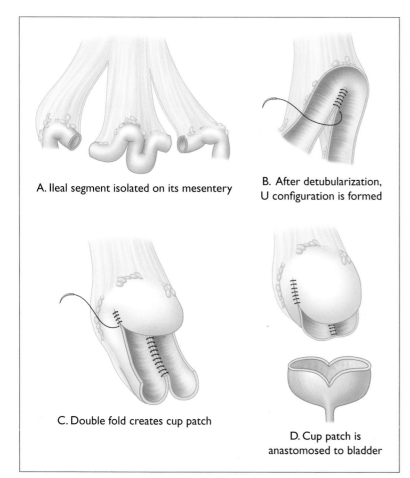

A. Ileal segment isolated on its mesentery

B. After detubularization, U configuration is formed

C. Double fold creates cup patch

D. Cup patch is anastomosed to bladder

Figure 4-21. The shape of the cystoplasty is important, mainly in the interruption of the strong circular bowel layer to prevent high-pressure situations. **A,** Use of the ileum allows preservation of the ileocecal valve, decreasing postoperative chronic diarrhea. **B–D,** The ileum may be formed into a "cup."

Research in artificial bladders is ongoing. Nearer to clinical application is the concept of tissue engineering with autologous urothelium and bladder muscle cells. The cells are grown by tissue culture on a polymer scaffold and then implanted in animal models; clinical trials are forthcoming [16].

Supravesical urinary diversion indications have decreased with the advent of intermittent catheterization, alone or with bladder augmentation. A group of patients with neurogenic bladder dysfunction are still candidates for diversion. The chief indications are: 1) persistent upper tract (ureterovesical) obstruction as in severe bladder overactivity or anatomic or functional subvesical obstruction and 2) vesicorenal reflux with renal deterioration and a small bladder capacity or detrusor hypertrophy that make ureteral reimplantation technically difficult.

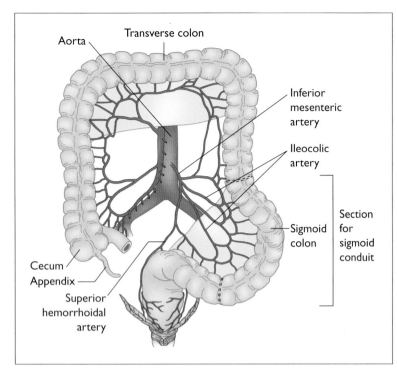

Figure 4-22. The more common procedures include ileal conduits and colonic conduits, most commonly using the sigmoid bowel segment. Complications include loop stenosis, ureteric–intestinal anastomosis stenosis, bacteriuria, stone formation, dilatation of the upper urinary tract, and renal deterioration, which occurs in 20% to 35% of patients after 10 years [17].

A "continent" urinary diversion means that the patient has a pathway for intermittent bladder emptying and an external storage apparatus for urine is not necessary. Improvement in the quality of life and social situations may be significant. The oldest form of continent urinary diversion is the ureterosigmoidostomy, which is indicated for bladder exstrophy, incontinent urogenital sinus, or traumatic loss of the urethral sphincter. The procedure is totally dependent on normal functioning of the anal sphincter. Other methods of continent diversion use the Mitrofanoff principle. Mitrofanoff originally used the appendix and developed the principle of burying a narrow tube within the wall of the bladder or urinary reservoir and bringing the distal end to the abdominal wall to form a catheterizable stoma

that is suitable for intermittent catheterization. Several narrow tubes are available for the Mitrofanoff conduit, although other methods of creating a continent urinary diversion are available. The ileocecal valve is an obvious sphincter to combine with the cecal reservoir and terminal ileum as the conduit. The Indiana system reinforces the valve with nonabsorbable placating sutures and a tailored terminal ileum conduit. The Mainz pouch intussuscepts a length of terminal ileum through the ileocecal valve as a "Kock" nipple. Continence rates with these procedures are good.

The ultimate and most invasive surgical option for lower urinary tract dysfunction is total cystectomy and urethrectomy. Commonly performed for painful bladder syndrome, the procedure may be simple or include continent urinary diversion. Simple diversion may be performed without cystectomy, but the latter is considered when bladder pain is persistent. It may follow unsuccessful augmentation and the bowel segment used in the augmentation may be converted to a conduit. Chronic inflammatory changes in the cystoplasty pouch may be seen [18].

Bladder outlet surgery may stand alone or may be done in conjunction with compliance surgical procedures. Bulking agents and the artificial urinary sphincter have advocates, but both have failure rates and complications. Mechanical failures are the most common type of failure with the artificial sphincter. Over time, reduced bladder compliance may develop, so long-term follow-up is necessary. Slings are also used in children; published results suggest that the artificial sphincter gives more consistent results in boys and that slings are equally effective in boys and girls. Bladder outlet reconstruction usually requires the problems to be anatomic rather than functional. Intermittent catheterization (IC) may be useful short term in anatomic corrections, but if the surgery is to create continence in an incontinent patient, reconstruction mandates IC. The most useful procedures for dryness utilize a flap valve or tunnel, and slings and "wraps" have also been used. A flap valve can be created by using a full-thickness anterior or posterior bladder flap to construct a tube that is placed in a submucosal tunnel. Areas of urethral stricture require differing surgeries depending on the particular circumstance, but all may include excision of the stricture and construction of a spatulated anastomosis. The success of ladder neck reconstruction is related to bladder function: bladder capacity, contractility, and outlet resistance are determinants of continence after bladder neck reconstruction.

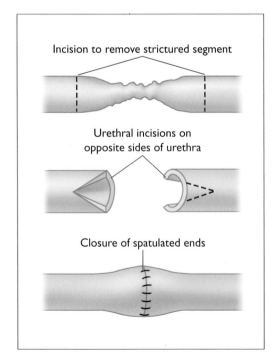

Figure 4-23. Excision of urethral stricture and anastomosis of spatulated ends. The cut ends of the mobilized urethra have dorsal and ventral incisions at opposite sides. They are anastomosal with interrupted sutures over an inlying urethral catheter.

Pathophysiologic Mechanisms of Anal Incontinence

Causes	Etiology	Effect
Anatomic		
Sphincter muscle	Obstetric, hemorrhoidectomy, anal dilation	Loss of sampling reflex due to neuropathy
Puborectalis	Trauma, sacral radiculopathy	Obtuse anorectal angle, sphincter weakness
Rectum	Inflammation, radiation	Lost accommodation
Pudendal nerve	Obstetric injury, perineal descent	Sphincter weakness, sensory loss
CNS	Injury, MS, diabetes, stroke	Lost sensation and lost accommodation
Functional		
Fecal impaction	Aging, defecation dysfunction	"Overflow" incontinence
Anorectal sensation	Obstetric injury, CNS, anal sphincter injury	Loss of stool awareness
Increased stool volume	Infection, irritated bowel, drugs, metabolism	Rapid stool transport
Irritants	Bile salt malabsorption	Diarrhea
Drugs	Anticholinergics, laxatives, antidepressants, caffeine	Constipation, diarrhea, altered sensation, decreased sphincter tone
Foods	Lactose, fructose, sorbitol	Diarrhea

CNS—central nervous system; MS—multiple sclerosis.

Figure 4-24. Pathophysiologic mechanisms of anal incontinence. Disruption of the normal anatomy or physiology of the anorectal unit leads to incontinence. Anal incontinence is virtually always due to multiple pathogenic mechanisms. The "sampling" reflex (see Chapter 3, Fig. 3-20) is intimately associated with anal continence and incontinence may involve variable pathogenic mechanisms.

Damage to the internal anal sphincter (IAS), most commonly caused by obstetric trauma, leads to a poor seal and impaired sampling reflex. Disruption of the external anal sphincter (EAS) causes urge-related or diarrhea-associated fecal incontinence. In most patients, both sphincters are affected. Symptoms commonly develop years after the precipitating event (obstetric delivery), probably due to ensuing neuropathy. The puborectalis muscle also is important in continence, probably due more to its effect on the anal canal pressure than on the rectoanal angle. The nerve supply to the upper puborectalis is by direct branches of anterior S3-4 and varies, then, from the pudendal supplied EAS. Incontinence can be produced either by a loss of sphincter function or by a loss of puborectalis muscle function.

Neuropathy may cause anal incontinence by dysfunctions involving the pudendal nerve (sphincter function), sacral nerve roots (as in cauda equina syndromes), and autonomic neural dysfunction, which affects bowel motility and IAS activity in the peripheral nervous system. Upper motor neuron dysfunction in the parasagittal cortical areas may be affected and nearby sensory areas can be affected as well, leading to incontinence secondary to loss of sensory awareness. Thus, the central nervous system has intimate involvement with anal continence, as with urinary continence.

Rectal reservoir function may have impairment secondary to radiation, Crohn's disease, ulcerative colitis, or tumor. Neurogenic causes of a loss of rectal compliance may be seen with radical hysterectomy, rectal surgery, and spinal cord injury. Prolonged stool retention in the rectum leads to prolonged relaxation of IAS tone and the loss of liquid seepage around the fecal impaction.

Long-standing constipation and excessive straining lead to progressive pelvic floor muscle denervation and possible anal incontinence. On examination, patients may have perineal descent and sphincter weakness.

Stool characteristics influence anal continence. Large-volume liquid stools may overwhelm continence mechanisms. Patients with bile salt malabsorption or lactose or fructose intolerance may have colonic transit that is too rapid for the patient's defenses.

The decrease in childbirth mortality and the increase in life expectancy of women demand attention to minimize morbidity. Eighty percent of women with "idiopathic" anorectal incontinence have evidence of denervation of the pelvic floor muscles, especially the puborectalis and the EAS [19].

Perineal Tears with Obstetric Deliveries: Royal College of Obstetrics-Gynecology Guidelines

First Degree	Second degree	Third Degree	Fourth Degree
Laceration of vaginal ephithelium or perineal skin only	Involvement of the perineal muscles but not the anal sphincter	Disruption of anal sphincter muscles 3a: < 50% 3b: > 50% 3c: Internal sphincter torn also	A third-degree tear with disruptions of the anal epithelium

Figure 4-25. Perineal tears with obstetric deliveries: Royal College of Obstetrics–Gynecology guidelines. Internal and external anal sphincter injury, with the recent advent of ultrasound studies, is now recognized not to be limited to patients with third- or fourth-degree tears. The classification of third-degree tears into three subclasses is advocated to better correlate with treatment plans. Fifty percent of patients who have a third- or fourth-degree tear have had an instrumental delivery, with vacuum extraction causing fewer tears than forcep deliveries. Restricting the use of episiotomies decreases posterior trauma, and midline episiotomies extend into the anal sphincter more than mediolateral episiotomies (12% vs 2%) [20].

The conclusions and recommendations of the Committee of the Third International Consultation on Incontinence include the following: 1) vacuum extractor is preferred over forceps (level I); 2) mediolateral episiotomy has a lower risk of anal sphincter rupture (level I); 3) the episiotomy rate should be about 30% (grade C); 4) the second stage of labor should not be prolonged (grade C); 5) cesarean delivery is advised for patients with compromised anal sphincter function or those who have previously had successful surgery for anal incontinence (grade C); 6) antenatal exercise values are currently being evaluated; 7) modifications in delivery techniques to reduce anal sphincter injury need further research; and 8) a focused training program for physicians and midwives must be implemented.

PELVIC ORGAN PROLAPSE

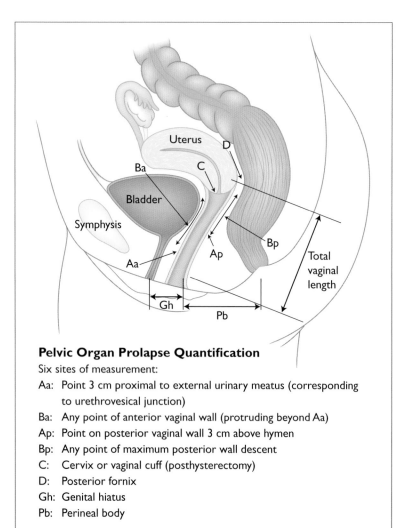

Pelvic Organ Prolapse Quantification

Six sites of measurement:

Aa: Point 3 cm proximal to external urinary meatus (corresponding to urethrovesical junction)

Ba: Any point of anterior vaginal wall (protruding beyond Aa)

Ap: Point on posterior vaginal wall 3 cm above hymen

Bp: Any point of maximum posterior wall descent

C: Cervix or vaginal cuff (posthysterectomy)

D: Posterior fornix

Gh: Genital hiatus

Pb: Perineal body

Figure 4-26. Vaginal delivery has been implicated as an important risk factor for pelvic organ prolapse (POP), and pregnancy itself is now recognized as having effects. Parity is the strongest risk factor for the development of POP. Age, hysterectomy, and large infants delivered vaginally are risks for POP. Constipation (and its link to pelvic floor denervation and neuropathy) is a risk, as are pelvic muscle weakness and neural abnormalities [21]. Occupational heavy lifting, obesity, and pulmonary dysfunction are risks. Previous surgery for prolapse is a risk factor, with controversial data regarding vaginal and abdominal routes of surgery related to reoperation rates.

Collagen synthesis abnormalities may be linked to POP. Differential gene expression in the pubococcygeus muscle related to actin, myosin, and extracellular matrix proteins has been shown in women with POP and controls [22]. On a genome-wide scale, a differential gene expression in patients with POP exists, affecting the connective tissue of the entire pelvis [23]. There also appears to be a link between POP and hernias.

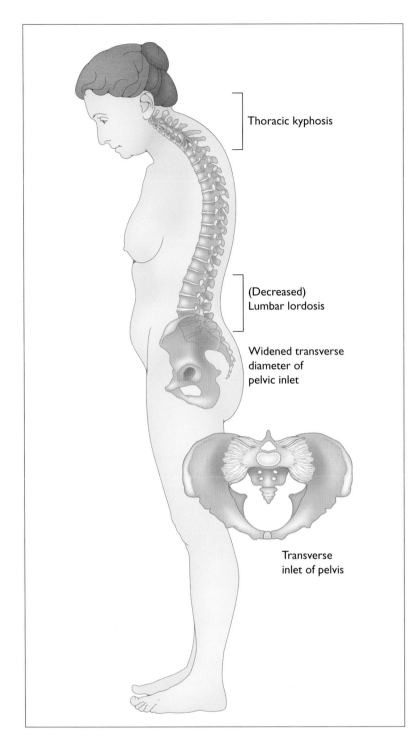

Thoracic kyphosis

(Decreased)
Lumbar lordosis

Widened transverse
diameter of
pelvic inlet

Transverse
inlet of pelvis

Figure 4-27. There is evidence that variations in pelvic and axial skeletal structures can be associated with pelvic organ prolapse. Thoracic kyphosis, lumbar lordosis decrease, and increased transverse diameter of pelvic inlet appear to be linked [24].

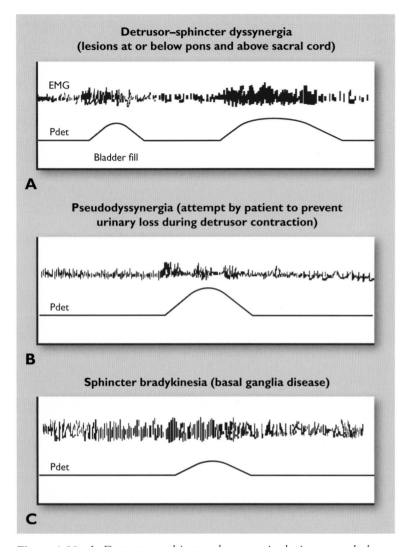

**Detrusor–sphincter dyssynergia
(lesions at or below pons and above sacral cord)**

EMG

Pdet

Bladder fill

A

**Pseudodyssynergia (attempt by patient to prevent
urinary loss during detrusor contraction)**

Pdet

B

Sphincter bradykinesia (basal ganglia disease)

Pdet

C

Figure 4-28. A, Detrusor–sphincter dyssynergia: lesions at or below
the pons and above the sacral cord. Intracranial lesions may affect
urinary storage and voiding directly, by dysfunction of the pathways
involved in urinary tract function, or indirectly, by changes in physical or mental status. Lesions located above the pons leave the pontine–spinal pathways intact so the neurogenic detrusor overactivity
that so often accompanies these lesions is coordinated with urethral
(outlet) relaxation. Because bladder–sphincter dyssynergia is not
present, as it is with lesions in or below the pons, bladder emptying
is usually adequate. Thus, there is a low incidence of upper urinary
tract complications in these patients. **B,** Attempts by the patient to
prevent urine loss during detrusor contractions create a "pseudodyssynergia." The pelvic floor may also fail to relax in the rigidity seen in
Parkinson's disease (*see* Chapter 3), a condition termed *bradykinesia*.
C, Spincter bradykinesia is shown as seen in basal ganglia disease.

Cerebrovascular accidents (CVAs) are the third most common
cause of disability in the United States. The most common urinary
problems are nocturia, urge incontinence, and trouble voiding. In
stroke patients, damage to the anteromedial frontal lobe and the
basal ganglia is mainly responsible for urinary symptoms, whereas
in patients with brainstem lesions, retention problems predominate.
Initially following a CVA, detrusor areflexia is present, followed in
days or weeks by detrusor hyperreflexia, likely resulting from a loss
of cortical inhibition. Experimental models have concluded that

N-methyl-D-aspartate receptors [25] have an essential role in bladder overactivity after CVA and glutamate receptor antagonists can
be expected to be beneficial in therapy. Although it was formerly
believed that right-sided lesions were associated with incontinence
more than left-sided lesions, further studies have not supported this
concept. Urinary retention has been described with brain lesions,
but this condition is less common. The involvement of cortical areas
related to awareness determines symptoms that are secondary to
bladder instability. Thus, the patient may have urgency and urge
incontinence, or incontinence without urge, or even incontinence
without social awareness, depending on the extent of the lesion.
Physical signs generally include pyramidal signs with hyperactive
muscle stretch reflexes and Hoffmann or Babinski reflexes (*see*
Chapter 3, Fig. 3-26). Urodynamic findings do not demonstrate
definitive patterns correlating with the lesion location.

Parkinson's disease is usually seen after age 50 and is associated
with a loss of pigmented neurons in the substantia nigra and a loss
of dopamine in caudate nucleus, putamen, and globus pallidus and
principal nuclei of the basal ganglia. Autonomic functions may be
altered, including urinary tract function, constipation, and hypo-
hidrosis. The basal ganglia play a major role in normal voluntary
movement. Unlike most components of motor systems, they do not
have direct input or output connections with the spinal cord, but do
have primary input from the cerebral cortex and output to the brainstem and via the thalamus back to the cortex. This "extrapyramidal"
system, characterized by involuntary movements, muscular rigidity,
and immobility without paralysis, has been distinguished from the
"pyramidal" tract syndrome, which is characterized by spasticity and
paralysis. Such distinction is no longer of value, however, because
the two motor systems are not truly independent and because other
parts of the brain participate in voluntary movement. The extrapyramidal motor system has an inhibitory effect on the micturition
reflex and loss of this effect results in detrusor hyperreflexia. Detrusor areflexia is seen in some patients and bladder outlet obstruction
or anticholinergic and α-adrenergic medications may be significant
factors in this condition. The external anal sphincter needle electromyographic studies demonstrate decreased voluntary control, pseudodyssynergia, and bradykinesia. The classic clinical presentation of
patients with Parkinson's disease reveals resting tremor, "cogwheel"
rigidity, and bradykinesia. Abnormalities in posture and equilib-
rium are frequent. Treatment is more complicated in male patients
because prostatic obstruction confuses the bladder-instability picture
and differentiating between the underlying causes is often difficult.

Other intracranial diseases tend to have detrusor instability, which
is coordinated with sphincter function. Of particular interest is Shy–
Drager syndrome, an autonomic disorder of intracerebral, cerebellar,
and spinal cord tracts that involves external sphincter denervation
and detrusor areflexia. Because of the involvement of the central
nervous system and the autonomic nerves, it may be called multiple-
system atrophy (MSA). Orthostatic hypotension, loss of sweating,
rigidity and tremor, and urinary and anal incontinence are features
of the syndrome. Studies of the brains of Parkinson's disease patients
reveal that one fifth have changes that are typical of MSA. The prognosis is poor, with patients rarely surviving more than 6 years after
diagnosis. The index of suspicion may be increased in patients with
Parkinson's disease, who have severe bladder symptoms.

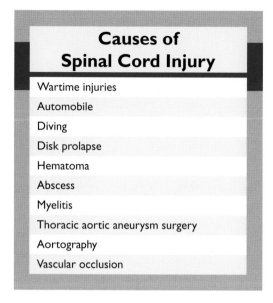

Causes of Spinal Cord Injury

Wartime injuries

Automobile

Diving

Disk prolapse

Hematoma

Abscess

Myelitis

Thoracic aortic aneurysm surgery

Aortography

Vascular occlusion

Figure 4-29. Causes of spinal cord injury. Despite modern advances in the care of patients with spinal cord injury, urologic complications continue to be problematic and the most common cause of death is renal failure.

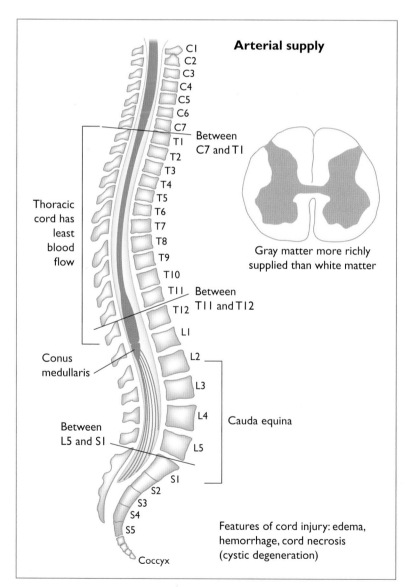

Figure 4-30. Vascular anatomy is important because it frequently relates to the locale of cord injury and, hence, the symptoms and signs. The principal arteries are end arteries and the gray matter is better supplied than the white. The thoracic cord segments receive the least amount of vascular supply, explaining why (with the

realization of the disproportionate growth of the vertebral column and spinal cord) extensive lower motor neuron (LMN) lesions may occur in low thoracic lesions. Cervical and upper thoracic lesions lead to partial or complete upper motor neuron (UMN) lesions with exaggerated muscle stretch reflexes and pathologic reflexes. (See the Hoffmann, Babinski, flexion spinal defense reflex, crossed extensor reflex, discussed in Chapter 3, Fig. 3-26.) Injuries in the lower thoracic and upper lumbar regions may lead to LMN lesions with areflexia or to mixed UMN and LMN findings. Sensory findings depend on the extent of the cord lesion. Findings with transverse, posterior, anterior, syringomyelia, and Brown–Séquard cord lesions are described in Chapter 3 (see Fig. 3-29). Almost all complete lesions sparing sacral cord segments produce a UMN hyperreflexic bladder and striated sphincter.

A particular event syndrome that is necessary to understand is autonomic dysreflexia. In spinal cord–injured patients with lesions above T5, with viable cord segments distal to the lesion that allow the thoracolumbar sympathetic outflow to be intact, the episodes may occur. These episodes are characterized by profound vasomotor disturbances with marked elevations of blood pressure, sweating, piloerection, and paradoxical bradycardia. The event is precipitated in response to a distended bladder, distended rectum, or acute skin irritation. Cerebrovascular accidents, convulsions, and death can occur. Management includes immediate bladder decompression, rectal disimpaction, and pharmacologic agents for the hypertension. Tetraethylammonium chloride (400 mg intramuscularly), sodium nitroprusside, and chlorpromazine have been used in the acute phase. Prophylaxis, as when surgical manipulation is necessary, may be performed with α-adrenergic blocking agents such as phenoxybenzamine.

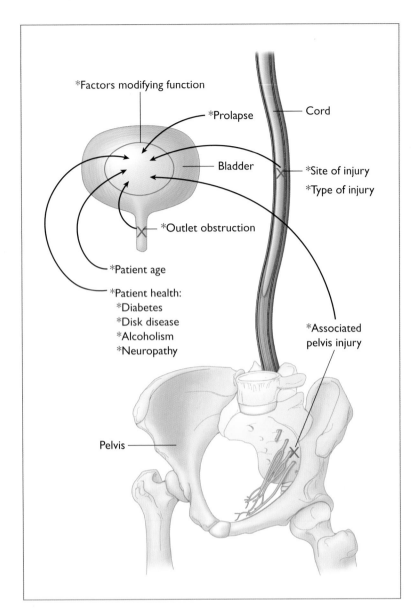

*Factors modifying function

*Prolapse

Cord

Bladder

*Site of injury

*Type of injury

*Outlet obstruction

*Patient age

*Patient health:
*Diabetes
*Disk disease
*Alcoholism
*Neuropathy

*Associated pelvis injury

Pelvis

Figure 4-31. The neurourologic aspects of spinal cord injury involve the consideration of many aspects of the individual patient. In the acute stage of injury, suprasacral cord–injured patients usually experience "spinal shock," in which there is the diminution or disappearance of the spinal skeletal and visceral reflexes innervated by cord segments distal to the injury occurs. This condition lasts for hours to weeks and the reflexes earliest to reappear with spinal shock recovery are the anal and genital reflexes. The bladder is completely areflexic, with overflow incontinence developing if not prevented. Typically, the bladder has a smooth contour, minimal trabeculation, and closed bladder neck, with some reports [26] indicating that there is a loss of tonic periurethral skeletal muscle activity. The detrusor reflex appears 6 to 8 weeks after the return of somatic reflexes. The supraspinal micturition reflex is lost in animals with spinal cord injuries (*see* Fig. 4-8).

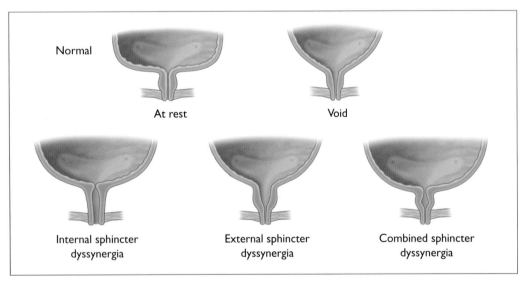

Normal

At rest

Void

Internal sphincter dyssynergia

External sphincter dyssynergia

Combined sphincter dyssynergia

Figure 4-32. With recovery from the spinal shock, patients may lose the sense of a desire to void (lost proprioception) although other indirect symptoms representing bladder filling may develop. The contractions usually have dyssynergia and incoordination with the outlet.

The establishment of voiding patterns after spinal shock recovery rarely shows detrusor areflexia in suprasacral lesions, but detrusor hyperreflexia is present in the vast majority. The hyperreflexia is associated with varying degrees of striated urethral sphincter overac-

tivity, causing detrusor–sphincter dyssynergia (DSD). Most complete suprasacral cord lesions have varying degrees of DSD. Persistent detrusor hyperactivity may result in a small, trabeculated, fibrotic bladder. Due to the structural changes in the bladder wall, upper tract deterioration may occur and is more prominent in patients with spinal cord injury than in patients with other cord pathologies, such as multiple sclerosis, for reasons that are not entirely clear.

Continued on the next page

Figure 4-32. *(Continued)* Urologic management principles include intermittent catheterization during the spinal shock phase to maintain bladder capacity, not allowing distention over 500 mL. After recovery from spinal shock, patients may develop various stimulatory measures (touching perineal area, stretching anus, etc.) to produce detrusor contractions. Even though patients may have low residual urine, the detrusor contractions may occur at high intravesical pressures and trabeculation, pseudodiverticula, and upper tract changes may occur. Thus, following the patient urodynamically is important. Anticholinergic medications may be necessary if such changes occur and, if residual urine increases, intermittent catheterization may become necessary. In minor degrees of smooth muscle sphincter dyssynergia, α-adrenergic antagonists may be used. In more severe cases of vesicosphincter dyssynergia, outlet surgical procedures or botulinum toxin therapy may be employed, although intermittent catheterization may be preferable. More radical outlet procedures may be necessary for the pronounced outlet obstruction seen in patients with complete cervical cord lesions, as well as patients with low-pressure vesicoureteral reflux and patients with acontractile bladders that are associated with spastic outlets.

Female patients with spinal cord injury have problems with appliances for urinary drainage. Self-catheterization should be encouraged. The hyperactive bladder should be converted into an acontractile bladder by pharmacologic or neurosurgical means (sacral root block, rhizotomies). Indwelling catheters as a permanent procedure should be reserved for those who cannot self-catheterize, cannot transfer to a toilet, and who have inadequate assistance. Urinary diversions are rarely indicated in spinal cord injury patients, the indications being chronic suppurative processes, small fibrotic bladder, severe vesicoureteral reflux, and neoplastic lesions.

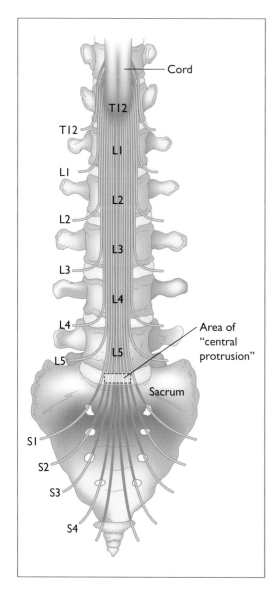

Figure 4-33. Cauda equina and conus lesions usually produce a lower motor neuron (LMN) type of vesicourethral dysfunction as well as LMN clinical findings. The conus medullaris, the terminal portion of the spinal cord, is located at the level of the T12 and L1 vertebral bodies. The detrusor and pudendal motor nuclei are both located in this small spinal cord area, the former in the intermediolateral cell column and the latter in the ventromedial ventral gray matter. Sacral cord neuropathology may be produced by trauma, tumor, disk disease, spondylosis, or multiple sclerosis. The most common etiologic factor in cauda equina dysfunction is spinal cord injury at the level of the T12 vertebra or below; for disk disease, it is the second most common cause, with disk protrusion leading to spinal root compression, usually in the L4–5 or L5–S1 disk space.

Because lower lumbar and sacral nerve roots occupy the central portion of the cauda equina, central disk prolapse is more often associated with lower urinary tract dysfunction. In partial lesions, some detrusor activity may be maintained. Lumbar spondylosis is more common than disk disease in older age groups, leading to spinal stenosis. This degenerative hypertrophy of the cartilage, ligaments, and osseous structures of the spine evolves slowly and symptoms become progressive. Intractable leg pain develops, which is increased by walking and constitutes a neurologic instead of a vascular "claudication" picture. Leaning forward tends to open the stenosed spinal canal, so patients have less pain walking uphill than down. A typical picture is a woman leaning over the shopping cart in a grocery store as she ambulates. Fifty percent of patients with spinal stenosis have bladder dysfunction. Lumbar decompressive laminectomy is the treatment of choice, done primarily for leg pain relief, but 75% of patients have reported improvement in bladder function after laminectomy [27]. The chief urodynamic signs of bladder dysfunction in patients with lumbar stenosis are increased residual urine and reduced flow rate. Conversely, patients found to have such findings should be asked about back and leg pain and, if these are present, they should be investigated for spinal stenosis.

Clinical Differentiation of Cauda Equina and Conus Medullaris Syndromes

	Pain	Sensory Deficit	Motor Deficit	Reflexes	Sphincter Dysfunction	Sexual Dysfunction
Cauda equina (lumbosacral roots)	Severe, asymmetric, radicular	Saddle, assymetric, no sensory dissociation	Assymetric, severe, more atrophy	Variable	Moderate	Severe
Conus medullaris (lowa sacral cord)	Uncommon, mild, bilateral, symmetric perineum, thighs	Saddle, symmetric, sensory dissociation	Symmetric, mild, no atrophy	Achilles absent, patellar normal, sacral absent	Severe	Impaired

Figure 4-34. Clinical differentiation of cauda equina and conus medullaris lesions. Electrodiagnostic assistance is gained with studies of sacral nerve–supplied muscle needle electromyogram and sacral reflexes (*see* Chapter 3, Figs. 3-32 and 3-39). Sphincter neuropathy is common. Bladder sensation is not entirely abolished because the afferent nerves following the thoracolumbar pathways are intact. The typical urodynamic dysfunction is areflexia with retention and a positive bethanechol denervation supersensitivity test (*see* Chapter 3, Fig. 3-7). Stress incontinence may occur. Patients with lower motor neuron bladder and outlet are best treated by intermittent catheterization (IC). Fibrosis of the external sphincter region may occur and sphincterotomy may be required. The bladder may become fibrotic and lose compliance, a situation that may be helped by augmentation cystoplasty. Cholinergic agents have not been proven beneficial. Anti-incontinence procedures for stress incontinence are indicated when IC is effective.

PELVIC PLEXUS INJURY

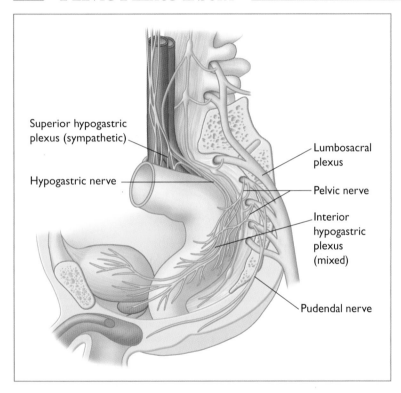

Superior hypogastric plexus (sympathetic)

Hypogastric nerve

Lumbosacral plexus

Pelvic nerve

Interior hypogastric plexus (mixed)

Pudendal nerve

Figure 4-35. The pelvic plexus. The plexus contains the sympathetic postganglionic nerves, parasympathetic preganglionic nerves, sacral somatic nerves, and visceral afferent nerves that follow the autonomic pathways. The pudendal nerve is not part of the plexus. Understanding this anatomy makes it clear that clinical findings relative to the pudendal nerve (*eg*, perineal sensory dysfunction) will not be seen with pelvic plexus injury. Likewise, the sacral reflex studies, as outlined in Chapter 3, will demonstrate involvement with the bladder–anal and urethral–anal reflexes, as the afferent arm of the reflexes is via the pelvic plexus, but the clitoral–anal (bulbo-cavernosus) reflex will be unaffected as the pudendal afferents and efferents are not involved in the plexus. The most common cause of pelvic plexus injury is iatrogenic, following such procedures as abdominoperineal resection for rectal cancer, proctocolectomy, radical hysterectomy, and low anterior resection. Malignancy and radiation may cause injury. (*Adapted from* Yalla and Andriole [28].)

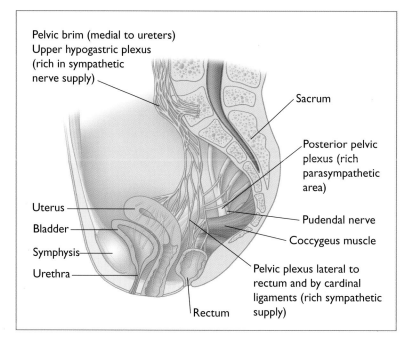

Pelvic brim (medial to ureters)
Upper hypogastric plexus
(rich in sympathetic
nerve supply)

Sacrum

Posterior pelvic
plexus (rich
parasympathetic
area)

Uterus

Bladder

Symphysis

Urethra

Pudendal nerve

Coccygeus muscle

Pelvic plexus lateral to
rectum and by cardinal
ligaments (rich sympathetic
supply)

Rectum

Figure 4-36. Pudendal nerve damage may occur during the perineal portion of abdominoperineal resection with mobilization of the anus, but this is not a component of the pelvic plexus. Direct damage to the parasympathetic nerves and the posterior part of the pelvic plexus may occur with dissection on the anterolateral, lower rectum, and the area inferolateral to the cervix. Sympathetic damage may occur at the pelvic brim, medial to the ureters, and in the region lateral to the rectum and the cardinal ligaments. Parasympathetic damage may cause detrusor areflexia and sympathetic damage may produce a loss of proximal urethral pressure. Many of the symptoms of pelvic plexus injury improve so that voiding may improve in 3 to 6 months. One third of patients, however, have a residual problem that requires treatment.

For the pelvic plexus, note the portions rich in parasympathetic and sympathetic neural supply. Note also that the pudendal nerve goes beneath the coccygeus muscle and is not a part of the pelvic plexus [29]. Uroflowmetry indicates detrusor hypoactivity. Parasympathetic dysfunction produces a decrease in detrusor function and dysfunction of the visceral afferents following the parasympathetics leads to the loss of urge sensation. After parasympathetic denervation, adrenergic influences result in an increase in bladder tone. Sympathetic β-adrenergic denervation leads to a decrease in bladder compliance, which may lead to upper tract problems if it persists. Early detection is necessary. The α-adrenergic denervation may lead to proximal sphincter (bladder neck) incompetence. Intermittent catheterization is a mainstay of therapy. If bladder pressures are increased, anticholinergic medication is indicated to help protect upper tracts. If bladder "tone" is elevated at the bladder neck, α-blocking agents may be indicated. In severe compliance problems, bladder augmentation may be necessary.

DIABETES AND PERIPHERAL NEUROPATHIES

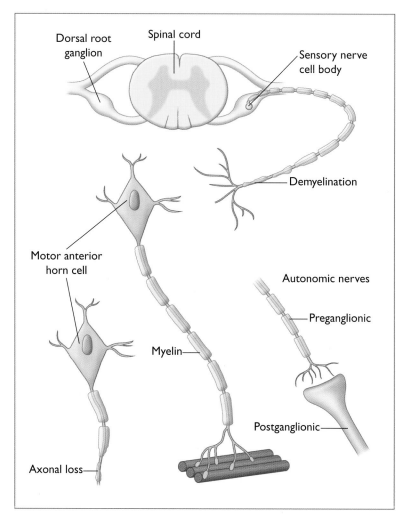

Dorsal root
ganglion

Spinal cord

Sensory nerve
cell body

Demyelination

Motor anterior
horn cell

Autonomic nerves

Preganglionic

Myelin

Postganglionic

Axonal loss

Figure 4-37. Diabetes is among the most common of the polyneuropathies. It is unique in the classification of polyneuropathies because, like uremia, it produces mixed pathophysiologic patterns of axonal loss and demyelination and affects both sensory and motor (including autonomic) nerves. Patients characteristically have paresthesias and disabling dysesthesias in the distal lower limbs. Vibratory sensation, two-point discrimination, and proprioception are reduced in a distal-to-proximal gradient. Thus, the larger sensory nerves are involved. Involvement of smaller nerves occurs in more severe disease and is evident from pain and temperature-sensation alteration and dysautonomia, including cystopathy.

Pathophysiology of Pelvic Visceral Dysfunction

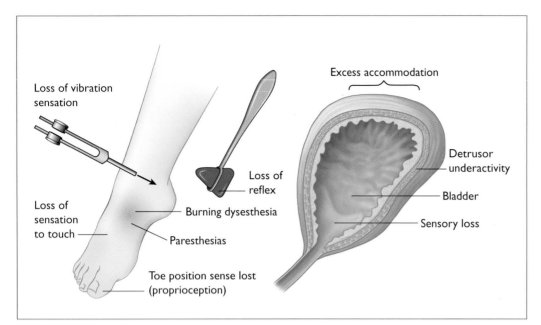

Figure 4-38. Cystopathy occurs in up to 80% of patients with insulin-dependent diabetes [30] and correlates with peripheral neuropathy in 75% to 100% of cases. Usually there is a reduced sensation of bladder fullness and decreased voiding frequency, with increased accommodation and decreased detrusor activity, reflecting the involvement of sensory and autonomic nerves. Urinary tract infections are common. Involuntary detrusor contractions are also seen in diabetic cystopathy, but the relationship with diabetes per se is not yet determined. Treatment modalities are as for other conditions with poor detrusor function.

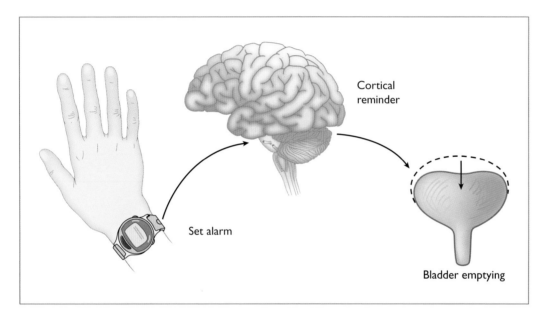

Figure 4-39. In patients with bladder sensory impairment, voiding "by the clock" is advisable to prevent recurring bladder overdistention. Relatively inexpensive devices are available at nonmedical electronic supply stores. They can be set at desired intervals to sound and remind patient to void. Postvoid residual urine determination and urine examination for infection are advised at least yearly in all patients with insulin-dependent diabetes. In patients with residual urine problems, intermittent catheterization remains the treatment of choice.

MULTIPLE SCLEROSIS

Multiple sclerosis, a disabling neurologic disease, appears to be due to an autoimmune process involving central nervous system (CNS) antigens, as suggested by an immunoglobulin response in the cerebrospinal fluid, a cellular immune response seen histologically, and by symptom improvement with steroids. A multiple sclerosis lesion is an area of focal demyelination called a plaque. Histologically, the plaques have an inflammatory reduction in oligodendroglia (the myelin-producing cells in the CNS) with abundant edema increasing the plaque size and causing more neurologic impairment. After the acute phase, the inflammation subsides and gliosis with scarring and an increase in fibrous astrocytes are seen. The edema lessens, allowing neurologic remission. Thus, many patients will have frequent exacerbations and remissions with minimal disease progression. Some, however, have severe progression from the disease onset.

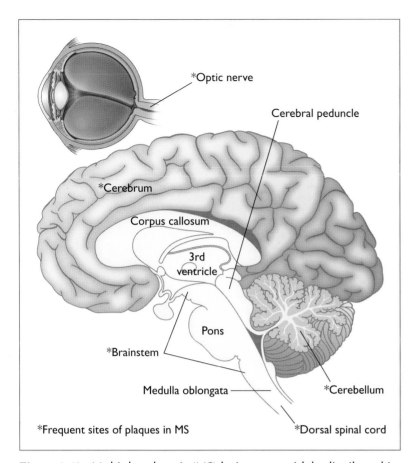

*Frequent sites of plaques in MS

Figure 4-40. Multiple sclerosis (MS) lesions are widely distributed in the central nervous system (CNS) white matter and have a predilection for the optic nerve, cerebrum, cerebellum, dorsal spinal cord, and brainstem. Approximately 75% of patients with MS have spinal cord involvement, generally affecting motor tracts before sensory. The incidence of MS increases with latitude. There is a familial predisposition for development of MS and women are affected more often than men and whites more often than blacks. Although this is not mentioned in textbooks, the vast majority of patients seem to have a calm demeanor of acceptance and are notably pleasant in their relationships.

For diagnosis, lesions at two or more sites and at two or more times must be demonstrated. Common conditions are lower limb weakness and spasticity, tremors, ataxia, incoordination, paresthesias, visual impairment, and lower urinary tract (LUT) dysfunction. Laboratory studies aid in the diagnosis, including visual, auditory, and somatosensory evoked potentials, and CT and MRI studies of brain and cord. MRI is more sensitive than CT for plaque demonstration and focal enhancement with gadolinium is considered to be evidence of an "active" plaque. Spinal fluid studies may show increase in protein and lymphocytes and immunoglobulin G and urodynamic studies may characterize the urologic status.

Approximately 75% of MS patients have LUT dysfunction and virtually 100% of MS patients whose disease has caused walking difficulties will have LUT dysfunction. In the Western world, urinary symptoms are chiefly filling symptoms, whereas Asians have more voiding symptoms. The common early complaints are irritative symptoms of frequency, urgency, urge incontinence, and nocturia related to the common finding of neurogenic overactive detrusor (detrusor hyperreflexia). Hesitancy, incomplete emptying, and retention occur in 25% of patients. Bowel and sexual symptoms are commonly associated. The degree of urologic dysfunction relates to the extent of neuropathology.

Neurologic signs and symptoms do not categorize the urologic function; hence, urgency and frequency, for example, are not necessarily a result of detrusor hyperreflexia but may be caused by areflexia. Generally, suprasacral plaques result in detrusor hyperreflexia and sacral plaques result in detrusor areflexia, but exceptions are common.

Genitourinary Dysfunction in MS

Plaque Location	Urodynamic Findings*	Sphincter EMG, Sacral Reflex	Voiding
Suprapontine	Overactive detrusor	Normal	Coordinated
Subpontine, suprasacral	Overactive detrusor	Normal	Not coordinated
	Poorly sustained contractions		Possible elevated residual urine
	Variable sensations		
	Small capacities		
	Possible detrusor–sphincter dyssynergia†		
Sacral	Areflexia	Abnormal	Strain to void
	Large capacity		Elevated residual urine
	Poor sensation		
	Nonrelaxing sphincter		
	Positive bethanechol denervation supersensitivity test		

*May change during the course of MS.
†More common in long-term MS and usually associated with more complete spinal lesions; frequently seen with lower limb pyramidal signs.

Figure 4-41. Genitourinary dysfunction in multiple sclerosis (MS) patients. Urinary signs and symptoms are important but are not accurate enough to categorize urologic function. Vesicosphincter dyssynergia is seen in 6% to 66% of cases with detrusor hyperreflexia. The corticospinal and the reticulospinal tracts controlling, respectively, the external sphincter and the detrusor are commonly impaired, producing an upper motor neuron type of vesicourethral dysfunction. Patients, then, with lower limb pyramidal signs (hyperactive reflexes, positive Babinski sign) are likely to have bladder dysfunction.

Continued on the next page

Figure 4-41. *(Continued)* The pattern of vesicosphincter dyssynergia can be mimicked by limb hyperreflexia and spasms, so the urethral or anal electromyogram (EMG) recording in urodynamic studies should be performed with needle, rather than surface, electrodes.

Patients with detrusor areflexia have large-capacity bladders, elevated residual urine, and poor bladder sensation, and most have a positive bethanechol supersensitivity test (*see* Chapter 3, Fig. 3-7). Patients with sacral cord plaques interfering with Onuf's nucleus have abnormal sphincter needle electromyographic findings associated with the lower motor neuron clinical findings and detrusor areflexia with involvement of the sacral intermediolateral cell column. During attempts to void, the sphincter is usually nonrelaxing. If a patient with denervation of the sphincter based on needle EMG study also has hyperreflexia, then there is urodynamic evidence of both suprasacral and sacral myelopathy, fulfilling the requisite two sites of involvement that are necessary for an MS diagnosis.

Different study designs have made the correlation of urodynamic patterns with MRI findings controversial. Urodynamic patterns can and do change in MS patients. Good data on the urodynamic changes with time are lacking. Detrusor areflexia and neurogenic overactive detrusor can change to vesicosphincter dyssynergia and vice versa. In patients with long-term progressive MS, the most common urodynamic pattern is vesicosphincter dyssynergia [31]. This pattern is seen in suprasacral spinal cord lesions, which tend to be complete. The potential for change makes urologic follow-up essential. The sacral reflex test (Chapter 3), in combination with anal sphincter needle EMG, is helpful in the diagnosis of sacral myelopathy. Uroflow studies and residual urine determinations are also helpful in patient follow-up, and study of urine is vital as MS patients frequently have urinary tract infections without symptoms.

In patients with elevated postvoid residual urine, urodynamic studies and sacral clinical neurophysiologic studies are recommended to define the cause. Thus, uroflow, residual urine, and urinalysis (or culture) are important to follow. There is controversy regarding periodic urodynamic studies and clinical neurophysiologic studies of the sacral reflex and sphincter needle EMG. With the poor relationship of symptoms to the urologic status, regular urodynamic studies may be advocated. The purpose of urodynamic study is to assess the presence of risk factors that would change therapy. In the majority of MS patients, risk factors for infection, incontinence, and voiding problems are frequently found to change markedly as time progresses. This and the changes in therapies for MS, which may have urologic consequences, make repeated evaluation more necessary.

One consideration not yet mentioned for repeated evaluation of urologic status is protection of the upper tracts. For reasons that are not clear, upper tract deterioration is less common in patients with MS than in spinal cord–injured patients. However, there still is a 10% to 20% incidence of upper tract pathology including pyelonephritis; stone disease; hydronephroses: reflux; renal insufficiency; and occasionally sepsis, uremia, and death [32]. Upper tract evaluation is then suggested when there is an increased risk, which is the situation with urinary tract infection and abnormal urodynamic patterns. The urodynamic patterns leading to high intravesical pressures are especially worrisome.

Therapies for the lower urinary tract dysfunction should be mainly for symptomatic relief, less than for upper tract protection as with spinal cord–injured patients. Thus, the therapies may be more conservative, especially because the patient's status has potential for change. Irreversible forms of therapy are not mandated until there is hopeless and permanent neurologic progression, conservative therapies have failed, or upper tract pathology has developed.

REFERENCES

1. Steers WD, Creedon D, Tuttle JB: Immunity to NGF prevents afferent plasticity following hypertrophy of the urinary bladder. *J Urol* 1996, 155:378–385.

2. DeGroat WC: Neurologic basis for the overactive bladder. *Urology* 1997, 50(Suppl 6A):36–52.

3. Elbadawi A, Yalla SV, Resnick NM: Structural basis of geriatric voiding dysfunction. *J Urol* 1993, 150:1657–1695.

4. Steers WD, De Groat WC: Effect of bladder outlet obstruction on micturition reflex pathways in the rat. *J Urol* 1988, 140:864–871.

5. Sui GP, Coppen SR, Dupont E, *et al.*: Impedance measurements and connexin expression in human detrusor muscle from stable and unstable bladders. *BJU Int* 2003, 92:297–305.

6. Yoshida M, *et al.*: Effects of age and muscle stretching on Ach release in isolated human bladder smooth muscle. *J Urol* 2002, 167:40.

7. McGuire EJ: Diagnosis and treatment of intrinsic sphincter deficiency. *Int J Urol* 1995, 2(Suppl 1):7–10.

8. Sanders RC, *et al.*: Imaging the female urethra. *Ultrasound Q* 1994, 12:167–183.

9. Arbuckle JB, Docherty RJ: Expression of tetrodotoxin-resistant sodium channels in capsaicin-sensitive dorsal root ganglion neurons of adult rats. *Neurosci Lett* 1995, 185:70–73.

10. Apodaca G, Kiss S, *et al.*: Disruption of bladder epithelium barrier function after spinal cord injury. *Am J Physiol* 2003, 284:F966.

11. Krane RJ, Siroky MB: *Clinical Neuro-Urology*, edn 2. Boston: Little, Brown; 1991.

12. King LR, Levitt SB: Vesicoureteral reflux, megaureter, and ureteral reimplantation. In *Campbell's Urology*, edn 5. Edited by Walsh PC, Gittes, Perlmutter, Stamey. Philadelphia: WB Saunders; 1986.

13. Stickler D, Dolman J, Rolfe S, Chawla J: Activity of antiseptics against Escherichia coli growing as biofilms on silicone surfaces. *Eur J Clin Microbiol Infect Dis* 1989, 8:974–978.

14. Pannek J: Transitional cell carcinoma in patients with spinal cord injury: a high risk malignancy? *Urolology* 2002, 59:240.

15. Dromerick AW, Edwards DF: Relation of postvoid residual to urinary tract infection during stroke rehabilitation. *Arch Phys Med Rehabil* 84:1369–1372.

16. Hutton KA, Trejdosiewicz LK, Thomas DF, Southgate J: Urothelial tissue culture for bladder reconstruction: an experimental study. *J Urol* 1993, 150:721–725.

17. Pernet F, Jonas U: Ileal conduit urinary diversion: early and late results of 132 cases in a 25 year period. *World J Urol* 1985, 3:140–144.

18. Messing EM, Stamey TA: Interstitial cystitis: early diagnosis, pathology and treatment. *Urology* 1978, 12:381–391.

19. Beersiek F, Parks AG, Swash M: Pathogenesis of anorectal incontinence: a histometric study of the anal sphincter musculature. *J Neurol Sci* 1979, 42:111–127.

20. Coats PM, Chan KK, Wilkins M, Beard RJ: A comparison between midline and mediolateral episiotomies. *Br J Obstet Gynaecol* 1980, 87:408–412.

21. Busacchi P, Perri T, Paradisi R, *et al.*: Abnormalities of somatic peptide containing nerves supplying the pelvic floor of women with genitourinary prolapse and stress urinary incontinence. *Urology* 2004, 63:591–595.

22. Visco AG, Yuan L: Differential gene expression in pubococcygeus muscle from patients with pelvic organ prolapse. *Am J Obstet Gynecol* 2003, 189:102–112.

23. Brizzolara GS, Okimoto J, Urschitz: Pathobiology of pelvic organ prolapse. *Int Urogynecol J* 2006, 17(Suppl 3):S361–S408.

24. Lind L, Lucente V, Kohn N: Thoracic kyphosis and the prevalence of advanced uterine prolapse. *Obstet Gynecol* 1996, 87:605–609.

25. Yokoyama O, Mizuno H, Komatsu K, Akino H: Role of glutamate receptors in the development and maintenance of bladder overactivity after cerebral infarct in the rat. *J Urol* 2004, 171:1709–1714.

26. Diokno AC, Koff SA, Bender LF: Periurethral striated muscle activity in neurogenic bladder dysfunction. *J Urol* 1974, 112:743–749.

27. Sharr MM, Garfield JS, Jenkins JD: Lumbar spondylosis and neurologic bladder: investigation of 73 patients with chronic urinary symptoms. *Br Med J* 1976, 1:695–697.

28. Yalla SV, Andriole G: Vesicourethral dysfunction following pelvic visceral ablative surgery. *J Urol* 1984, 132:503.

29. Eickenberg HU, Amin M, Klompus W, Lich R Jr: Urologic complications following abdominoperineal resection. *J Urol* 1976, 115:180–182.

30. Frimodt-Møller C: Diabetic cystopathy: epidemiology and related disorders. *Ann Intern Med* 1980, 92:318–321.

31. Wheeler JS, Siroky MB, Pavlakis AJ, *et al.*: The changing neurourologic pattern of multiple sclerosis. *J Urol* 1983, 130:1123–1126.

32. Andersen JT, Bradley WE: Abnormalities of detrusor and sphincter function in multiple sclerosis. *Br J Urol* 1976, 48:193–197.

5

Diagnosis of Urinary Incontinence and Retention

Mary T. McLennan and Alfred E. Bent

It is estimated that up to 35% of adult women have urinary incontinence [1]. Factors including genetics, vaginal delivery, age, smoking, and obesity contribute to the risk of developing urinary incontinence. The estimated societal cost in the United States is in excess of $20 billion [2].

The initial assessment should establish a presumptive diagnosis and exclude related or unrelated conditions that require intervention, assess the level of bother, allow for specific therapy based on a risk–benefit ratio, and prompt additional testing or a referral if indicated [3]. Differential diagnosis involves the diagnoses of stress urinary incontinence, urge urinary incontinence, and mixed incontinence (a combination of the two other types) almost 95% of the time (*see* Figure 5-1). The proportion of women with stress urinary incontinence predominates (close to 50% of cases), while urge urinary and mixed incontinence are equally divided in the remainder. With age, the number of patients with mixed incontinence increases and the number of those with stress incontinence declines. Reversible conditions must be diagnosed and managed in the elderly (*see* Figure 5-2).

A basic evaluation includes history, physical examination, urinary diary (frequency volume chart), postvoid residual urine determination, and urinalysis. The history and general assessment includes the presence, severity, duration, and bother of urinary symptoms. Further inquiry is directed to the effect of symptoms on sexual function; previous conservative, medical, or surgical treatment; environmental issues; mental status; physical abilities; coexisting disease; medications; obstetric and menstrual history; lifestyle; goals of treatment; and support systems. The physical examination includes a simple neurologic screen and abdominal, pelvic, and rectal examinations. The voluntary pelvic floor muscles are assessed for strength. If appropriate, a cough stress test may be performed to demonstrate stress incontinence. Urine is collected and tested by dipstick, examined by microscopy, or sent for culture. Symptoms may be quantified using a frequency volume chart (urinary diary). Postvoid residual urine should be determined in any patient with voiding dysfunction [4].

Empiric treatment may commence from this point unless a complicated condition exists. These would include recurrent incontinence or incontinence associated with pain, hematuria, recurrent infection, pelvic irradiation, radical pelvic surgery, or suspected fistula. Additional testing would be required for diagnosis in this group of patients. Imaging is highly recommended for patients with neurogenic urinary incontinence such as myelodysplasia or spinal cord trauma, incontinence associated with a significant postvoid urinary residual, coexistent kidney pain, severe untreated pelvic organ prolapse, and suspected extraurethral urinary incontinence. Endoscopy is recommended in patients with failed prior surgery, recurrent urinary tract infections, suspected interstitial cystitis, hematuria, pain in the urinary tract, and suspected fistula.

High-quality questionnaires may be recommended for the assessment of the patient's perspective on symptoms of incontinence and their impact on quality of life. Urodynamic testing is recommended prior to most invasive treatments, after treatment failures, and in complicated incontinence. Routine urodynamics evaluate bladder sensation, detrusor overactivity, urethral competence during filling, and detrusor function during voiding. Uroflowmetry is recommended for screening patients with concomitant voiding dysfunction. Additional tests of urethral function such as urethral closure pressure profile, leak point pressure, videourodynamics, and electromyography are considered to be optional. Neurophysiological testing of striated muscle and nervous pathways may be considered in patients with peripheral lesions prior to treatment of the lower urinary tract or anorectal dysfunction. Pudendal nerve latency testing is not recommended. Imaging techniques including cystourethrography, ultrasound, CT, or MRI may be indicated in suspected pelvic floor dysfunction, failed surgery, urethral diverticulum, and in the assessment of urethral mobility [4].

DIFFERENTIAL DIAGNOSIS OF INCONTINENCE

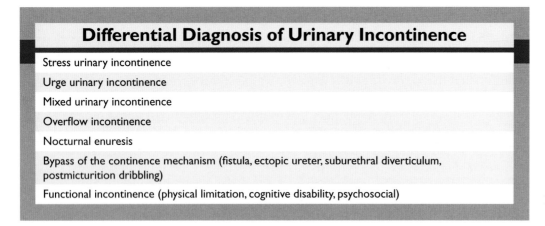

Differential Diagnosis of Urinary Incontinence

Stress urinary incontinence

Urge urinary incontinence

Mixed urinary incontinence

Overflow incontinence

Nocturnal enuresis

Bypass of the continence mechanism (fistula, ectopic ureter, suburethral diverticulum, postmicturition dribbling)

Functional incontinence (physical limitation, cognitive disability, psychosocial)

Figure 5-1. Differential diagnosis of urinary incontinence [5].

Causes of Transient Incontinence in the Elderly—DIAPPERS

D	Delirium
I	Infection
A	Atrophic urethritis, vaginitis
P	Psychologic (depression, neurosis)
P	Pharmacologic
E	Excess urine output
R	Restricted mobility
S	Stool impaction

Figure 5-2. Causes of transient incontinence in the elderly.

PATIENT HISTORY

Although a careful history is valuable, the patient's recall of symptoms alone may be misleading for the appropriate diagnosis of the type of incontinence. The positive predictive value for a diagnosis of genuine stress incontinence via extensive questionnaires was 80% and only 20% for overactive bladder [6]. This is important as a more definitive diagnosis should be obtained before embarking on invasive treatments such as surgery. In addition, patients with severe prolapse may not complain of incontinence due to anatomic changes that may mask stress incontinence, but clinicians need to be aware of this condition and evaluate the patient appropriately. Although history does not predict the diagnosis 100% of the time, it is useful to plan further evaluation as well as treatment. For this reason, it is useful for the patient to complete a questionnaire prior to being seen in the office, as it allows her to examine more closely the factors that may precipitate leakage, severity of the leakage, and the effect of previous treatments. New questionnaires are used to measure the severity of the condition and the effect on the patient's quality of life.

Patient Questionnaire

Please bring this completed form with you at the time of your first visit.

Name _____ Date _____
Birthdate _____ Age _____
Please describe your current medical problem: _____
_____

OBSTRETIC AND GYNECOLOGIC HISTORY

Number of pregnancies	_____	Number of children born alive _____
Number of miscarriages	_____	Current birth control method _____
Onset of first menstrual period	_____	Last menstrual period _____
Length of menstrual cycle	_____	Duration between menstrual cycles _____
Are your periods regular? Yes _____ No _____		Have you been through menopause? _____

Have you had any treatment to your cervix? Yes _____ No _____
Cautery _____ Other _____
Cryosurgery _____ If yes, when? _____

Do you have any of the following?
    Bleeding between periods; if yes, duration _____
    Bleeding after intercourse; if yes, duration _____
    Heavy menstrual periods; if yes, duration _____
    Pain with periods; if yes, duration _____
    Uncontrolled loss of urine; if yes, duration _____

Have you ever had any of the following:
    Herpes   _____
    Venereal warts   _____
    Sexually transmitted diseases _____

Are you sexually active at this time? Yes _____ No _____
Is your sex life satisfactory for you? Yes _____ No _____

PAST MEDICAL HISTORY — PLEASE ANSWER YES OR NO
As a child did you have:
_____ Rheumatic fever   _____ Rubella (measles)
_____ Scarlet fever   _____ Other

As an adult have you had:
_____ Bladder infections   _____ Asthma
_____ Chronic fatigue syndrome   _____ Heart disease
_____ Diabetes   _____ Epstein-Barr virus
_____ Kidney disease   _____ High blood pressure
_____ Kidney infection   _____ Jaundice
_____ Liver disease   _____ Mononucleosis
_____ Pneumonia   _____ Serious injuries or accident
_____ Stroke   _____ Tuberculosis

Please list all medicines which you are currently taking including contraceptives and vitamins; include dose and frequency. _____
_____

Do you have any allergies? If so, please list: _____

SURGICAL HISTORY
Have you had any operations?   Yes _____ No _____
If yes, please list type, and date or age when performed _____
_____

Have you had any blood transfusions?   Yes _____ No _____

HEALTH HABITS
Do you consider yourself healthy?
Do you smoke?   _____ Yes _____ No   How many packs a day? _____
Do you use alcohol?   _____ Yes _____ No   Do you use any street drugs? _____

Figure 5-3. A generic general medical questionnaire gives the clinician an overview of the patient's general health, expedites the first visit, and fulfills the need for documentation for the level of service. It is reviewed with the patient at the first visit and addendums are made as necessary.

Diagnosis of Urinary Incontinence and Retention **83**

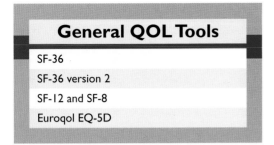

General QOL Tools
SF-36
SF-36 version 2
SF-12 and SF-8
Euroqol EQ-5D

Figure 5-4. General quality of life (QOL) tools. Research into the success of various interventions now includes aspects of QOL, not just cure or improvement of incontinence. These forms are validated general QOL instruments and have been translated into multiple languages. There is a fee for use and for scoring of these. SF—short form.

Commonly Used Incontinence-Specific Questionnaires
Urogenital Distress Inventory (UDI)
Urogenital Distress Inventory Short Form (UDI-6)
Incontinence Impact Questionnaire Short Form (IIQ-7)
Kings Health Questionnaire
Bristol Female Lower Urinary Tract Symptom Questionnaire (BFLUTS)

Figure 5-5. Condition-specific questionnaires. A number of validated urinary incontinence–specific questionnaires are available. However, no single tool has been shown to be superior and the clinician will need to evaluate which is most applicable to his or her population [7]. The American Urogynecologic Society website (www.augs.org) is a good source of information on questionnaires and indicates which require permission and a fee, as well as the sources to access them [8].

Subjective Questionnaires	
Urogenital Distress Inventory—Short Form UDI-6	**Incontinence Impact Questionnaire—Short Form IIQ-7**
Do you experience and, if so, how much are you bothered by:	Has urine leakage and/or prolapse affected your:
Frequent urination?	Ability to do household chores (cooking, house cleaning, laundry)?
Urine leakage related to the feeling of urgency?	Physical recreation such as walking, swimming, or other exercise?
Urine leakage related to physical activity, coughing, or sneezing?	Entertainment activities (movies, concerts, etc.)?
Small amounts of urine leakage (drops)?	Ability to travel by car or bus more than 30 minutes from home?
Difficulty emptying your bladder?	Participation in social activities outside your home?
Pain or discomfort in the lower abdominal or genital area?	Emotional health (nervousness, depression, etc.)?
	Feeling frustrated?

Figure 5-6. Short forms minimize the patient burden and are useful as a means to assess not only symptoms but also their severity. The forms may also aid in diagnosis and help to direct treatment [9].

Date	Time	Amount Voided	Accidents?	Reason for accident	Amount of fluid I drank
10/23	6:30 a.m.	300 mL	Yes	Getting to bathroom	
	9:15 a.m.	300 mL			8 oz
					8 oz
					4-6 oz
	9:45 a.m.	100 mL	Yes	Urge	
	11 a.m.	150 mL			
	12:45 p.m.	200 mL			8 oz
	2:15 p.m.	200 mL	Yes	Sitting	6 oz
	3:30 p.m.	100 mL	Yes	Urge	
	5:00 p.m.	150 mL			
	8:00 p.m.	200 mL	Yes	Eating	8 oz
	10:45 p.m.	100 mL	Yes	Prepare for bed	8 oz

Number of pads I used today: ____4____

A

Figure 5-7. Urinary diary. These forms provide an accurate assessment of urinary symptoms and provide information for behavioral intervention and response to therapy. They assess intake (volume and type), output (volume and timing), and activities or symptoms that are related to leakage. There is good test–retest reliability. A 7-day diary performed with limited instruction has been shown to reliably reflect frequency and incontinence [10]. There are diverse opinions on appropriate fluid intake and these forms provide an accurate assessment, as well as possibly being helpful for counseling. **A,** Overactive bladder.

Continued on the next page

Time	Amount Voided	Leak Volume	Urge Present	Activity	Amount/Type of Intake
6:00 a.m.	2.5 oz			Awakening	
7:01 a.m.	2 oz			Awakening	
8:02 a.m.	3 oz			Awakening	
8:45 a.m.				Resting in chair	6 oz prune juice
9:15 a.m.					8 oz milk, 8 oz water
9:45 a.m.	2 oz				
11:00 p.m.	22 oz			Sitting in chair	4 oz water
11:10 a.m.					10 oz water
11:15 a.m.	1 oz			Walking	
11:20 a.m.	drops			Bowel mvmt	
11:55 a.m.	1.75 oz			Reading	
12:45 p.m.	1.5 oz			Standing	
1:15 p.m.	1.5 oz			Doing laundry	
2:00 p.m.					8 oz water
2:30 p.m.					16 oz iced tea
2:30 p.m.	2 oz			Eating lunch	
2:55 p.m.	2 oz			Bowel mvmt	42 oz water
3:10 p.m.	3 oz			Reading	
3:50 p.m.				Ironing	10 oz water
4:00 p.m.	3 oz			Ironing	
5:05 p.m.	2 oz			Ironing	
6:15 p.m.	2.75 oz			Ironing	
6:30 p.m.				Eating dinner	12 oz iced tea
7:20 p.m.	3 oz			Sitting	
7:37 p.m.	2 oz			Walking	
8:15 p.m.	2 oz			Resting in chair	
9:00 p.m.	2 oz			Folding laundry	
10:00 p.m.				Crocheting	1 oz water (with medication)
10:30 p.m.	3 oz			Crocheting	
12:15 a.m.	3 oz			Resting in chair	
12:35 a.m.	2 oz			Folding laundry	
1:50 a.m.	2.5 oz				
2:35 a.m.	2 oz			Sleeping	
3:00 a.m.	2 oz			Sitting in chair	8 oz milk
4:25 a.m.	3 oz			Sleeping	
6:00 a.m.	3 oz			Awakening	

B

Figure 5-7. *(Continued)* **B**, Interstitial cystitis.

PHYSICAL EXAMINATION

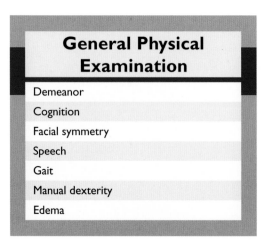

General Physical Examination

Demeanor

Cognition

Facial symmetry

Speech

Gait

Manual dexterity

Edema

Figure 5-8. Physical examination. The general physical examination should attempt to identify neurologic abnormalities and factors that affect toileting such as cognition, dexterity, and mobility. The examiner should observe the patient's demeanor, facial symmetry, speech, and gait. The presence of edema should be ascertained. Seeing the patient walk into the examining room provides valuable information on her general status.

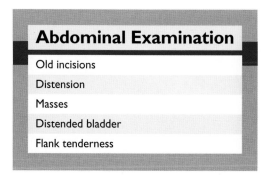

Abdominal Examination

Old incisions

Distension

Masses

Distended bladder

Flank tenderness

Figure 5-9. Abdominal examination. Abdominal examination may provide information on previous incontinence surgeries and possible contributors to increased intra-abdominal pressure or irritative bladder symptoms such as masses or a distended bladder. The examiner should also assess flank tenderness.

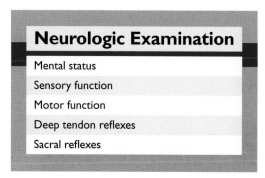

Neurologic Examination

Mental status

Sensory function

Motor function

Deep tendon reflexes

Sacral reflexes

Figure 5-10. Neurologic examination. Screening for mental status changes can be done rapidly in an informal manner by noting the patient's orientation, recent and past memory, speech and comprehension, sensory and motor function, and deep tendon and sacral reflexes. Patients with altered mental status often present with detrusor instability or overflow incontinence.

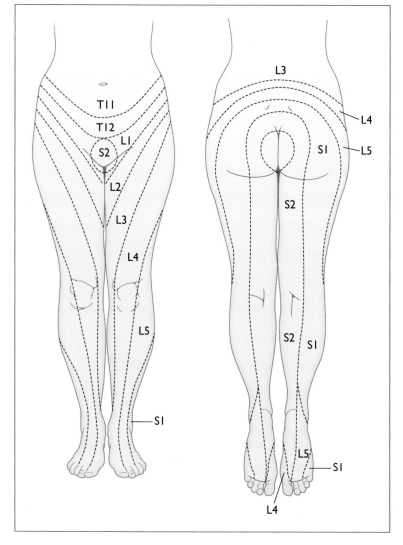

Figure 5-11. Extremity assessment. The proximal and distal extremities and perineum should be tested for light touch and pinprick. The presence or absence and symmetric nature of responses are noted. (*Adapted from* Lind *et al.* [11].)

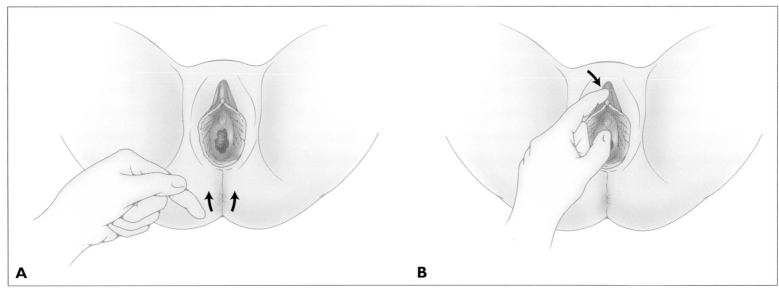

A   **B**

Figure 5-12. Sacral reflexes. Parasympathetic innervation of the detrusor arises from S2–3 with minor contribution from SI–2 traveling as the pelvic nerve. Stimulation results in detrusor contraction. Sympathetic fibers travel in the hypogastric nerve and regulate storage. The periurethral striated muscles are innervated by SI–4 via the pudendal nerve. Rectal examination enables assessment of the tone and voluntary contraction. In the absence of a sphincter tear, the preservation of tone but absent volume contraction indicates a suprasacral lesion and decreased tone implies a sacral nerve abnormality. Stroking the skin lateral to the anus results in a contraction (**A**). Similarly, tapping the clitoris and seeing the anal sphincter and perineal muscles contract tests the bulbocavernosus reflex (**B**). Pulling on a Foley catheter will result in a similar reflex. Note that these reflexes are absent in up to 30% of neurologically normal women [12]. (*Adapted from* Lind *et al.* [11].)

Pelvic Examination

Gross evidence of prolapse with/without Valsalva with any associated skin changes

Hypoestrogenism (urethral caruncle, urethral prolapse, erythema, petechial hemorrhages, thin mucosa, loss of rugae)

Supine empty stress test (have patient do Valsalva and cough)—result is positive if there are leaks and may indicate intrinsic sphincter deficiency [13]

Speculum examination

  Using bivalve speculum, observe for any pooling indicative of fistula or ectopic ureter

  Ask patient to strain and assess the apex for prolapse (*ie*, uterus or cuff)

  Anterior wall—split the speculum and place the posterior blade posteriorly and have the patient strain

    If cystocele is present, attempt to determine if there is a central or lateral defect

    If rugae are still present it may indicate a lateral defect; if absent, a central one. A lateral wall elevator or ring forceps may be used to elevate the lateral sulcus and, if the cystocele reduces, it may be indicative of a lateral defect. However, compared with the surgical detection of a defect, clinical evidence was sensitive (92%) but not very specific (53%) [14].

    If the cystocele does not reduce, this is indicative of a central defect

  Posterior wall—place the half speculum anteriorly and ask patient to strain; determine if there is protrusion from the posterior wall

Bimanual examination

  General examination of uterus and adnexa

  Specific palpations for tenderness of the bladder base as in urethral syndrome

  Palpation of the anterior vaginal wall and urethra to elicit discharge or a mass suggestive of local pathology

Pelvic floor squeeze

  The index finger is placed at the 4 then 8-o'clock position and the patient is asked to squeeze "like you are holding in gas or urine." The response can be graded from 1 to 4: 0, no contraction; 1, slight contraction; 2, stronger contraction; 3, contraction with some elevation; 4, contraction and elevation with resultant closure of the vagina

Rectal examination

  Assess resting tone and integrity of the sphincter, especially anteriorly

  Ask the patient to contract "as if holding in gas" and assess the pelvic floor muscles and neurologic integrity

Rule out masses and impaction

  A bidigital rectal/vaginal examination with the patient straining may detect an enterocele

Figure 5-13. Pelvic examination. Examination should assess for the all the elements listed. It should focus on evidence of pelvic floor dysfunction (loss of support, incontinence), exclude pelvic pathology, and assess muscle function (levator complex, rectal sphincter). It is useful to have the patient void prior to the examination.

Pelvic Organ Prolapse Quantification. This standardized measurement of prolapse was developed by the International Continence Society and adopted in 1996 [15]. It allows for reproducible and quantifiable measurement of the various segments involved in prolapse and is easily learned and reproducible between observers [16]. This technique will be discussed elsewhere in the atlas. (*See* Figure 4-28.)

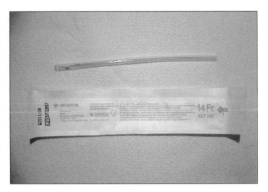

Figure 5-14. Assessment for postvoid residual. A short female self-catheter or a simple red rubber catheter can be used to determine the residual. Simple catheterization with a 12 or 14 F red rubber catheter can be performed shortly after voiding to assess the postvoid residual. Most clinicians consider 50 to 100 mL as indicative of normal emptying. An elevated postvoid residual is more difficult to interpret and should be repeated on several occasions because environment, amount in the bladder prior to voiding, and time lapse to catheterization all affect volume. The incidence of a positive urine culture after a single in–out catheterization ranges from 1% to 20% [17].

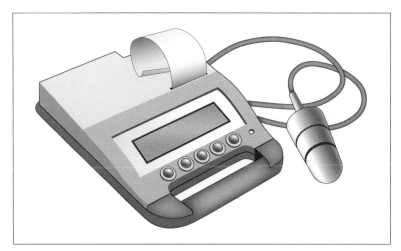

Figure 5-15. Sector ultrasound machines provide cross-sectional images of the bladder and automatically calculate bladder volume. With the patient supine, a small amount of gel is placed above the symphysis and the bladder scanner is placed firmly and directed toward the bladder. The scanner rotates 360° for 3 seconds and the volume is calculated. Correlation is excellent between catheterized and scanned volumes. This noninvasive instrument avoids the risk of catheterization [18].

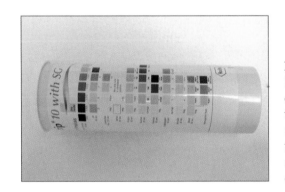

Figure 5-16. Testing methods. Urine "dip" testing is useful for rapid diagnosis but generally is less accurate than microscopy in the detection of infection. The esterase test relies on a color change caused by leukocyte esterase. The nitrate test detects the conversion of nitrate to nitrite by bacteria. Certain bacteria do not convert nitrates and also depend on bacterial concentrations and are less accurate with decreasing numbers of colonies per milliliter. These tests should be reserved for situations in which an experienced staff member is unavailable to do microscopy. False-positive tests for blood can result from dyes. About 3% of normal individuals will excrete more than three erythrocytes per high-power field [19].

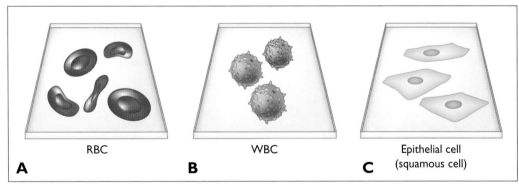

Figure 5-17. Microscopic investigation. Urine microscopy is useful in the detection of hematuria, pyuria, and bacteriuria. These conditions do not typically cause incontinence but may suggest aggravating factors (**A** and **B**). Microscopy of unspun urine is inexpensive and easy. Evidence of pyuria should not be used as a basis for treatment in elderly asymptotic patients. Several studies have shown no increased morbidity or mortality from nontreatment in this group [20]. No evidence in the literature supports routine urine cytology in the incontinent patient. Cytology should be limited to high-risk groups (those with a history of cervical cancer treated with radiation, exposure to aromatic amines, long-term catheter use, or previous cyclophosphamide treatment). **C,** Microscopy is a poor screening tool and well-differentiated tumors often shed minimally. Cells may appear to be normal, while the false-negative rate may be as high as 20% even with high-grade lesions [19]. RBC—red blood cell; WBC—white blood cell.

Diagnosis of Urinary Incontinence and Retention

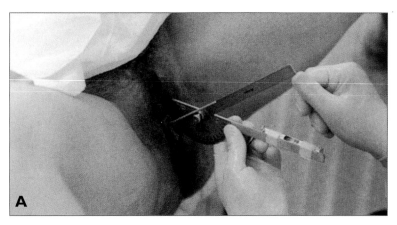

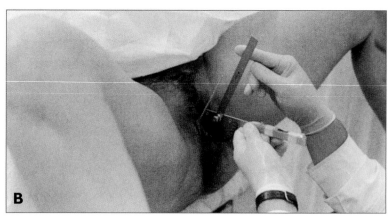

Figure 5-18. Mobility of the urethrovesical junction. The cotton swab test is the simplest means of assessing mobility. With the patient supine, the external urethral meatus is cleansed with povidone-iodine. The sterile swab is lubricated with 1% lidocaine jelly, introduced through the urethra into the bladder, then slowly withdrawn until resistance is met. **A**, The swab is now at the urethrovesical junction (UVJ). The patient is asked to strain and the degree of deflection from the horizontal is recorded using a goniometer. **B**, An angle greater than 30° indicates mobility. Mobility has been noted to be a prognostic factor for success with both retropubic and sling procedures [21,22]. (*From* Agosta [23]; with permission.)

SIMPLE OFFICE TESTS

A	Pad-Weight Test Kit Instructions for Patients
	1. Use the pads in the order in which they are numbered (from 1 to 6).
	2. When placing a pad, remove the paper backing from the adhesive strip on the pad and put the paper backing in the bag.
	3. Wear each pad for 2 h only.
	4. Record the time the pad was in place. (*See* examples given in Figure 5-19B.)
	5. After removing each pad, store it in the original bag, making sure that it is sealed.
	6. Store the sealed bags in the box provided. Keep the box in a cool, dry place until you return to the doctor's office the next day.
	7. Record any unusual activities or summarize your routine activities.
	8. If you need to change one of the pads before 2 h have passed (due to a large-volume leakage episode), you may use the next numbered pad and indicate the time you changed.
	9. Remember to begin early since the test lasts for 12 h. If you begin at noon, you will not finish until midnight.
	10. Return the pads to the office the next day.

B	12-Hour Pad Test						
Time	**Activity**	**Leaks**	**Urgency**	**Intake**	**Void Volume**	**Leak Volume**	**Weight**
Pad #1							
8:00 AM	Breakfast			Coffee (1 cup)	10 oz		Pre
8:30 AM	Walk to work	X				Small	Post
9:30 AM	Sitting at desk		X		7 oz		
Pad #2							
10:00 AM	Meeting	X	X			Medium	Pre
11:30 AM	Lunch			Iced tea (12 oz)			Post
11:45 AM	Climbing stairs	X				Small	

Figure 5-19. Pad tests. A pad test is useful to grade the severity of incontinence and to demonstrate leakage when other tests have failed to demonstrate incontinence. Tests are designed to measure the amount of urine leakage (incontinence) that a patient experiences at home, during normal daytime activities. The test can be done 1 day prior to the patient's next office visit. The test kit contains six preweighed, numbered sanitary pads in individual sealed bags. The 1-hour pad test has been standardized by the International Continence Society and is diagrammatically represented in this figure. Important points to remember are listed. **A** and **B**, The 12-hour test is performed at home and may provide additional benefits by demonstrating how factors may be precipitating events, relationship to activity, impact, or other clues as to the cause of incontinence or possible interventions. A pad-weight increase of greater than 1 g/h is abnormal. (*From* Pierson [24]; with permission.)

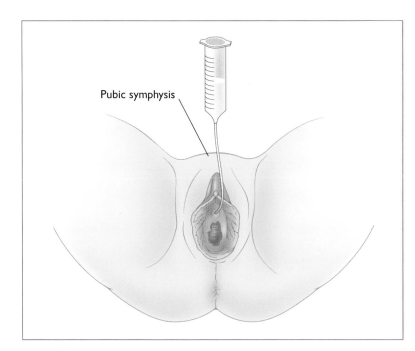

Pubic symphysis

Figure 5-20. Cystometry. Informal simple office cystometry can be performed at the time of the initial consultation to provide additional information. With the patient in the supine position, a bulb syringe can be attached to the catheter that is used to determine the postvoid residual. Room temperature sterile water is added in 50-mL increments. The syringe is elevated so the 50-mL mark is about 15 cm above the symphysis. The meniscus represents the intravesical pressure. The patient is asked to report her first sensation, fullness, and maximum capacity as the syringe is filled. A sudden rise in the meniscus associated with an urge or leakage indicates a detrusor contraction. The abdomen should be palpated to ensure that abdominal strain is absent. Several studies have found reasonable sensitivity (75%–88%) and specificity (75%) for the diagnosis of detrusor instability as compared with multichannel urodynamics [25]. Be aware that small contractions may be missed and that the supine position is less provocative for detrusor instability.

On completion of filling, the catheter is removed and the patient is asked to cough while supine. Instantaneous leakage represents a positive stress test. Leakage that continues after the cough may indicate the need for more detailed testing. If incontinence is not demonstrated, provoking maneuvers should be done with the patient in the standing position. This simple procedure may provide sufficient information to assist in conservative management decisions. Patients who require surgical intervention require more detailed testing. (*Adapted from* Bent and McLennan [26].)

MULTICHANNEL URODYNAMICS

Criteria for Urodynamic Testing

Patient complains of incontinence but none is demonstrated

Objective findings do not correlate with symptoms

Prior screening is normal or inconclusive

Not responding to conservative therapy

Surgical intervention, especially if previous surgery failed

Mixed incontinence where clinically difficult to determine which is a major contributor to symptoms

Patient with previous radical pelvic surgery

Patient with known or suspected neurologic disorders (such as multiple sclerosis, herniated disk, spinal cord injury, myelodysplasia)

Pelvic organ prolapse to hymen or beyond

Elevated postvoid residual

Figure 5-21. Urodynamic testing. This type of testing is not necessarily part of the initial evaluation of incontinence. Many patients can be successfully treated conservatively without initial testing. The criteria are guidelines for patients in need of a more specific diagnosis. Urodynamic testing is made up of several parts.

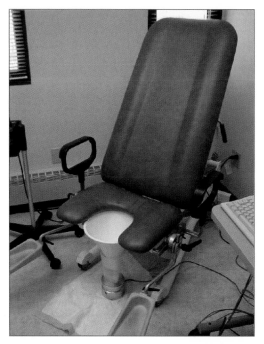

Figure 5-22. Uroflowmetry. The patient is asked to present with a comfortably full bladder, then to void as normally as possible in a chair, as seen here. The following measurements are obtained: maximum flow rate (milliliter/second); average flow rate (milliliter/second); flow time (seconds); and voided volume (milliliters). Flow time and the maximum and average flow rates increase with increasing voided volume up to 200 mL. There is no consensus on normal voiding parameters; however, most clinicians believe a normal voiding study consists of a voided volume of at least 200 mL, voided over 15 to 20 seconds with a maximum flow rate of 20 mL/s or greater with a smooth continuous curve. Uroflowmetry is used to identify patients with voiding dysfunction and is not useful in the diagnosis of incontinence.

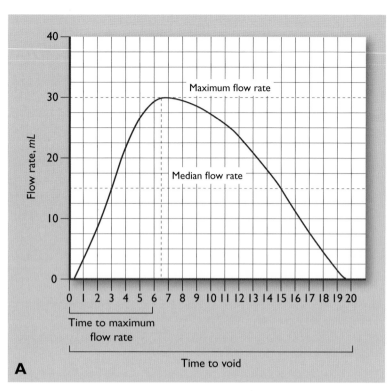

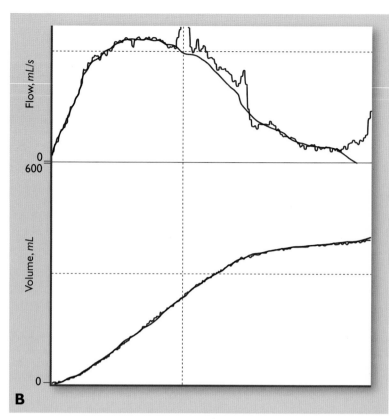

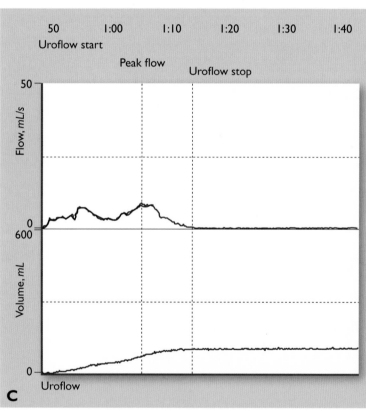

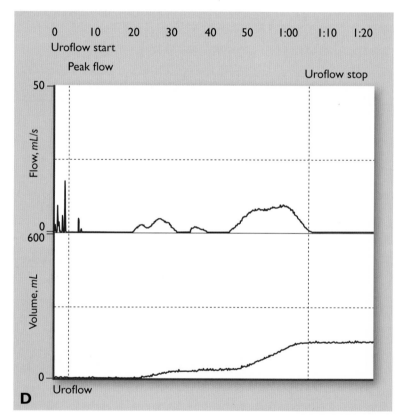

Figure 5-23. Uroflowmetry. **A** and **B**, Normal uroflow curves show continuous flow with minimal fluctuations with the maximal flow reached within one third of the total voiding time.

C, Rather than absolute values, the shape of the curve may be a better indicator of voiding dysfunction. Intermittent and interrupted flow patterns characteristically show increasing and decreasing flow rates as manifested by multiple peaks and valleys on the tracing. With the "intermittent" pattern, the downward deflection does not drop below 2 mL/s. **D**, If the deflection falls below this level, it is referred to as "interrupted." (Part A *adapted from* Karram [27].)

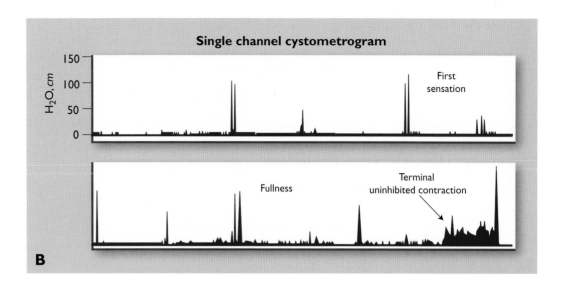

Single channel cystometrogram

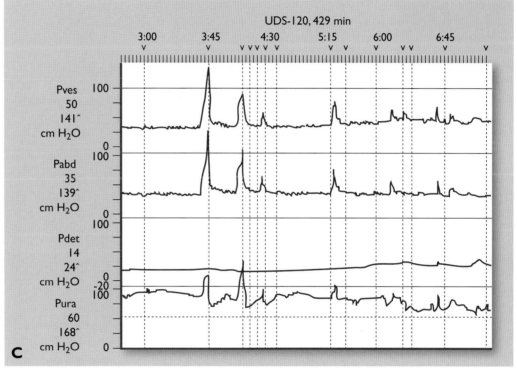

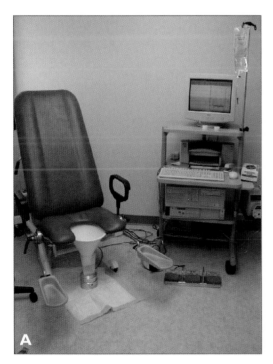

Figure 5-24. Cystometry. **A,** Urodynamic unit. Even a good history may be inadequate for the diagnosis of a particular type of incontinence. A meta-analysis study on the role of patient history in the diagnosis of urinary incontinence found that relying on history alone for the diagnosis of stress incontinence resulted in misdiagnosis in 25% of patients. The incidence of stress-induced detrusor contractions was between 9% and 52% [28]. Symptoms of urge incontinence were even worse predictors, with a diagnosis rate of 45%. Other authors have found surgical failure due to persistent detrusor instability [29]. Identifying these patients allows the physician to counsel the patient regarding her chance of cure and persistence of symptoms postoperatively.

B, This figure shows schematically the tracing from a single catheter placed in the patient's bladder. The spikes typically note a cough and the patient's first sensation and fullness are annotated. At the end of the tracing a rise in bladder pressure is noted, representing a bladder contraction.

C, This figure represents a multichannel study in which the bladder pressure (Pves), abdominal pressure (Pabd), and urethral pressure (Pura) are measured separately. The Pdet is the true pressure in the bladder wall and is calculated electronically by subtracting the abdominal pressure from the bladder pressure, allowing any increase in intra-abdominal pressure to be negated and not to be misinterpreted as a detrusor contraction.

Several investigators have compared single- (**B**) with multichannel (**C**) urodymanic studies. Although the specificity of a single-channel study has been consistently high (82%–100%), the sensitivity has been inconsistent [30]. The single-channel study is more difficult to interpret because increases in intra-abdominal pressure may be interpreted as detrusor contractions. Any movement will be shown as an increase in intra-abdominal pressure. It relies more on the operator's technical and interpretive skills.

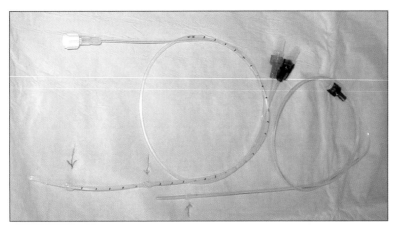

Figure 5-25. Urodynamic catheters (transducers). Various types of catheters have been used, but most recently air-charged catheters have gained favor as they are less costly at initial purchase and are disposable, cost effective, and accurate. They have a circumferential balloon that, in theory, should make them more accurate. Studies comparing them with the microtransducers have shown good con-

cordance in measurements of leak point pressure (LPP) and maximal urethral closure pressure [31].

The dual-balloon catheter is placed with the distal balloon in the bladder and the proximal one at the midurethra. The single-balloon catheter is typically placed in the vagina as this is more comfortable for the patient, but in the case of stage 3 or 4 prolapse, it may be placed rectally. The urodynamics chair is placed in an upright 45° angle and a resting 2-minute tracing is performed to detect fluctuations in resting urethral pressure, designated by some researchers as urethral instability [32]. Medium fill (80–100 mL/s) cystometry is performed. The patient is asked to report her first sensation to void, fullness, and maximum capacity. Provocative maneuvers (eg, handwashing, running water, and heel bounce) at maximum capacity may be useful in precipitating detrusor instability. Valsalva leak point pressures are performed at 150 and 200 mL by asking the patient to slowly perform the Valsalva maneuver and recording the exact point at which leakage occurs. If there is no leakage, then the patient can be asked to cough incrementally. The lowest change in vesical pressure needed to cause leakage is the LPP.

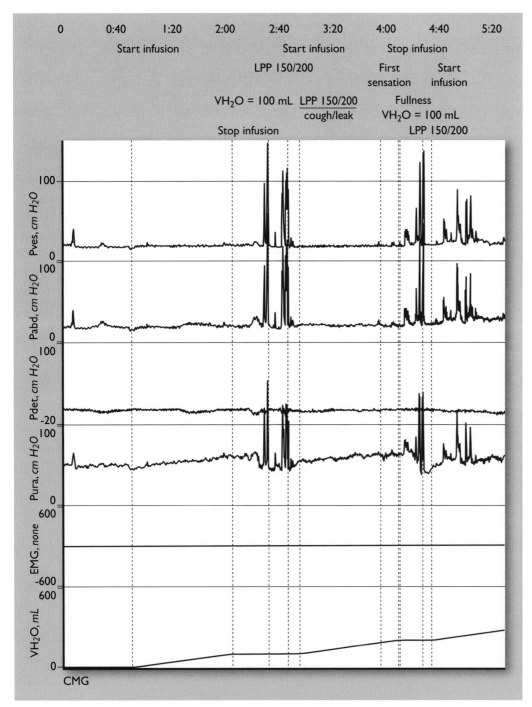

Figure 5-26. Leak point pressure (LPP). This 66-year-old woman (P2002) has a 12-month history of leakage with cough, sneezing, and walking that became more severe after an anterior repair that was performed for prolapse. She has a postvoid residual of 60 mL and a cotton swab strain angle of 50°. Cystometry shows an LPP of 119 cm (137 cm of vesical pressure at the moment of leakage; 18 cm, which is the resting vesical pressure). CMG—cystometrogram; EMG—electromyographic; Pves—bladder pressure; Pabd—abdominal pressure; Pdet—true pressure in the bladder wall; Pura—urethral pressure; VH_2O—volume of water.

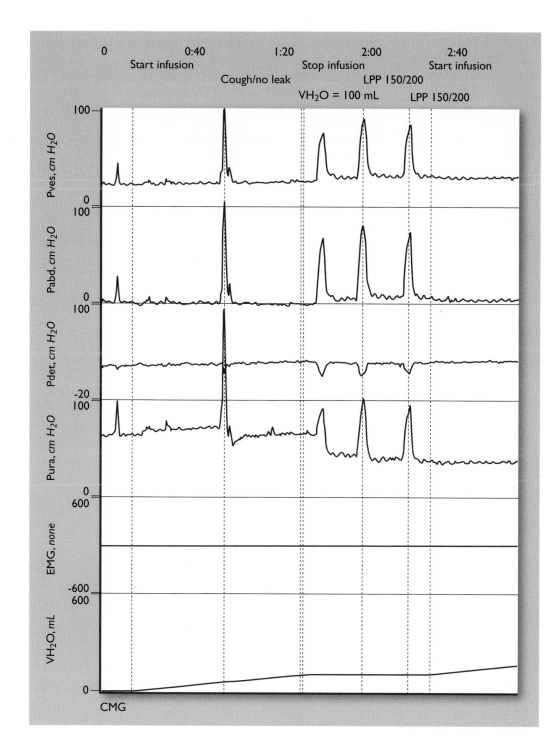

Figure 5-27. Low leak point pressure (LPP). This 78-year-old woman (P1001) has a history of leakage not only with coughing but also with walking and getting up out of a chair, even when her bladder is essentially empty (*ie*, immediately after voiding). She has a cotton swab angle of 30° and has tried three previous collagen treatments, which lasted only 3 months. She is desirous of further intervention. Her tracing shows a low leak point of 53 cm (*ie*, vesical pressure at strain of 78–25 cm resting). An LPP of less than 60 cm is considered by many urogynecologists and urologists as representing intrinsic sphincter deficiency [33]. CMG—cystometrogram; EMG—electromyogram; Pves—bladder pressure; Pabd—abdominal pressure; Pdet—true pressure in the bladder wall; Pura—urethral pressure; VH_2O—volume of water.

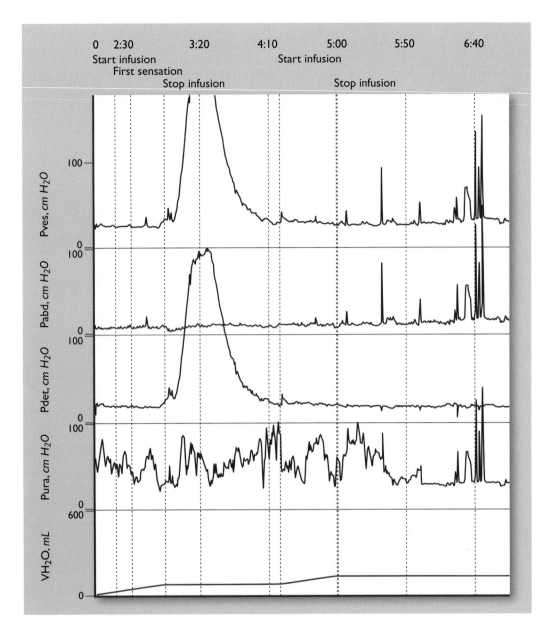

Figure 5-28. Detrusor overactivity. This 32-year-old woman (P2001) has a lifelong history of frequency. Over the past 12 months, she has had increasing incontinence in addition to voiding every 30 minutes. She has lost her job as she cannot sit at the telephone long enough to finish with a client. Clinically, a diagnosis of severe detrusor overactivity (overactive bladder) is made and confirmed by cystometry. The tracing shows that at 68 mL she had a large detrusor contraction measuring 182 cm of water. Also note the wide fluctuations in her urethral pressure. Pves—bladder pressure; Pabd—abdominal pressure; Pdet—true pressure in the bladder wall; Pura—urethral pressure; VH_2O—volume of water.

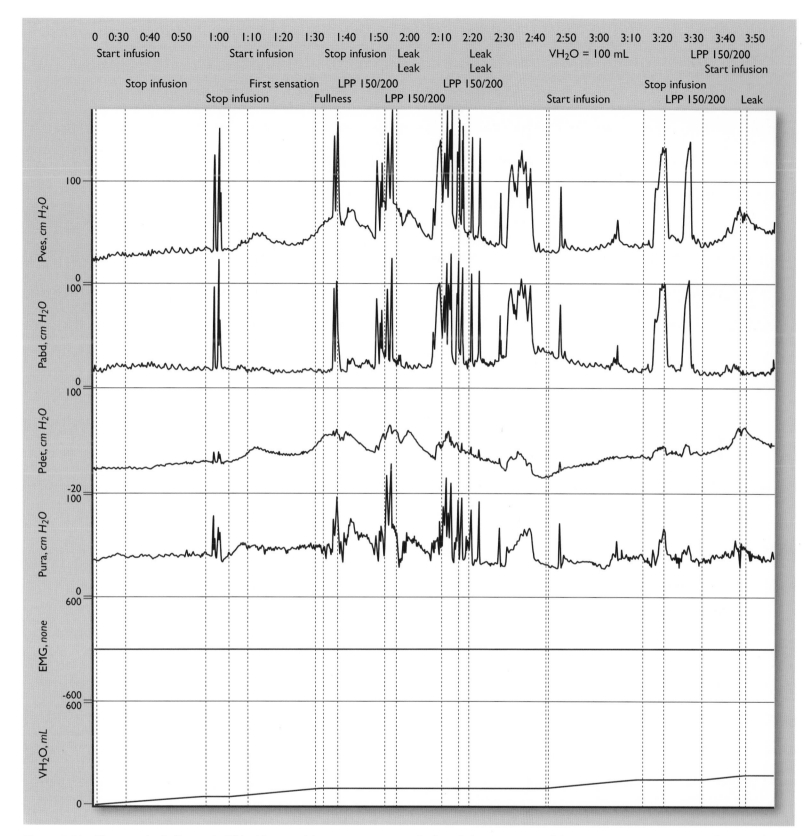

Figure 5-29. Chance of misdiagnosis. This 48-year-old woman (P4003) presented with a history of leakage with coughing. She stated that the leakage was severe as it soaked her clothing and she could not stop it once it started. Her tracing is unusual in that at 50 mL a detrusor contraction can be seen after a cough. Similarly, an attempted measurement of leak point pressure (LPP) at 150 mL shows multiple contractions after each cough. In this case, she has cough-induced detrusor overactivity, not stress incontinence. This correlates with the symptoms she describes in that she cannot stop the leakage once it starts and it is of a large volume. Typically, stress incontinence is an immediate loss of urine concomitant with the cough and stops once the Valsalva stops. EMG—electromyogram; Pves—bladder pressure; Pabd—abdominal pressure; Pdet—true pressure in the bladder wall; Pura—urethral pressure; VH_2O—volume of water.

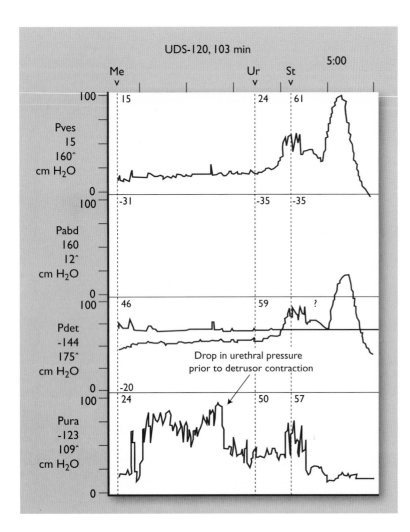

Figure 5-30. Urethral instability. This 52-year-old nulliparous patient presented with urgency and frequency. A 6-week course of anticholinergic medication improved her frequency but failed to significantly relieve the urgency. A cystometrogram showed an acute drop in her urethral pressure that just preceded an increase in detrusor pressure. These urethral pressure changes would have been missed on a single-channel study. These patients are challenging as they typically do not respond well to standard anticholinergic medication. The addition of an α-agonist may help, but unfortunately these are no longer available in cold preparations. Pves—bladder pressure; Pabd—abdominal pressure; Pdet—true pressure in the bladder wall; Pura—urethral pressure.

URETHRAL PRESSURE PROFILE

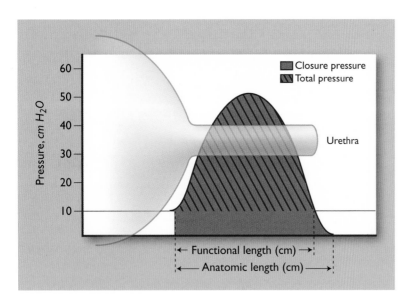

Figure 5-31. Urethral pressure. This measurement was challenging to obtain in the past, as the pressure is not uniform around its circumference and, therefore, orientation of the microtransducer was critical. With the air-filled catheters, this is no longer a concern. On completion of cystometry, the catheter is advanced so that both balloons are in the bladder. If a measurement of urethral length is desired, the catheter must be connected to a pulley arm and withdrawn at a known constant speed. Most clinicians find no clinical utility in this measurement. To save the cost of an expensive pulley arm, the catheter can be slowly withdrawn by hand and maximal urethral pressure and, more importantly, a maximal urethral closure pressure (MUCP) is measured. The MUCP is calculated by subtracting the vesical pressure from the maximal urethral pressure. (*Adapted from* Karram [34].)

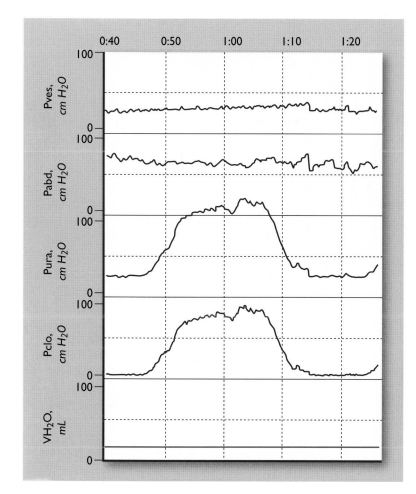

Figure 5-32. Normal-pressure urethra. This 62-year-old woman (G1001) presented with a 12-year history of stress incontinence. Cystometry showed a leap point pressure of 70 cm and a maximal urethral closure pressure (Pclo) of 75 cm (maximal urethral pressure [Pura] of 112 cm minus bladder pressure [Pves] of 37 cm). Pabd—abdominal pressure; VH$_2$0—volume of water.

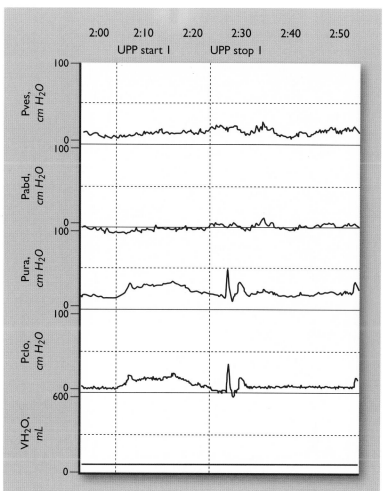

Figure 5-33. Low-pressure urethra. The definition of intrinsic sphincter deficiency remains controversial, with some physicians still favoring a definition of a low maximal urethral closure pressure (MUCP) less than 20 cm. This MUCP was chosen because it was found in a retrospective study that those with a measurement of less than 20 cm had a higher failure rate for a retropubic incontinence procedure. This 83-year-old nulliparous patient has a 12-year history of leakage with coughing and clearing her throat. Her cotton swab test showed poor mobility with an angle of 25°. Her MUCP was low, at 17 cm. Pabd—abdominal pressure; Pclo—urethral closure pressure; Pura—urethral pressure; Pves—bladder pressure; UPP—urethral pressure profile; VH$_2$0—volume of water.

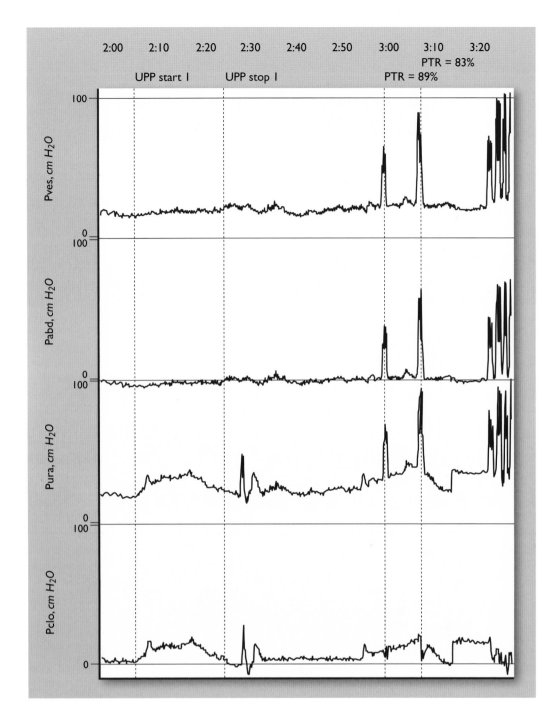

Figure 5-34. Cough profile. Genuine stress incontinence (GSI). The diagnosis of GSI can be further improved by the use of cough profiles. Here, the patient is asked to cough at the various quartiles as the transducer is withdrawn. The test provides an objective assessment of the transmission of abdominal pressure along the urethra during stress. For continence, the urethral pressure must remain higher than the bladder pressure. The profile is positive if there is equalization of pressure along the urethra with each cough. The pressure transmission ratio (PTR) is calculated by dividing the amplitude of the urethral pressure increase by the amplitude of the bladder pressure increase and multiplying by 100. The cough profile of the previous patient demonstrates that, with each cough, the PTR is less than 100% (89% in the proximal urethra and 83% in the midurethra). This patient had urodynamic stress incontinence. Pabd—abdominal pressure; Pclo—urethral closure pressure; Pura—urethral pressure; Pves—bladder pressure; UPP—urethral pressure profile.

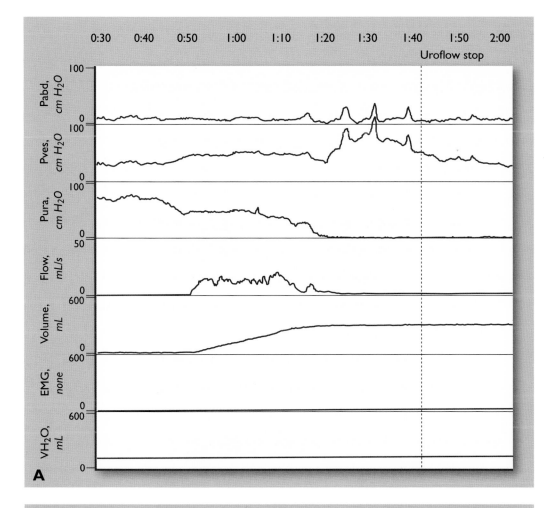

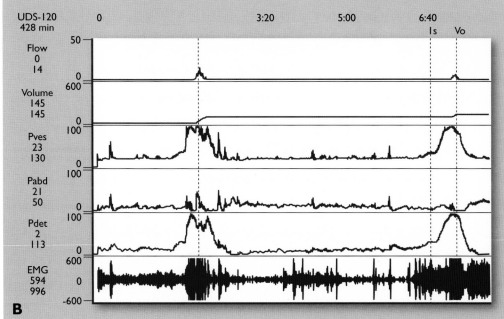

Figure 5-35. Pressure voiding study. The multichannel pressure voiding study simultaneously measures vesical, urethral, and abdominal pressure and electromyographic (EMG) and flow parameters. It objectively demonstrates the patient's voiding mechanism and is performed at maximum capacity after completion of the urethral pressure profiles. The patient is asked to void with the catheters in place.

A, Normal voiding study. This is a 45-year-old woman (P4004) with a history of frequency every 1 to 2 hours with a sense of incomplete emptying. A postvoid residual was 20 mL. Her pressure flow study shows that she empties with urethral relaxation and detrusor

contraction. Note there is an absence of abdominal straining. There is no electromyogram (EMG) attached to this patient. A significant percentage of patients (20%–30%) are unable to void with the catheter in place. It is also very difficult to know whether voiding in a strange place, in a strange chair with a "tube" in the urethra, represents normal voiding for the patient. During normal micturition, urethral relaxation is followed by a detrusor contraction.

B, Detrusor–sphincter dyssynergia. In a patient with complaints of emptying difficulty in the absence of an anatomic reason (*ie,* previous anti-incontinence surgery, stage 4 prolapse), the use of EMG may enhance the study. Surface EMG electrodes may be placed at 3 ,9, and 12 o'clock positions around the anus or a needle can be placed periurethrally in the urethral sphincter. In patients without neurologic dysfunction, the urethral sphincter and pelvic floor (perianal patches) relax just prior to detrusor contraction. It is often difficult to void in a strange place, in an unusual chair and with a catheter, so patients may tend to contract their pelvic floor during the study when in fact they are "normal voiders" at home. Therefore, it is important to take the result in context, *eg,* history suggestive of multiple sclerosis, spinal cord lesion. This study shows a 32-year-old woman (P1001) who presented after three separate episodes of acute urinary retention. At one of the episodes she was catheterized for 2000 mL. The voiding study shows that she appeared to mount a detrusor contraction of approximately 100 cm with minimal abdominal strain, but with each attempt at voiding the EMG activity increased at the same time as the detrusor contraction. The addition of EMG at this time is valuable only in the patient with unexplained voiding dysfunction in whom a neurologic cause is suspected. Other mechanisms are considered normal, but they should always include a component of urethral relaxation (*ie,* urethral relaxation alone, urethral relaxation with a detrusor contraction with or without Valsalva maneuver). Bhatia and Bergman [35] defined normal voiding parameters as adequate detrusor contraction, an increase in detrusor pressure of at least 15 cm of water, Valsalva voiding, an increase in abdominal pressure of at least 10 cm, adequate urethral relaxation, and a decrease in urethral pressure of at least 25 cm. The prime role for the test is in patients with symptoms of emptying dysfunction. Pabd—abdominal pressure; Pdet—true pressure in the bladder wall; Pura—urethral pressure; Pves—bladder pressure; VH_2O—volume of water.

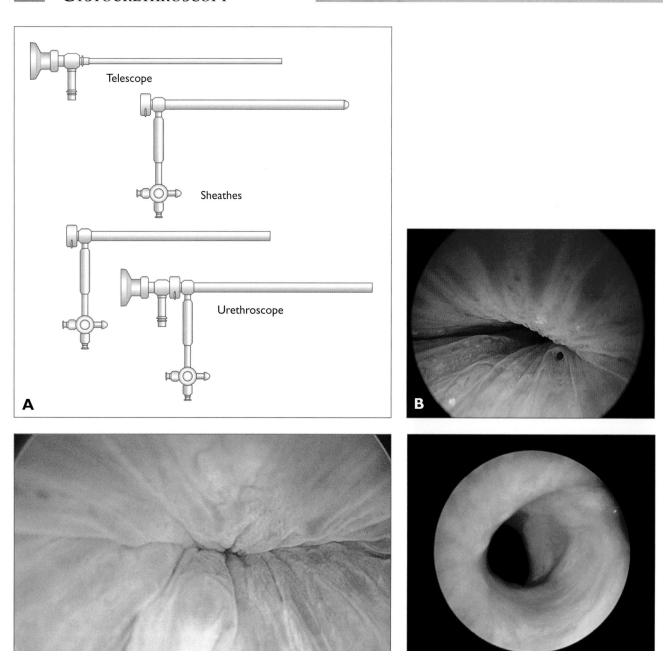

Figure 5-36. Bladder and urethra assessment. Cystourethroscopy allows anatomic assessment of the bladder and urethra. Not all incontinent patients require endoscopic assessment, but patients with failed prior surgery, history suggestive of intrinsic sphincter deficiency, irritative symptoms, or complicated urinary incontinence merit evaluation [36]. **A**, Urethroscopy is performed with a short 0° urethroscope. The sheath sizes for this telescope lens are 15 and 24 F. **B**, The urethral meatus is cleansed with antiseptic and the instru- ment is introduced with sterile water flowing. The urethral lumen is visualized to the urethrovesical junction (UVJ). **C**, The urethroscope is withdrawn approximately 0.5 to 1.0 cm distal to the UVJ and the patient is asked to strain down, cough, hold her urine, and squeeze her rectum. The UVJ should close with all maneuvers, but with a mobile bladder neck it opens with strain and cough. **D**, It may sit widely open if there is intrinsic sphincter dysfunction.

Continued on the next page

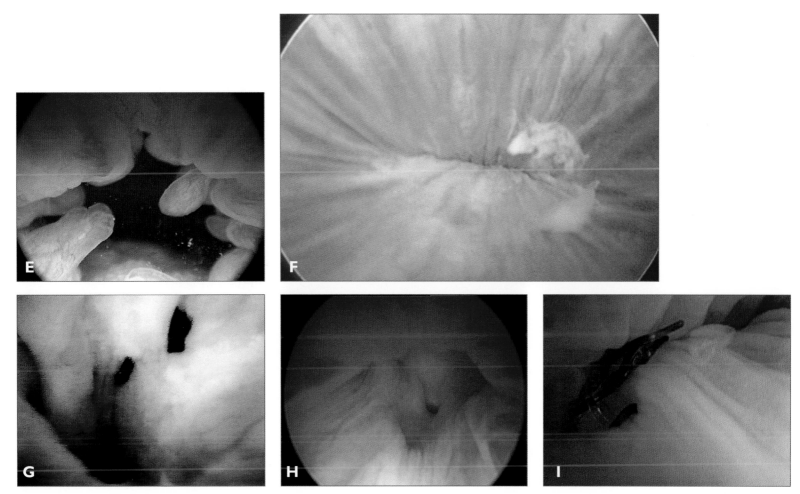

Figure 5-36. *(Continued)* **E**, Polyps are an incidental finding at the bladder neck and are not related to pathology or incontinence. **F**, With the instrument back in the bladder, the surgeon's index finger compresses the bladder neck against the urethroscope, which is then gradually withdrawn, allowing the finger to occlude the urethral lumen proximal to the lens. This allows maximum distension of the lumen while looking for debris from urethral glands or (**G**) diverticular openings. **H**, Withdrawal of the urethroscope will also reveal urethrovaginal fistula in rare cases. **I**, Conversely, postoperative voiding dysfunction after a tension-free tape procedure may reveal tape within the urethra on insertion of the urethroscope.

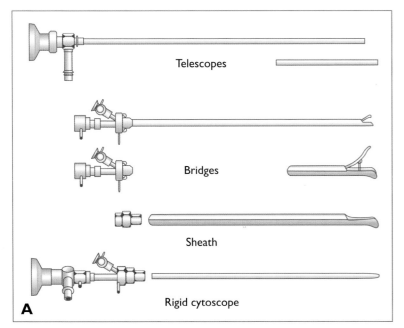

Telescopes

Bridges

Sheath

Rigid cytoscope

Figure 5-37. Cystoscopy examination. **A**, Cystoscopy is performed with a 30° or 70° telescope connected by a bridge to a sheath, usually 17 F in size, which is more readily tolerated in the outpatient setting. Lidocaine gel 2% will anesthetize the urethral mucosa somewhat and provide lubrication for movement of the sheath in the urethra. Sterile water is infused to a volume of 250 to 500 mL for adequate visualization.

Continued on the next page

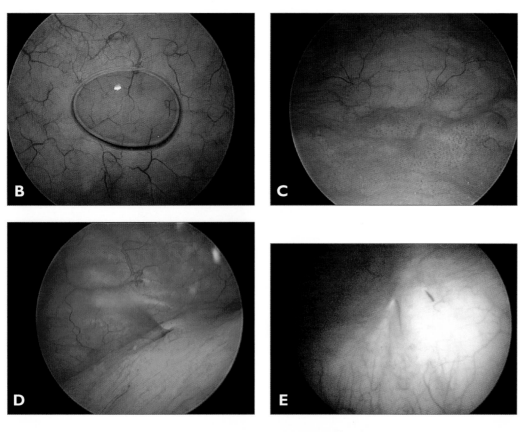

Figure 5-37. *(Continued)* **B,** The air bubble at the bladder dome allows proper orientation in order to examine the bladder completely by looking at each hour of an imaginary clock face. **C,** Looking down at the 6 o'clock position allows examination of the bladder base and trigone, as well as the ureters. **D,** The patency of the ureters is observed as urine escapes in a jet from each side. In this case, the patient had taken phenazopyridine, which stained the urine an orange color. **E,** A double ureter is an important consideration during surgical intervention and the upper pole kidney drains into the lower ureter, which can at times insert below the bladder neck and be a very rare cause of incontinence.

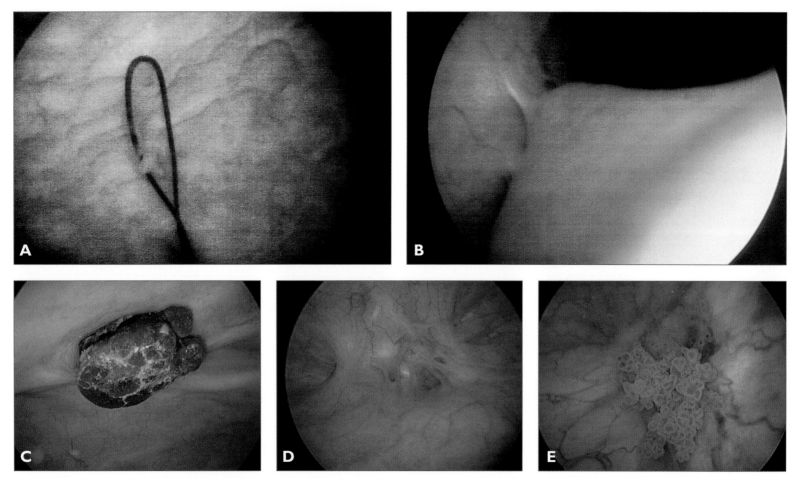

Figure 5-38. Mucosal lesions. These abnormalities can be diagnosed only by visualization, and in one study of women selected for urodynamics and cystoscopy, endoscopy was considered to be important to the final diagnosis in 19% of patients [1]. The types of mucosal abnormalities visualized include intravesical suture (**A** and **B**) and bladder stone (**C**), in this case formed on a suture placed into the bladder wall during bladder neck suspension. One very important cause of incontinence is a vesicovaginal fistula (**D**). Most bladder tumors (**E**) are easy to spot during cystoscopy, although the discovery is usually totally unexpected, as these incontinent patients usually have no symptoms related to the tumor.

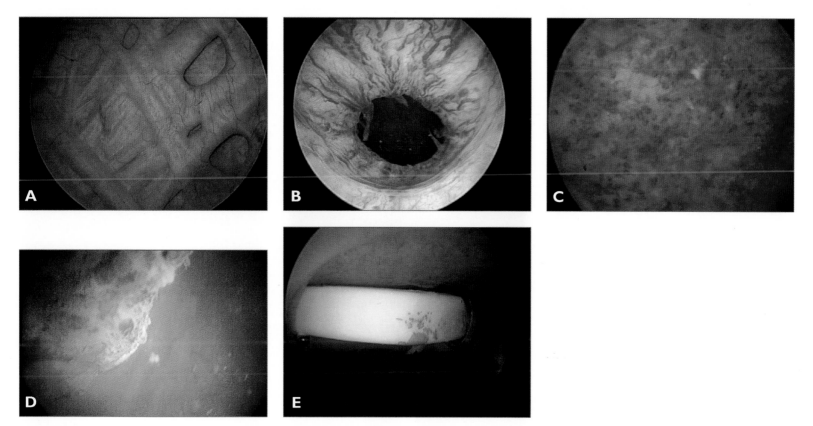

Figure 5-39. Detrusor overactivity and irritative voiding symptoms. There are few visible anatomic changes in a patient with an overactive bladder. **A**, Trabeculations in the lining of the bladder represent the bladder musculature on tension. They may be present in patients with detrusor overactivity but are not diagnostic. **B**, The urethra is relaxed and opened widely in this patient having an unexpected bladder contraction. **C**, Acute bladder inflammation from infection or chemical irritant can cause marked irritability of the bladder lining and lead to symptoms of detrusor overactivity. **D**, This patient presented with symptoms of urgency, frequency, and urge incontinence but on cystoscopy was found to have an aggressive grade III, stage III tumor. **E**, This large foreign body, originally placed as a type of sling under the bladder neck for stress urinary incontinence, eroded into the bladder and caused numerous irritative symptoms until it was surgically removed.

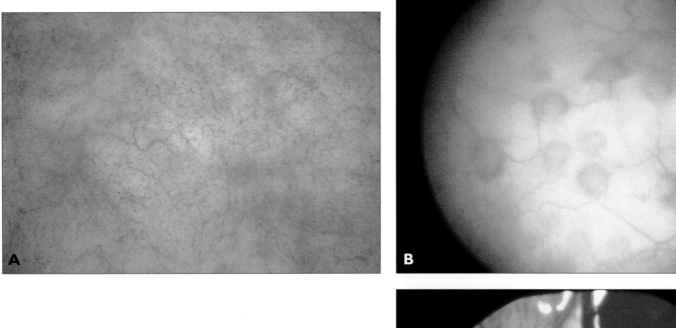

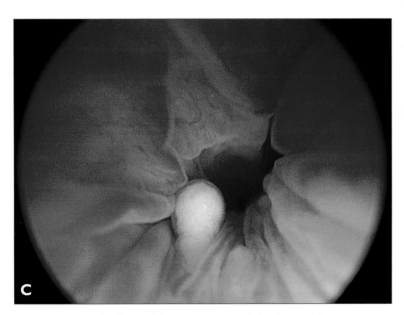

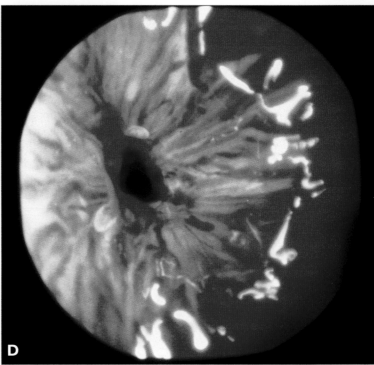

Figure 5-40. Irritative voiding symptoms. Irritative voiding symptoms classically present as frequency, urgency, urge incontinence, and nocturia. Both acute (**A**) and chronic (**B**) cystitis are included in the differential diagnosis of irritative voiding. Other conditions that have similar symptoms include urethritis (**C**) and interstitial cystitis (**D**).

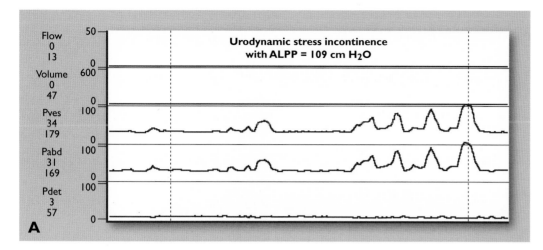

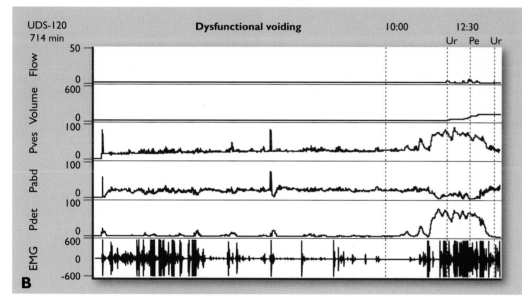

Figure 5-41. A, Videourodynamics combines fluoroscopy with urodynamics. It allows assessment of mobility, which may aid clinicians in assessing mobility and in categorizing incontinence as types 1, 2, or 3 depending on the presence or absence of bladder and urethral descent at rest and with Valsalva. The bladder is infused at a rate of 50 to 100 mL/min with contrast material. Some clinicians advocate not using a rectal catheter as it is not helpful and adds to patient discomfort. The patient is asked to perform a Valsalva as with standard cystometry and a leak point pressure can be measured. Studies have shown no significant difference in diagnosis between multichannel cystometry and videourodynamics [37].

B, Dysfunctional voiding. The cystometry demonstrates that the patient voids by detrusor contraction but does not relax her urethral sphincter and the pelvic floor, as seen with the increased electromyogram (EMG) activity. The addition of video demonstrates this condition well but does not provide the clinician with any additional information, just confirmation that the bladder neck opens but urethra fails to relax. ALPP—abdominal leak point pressure; Pabd—abdominal pressure; Pdet—true pressure in the bladder wall; Pves—vesical pressure; UDS—urodynamic study; VH_2O—volume of water.

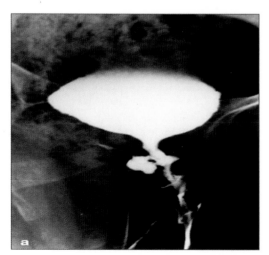

Figure 5-42. Voiding cystogram. This study may be useful for the diagnosis of urethral diverticulum and is more comfortable for the patient than a double-balloon catheter study (positive-pressure urethrography); however, it has a lower sensitivity for detection and may miss 7% to 70% of diagnoses [38,39]. This image shows a complex or multiple diverticulum.

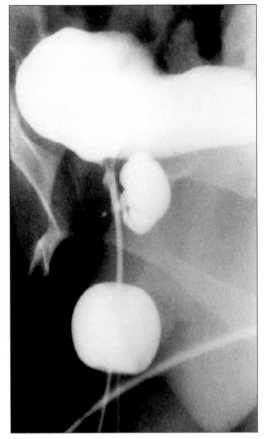

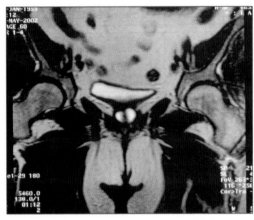

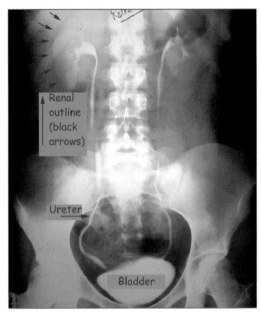

Figure 5-43. Double-balloon catheter study. This study involves placing a Foley catheter with two balloons into the bladder. One balloon is inflated inside the bladder and the larger one is inflated and compressed against the external urethral meatus to prevent spillage of dye. Dye is injected into the Foley lumen and exits a hole situated within the urethra. With steady pressure, the dye will enter the urethral lumen and hopefully outline any diverticula. The test has good sensitivity and specificity [40]. The image displays contrast in the bladder, the large external balloon, and a large proximal diverticulum.

Figure 5-44. MRI. This tool is useful for the diagnosis of urethral diverticulum. The fluid-filled bladder and diverticulum provide a high-density signal compared with the soft tissues. MRI is more costly and, therefore, should be considered when the diagnosis is highly suspected but more routine examinations (*ie*, clinical palpation, urethroscopy) are negative. The image shows signals from the bladder and a complex diverticulum [40].

Figure 5-45. Intravenous pyelogram (IVP). An IVP is not routinely performed in the assessment of incontinence; it should be performed only to assess the upper tracts in patients with hematuria, persistent bacteriuria, recurrent urinary tract infections, impaired compliance, and markedly reduced bladder capacity. This IVP demonstrates normal anatomy.

REFERENCES

1. Hannestad YS, Rotveit G, Sandvik H, *et al.*: A community-based epidemiologic survey of female urinary incontinence: the Norwegian EPINCOT study. *J Clin Epidemiol* 2000, 53:1150–1160.

2. Hu TW, Wagner TH, Bentkover JD, *et al.*: Costs of urinary incontinence and overactive bladder in the United States: a comparative study. *Urology* 2004, 63:461–465.

3. Staskin D, Hilton P, Emmanuel A, *et al.*: Incontinence. In *Proceedings of the 3rd International Consultation on Incontinence*. Edited by Abrams P, Cardozo L, Khoury S, Wein A. June 26–29, 2004. Auckland, New Zealand: Health Publications; 2005.

4. Abrams A, Anderson KE, Brubaker L, *et al.*: Evaluation and treatment of urinary incontinence, pelvic organ prolapse, and faecal incontinence. *Proceedings of the 3rd International Consultation on Incontinence*. June 26–29, 2004. Auckland, New Zealand: Health Publications, 2005.

5. Abrams P, Cardozo L, Fall M, *et al.*: The standardisation of terminology of lower urinary tract function: report from the standardisation sub-committee of the International Continence Society. *Neurourol Urodyn* 2002, 21:167–178.

6. Cundiff GW, Harris RL, Coates KW, Bump RC: Clinical predictors of urinary incontinence in women. *Am J Obstet Gynecol* 1997,177:262–266; discussion 266–267.

7. Graham CW, Dmochowski RR: Questionnaires for women with urinary symptoms. *Neurourol Urodyn* 2002, 21:473–481.

8. Shumaker SA, Wyman JF, Uebersax JS, *et al.*, Continence Program in Women (CPW) Research Group: Health-related quality of life measures for women with urinary incontinence: the Incontinence Impact Questionnaire and the Urogenital Distress Inventory. *Qual Life Res* 1994, 3:291–306.

9. Uebersax JS, Wyman JF, Shumaker SA, *et al.*, Continence Program for Women Research Group: Short forms to assess life quality and symptom distress for urinary incontinence in women: the Incontinence Impact Questionnaire and the Urogenital Distress Inventory. *Neurourol Urodyn* 1995, 14:131–139.

10. Brown JS, McNaughton KS, Wyman JF, *et al.*: Measurement characteristics of a voiding diary for use by men and women with overactive bladder. *Urology* 2003, 61:802–809.

11. Lind LL, Rosenzweig BA, Bhatia NN: Urologically oriented neurological examination. In *Urogynecology and Urodynamics*. Edited by Ostergard DR, Bent AE. Baltimore: Williams & Wilkins; 1996:102.

12. Blaivas JG, Zayed AA, Labib KB: The bulbocavernosus reflex in urology: a prospective study of 299 patients. *J Urol* 1981, 126:197–199.

13. McLennan MT, Bent AE: Supine empty stress test as a predictor of low Valsalva leak point pressure. *Neurourol Urodyn* 1998, 17:121–127

14. Barber MD, Cundiff GW, Weidner AC, *et al.*: Accuracy of clinical assessment of paravaginal defects in women with anterior vaginal wall prolapse. *Am J Obstet Gynecol* 1999, 18:87–90.

15. Bump RC, Mattiasson A, Bo K, *et al.*: The standardization of terminology of female pelvic organ prolapse and pelvic floor dysfunction. *Am J Obstet Gynecol* 1996, 175:10–17.

16. Hall AF, Theofrastous JP, Cundiff GW, *et al.*: Interobserver and intraobserver reliability of the proposed International Continence Society, Society of Gynecologic Surgeons, and American Urogynecologic Society pelvic organ prolapse classification system. *Am J Obstet Gynecol* 1996, 175:1467–70.

17. Fowler JE Jr: Nosocomial catheter-associated urinary tract infection. *Infect Surg* 1993, 2:43–53.

18. Bent AE, Nahhas DE, McLennan MT: Portable ultrasound determination of urinary residual volume. *Int Urogynecol J Pelvic Floor Dysfunct* 1997, 8:200–202.

19. Messing EM: Urothelial tumors of the bladder. In *Campbell-Walsh Urology*, edn 9. Edited by Wein AJ, Kavoussi LR, Novick AC, *et al.* Philadelphia: Saunders Elsevier; 2007:2407–2447.

20. Eberle CM, Winsemius D, Garibaldi RA: Risk factors and consequences of bacteriuria in non-catheterized nursing home residents. *J Gerontol* 1993, 48:266–271.

21. Summitt RL, Bent AE, Ostergard DR, Harris TA: Stress incontinence and low urethral closure pressure: correlation of preoperative urethral hypermobility with successful suburethral sling procedures. *J Reprod Med* 1990, 35:877–880.

22. Bergman A, Koonings PP, Ballard CA: Negative Q-tip test as a risk factor for failed incontinence surgery in women. *J Reprod Med* 1989, 34:193–197.

23. Agosta AM: Clinical evaluation. In *Female Pelvic Floor Disorders: Investigation and Management*. Edited by Benson JT. New York: Norton; 1992:64.

24. Pierson CA: Pad testing, nursing interventions and urine loss appliances. In *Urogynecology and Urodynamics*, edn 4. Edited by Ostergard DR, Bent AE. Baltimore: Williams & Wilkins; 1996:252.

25. Ouslander J, Leach G, Abelson S, *et al.*: Simple versus multichannel cystometry in the evaluation of bladder function in an incontinent geriatric population. *J Urol* 1988, 140:1482–1486.

26. Bent AE, McLennan MT: Geriatric urogynecology. In *Urogynecology and Urodynamics*, edn 4. Edited by Ostergard DR, Bent AE. Baltimore: Williams & Wilkins; 1996.

27. Karram MM: Evaluation of incontinence. In *Clinical Urogynecology*. Edited by Walters MD, Karram MM. St. Louis: Mosby; 1993.

28. Jensen JK, Neilsen FR Jr, Ostergard DR: The role of patient history in the diagnosis of urinary incontinence. *Obstet Gynecol* 1994, 83:904–910.

29. Sand PK, Bowen LW, Ostergard DR, *et al.*: The effect of retropubic urethropexy on detrusor stability. *Obstet Gynecol* 1988, 7:818–822.

30. Sutherst JR, Brown MC: Comparison of single and multichannel cystometry in diagnosing bladder instability. *Br Med J (Clin Res Ed)*1984, 288:1720–1722.

31. Pollak JT, Neimark M, Connor JT, Davila GW: Air-charged and microtransducer urodynamic catheters in the evaluation of urethral function. *Int Urogynecol J Pelvic Floor Dysfunct* 2004, 15:124–128.

32. McLennan MT, Melick CF, Bent AE: Urethral instability: clinical and urodynamic characteristics. *Neurourol Urodyn* 2001, 20:653–660.

33. McGuire EJ, Fitzpatrick CC, Wan J, *et al.*: Clinical assessment of urethral sphincter function. *J Urol* 1993, 150:1452–1454.

34. Karram MM: Manometric investigation: urodynamics. In *Female Pelvic Floor Disorders: Investigation and Management*. Edited by Benson JT. New York: Norton; 1992:110.

35. Bhatia NN, Bergman A: Urodynamic predictability of voiding following incontinence surgery. *Obstet Gynecol* 1984, 63:85–91.

36. Cundiff GW, Bent AE: The contribution of urethrocystoscopy to evaluation of lower urinary tract dysfunction in women. *Int Urogynecol J Pelvic Floor Dysfunct* 1996, 7:307–311.

37. Stanton S, Krieger M, Ziv E: Videocystourethrography: its role in assessment of incontinence in the female. *Neurourol Urodyn* 1988, 7:712–713.

38. Wang AC, Wang CR: Radiologic diagnosis and surgical treatment of urethral diverticulum in women: a reappraisal of voiding cystourethrography and positive pressure urethrography. *J Reprod Med* 2000, 45:377–382.

39. Jocoby K, Rowbotham RK: Double balloon positive pressure urethrography is a more sensitive test than voiding cystourethrography for diagnosing urethral diverticulum in women. *J Urol* 1999, 162:2066–2069.

40. Fortunato P, Schettini M, Gallucci M: Diagnosis and therapy of the female urethral diverticula. *Int Urogynecol J Pelvic Floor Dysfunct* 2001, 12:51–57.

6

Management of Urinary Incontinence and Retention

*Karen L. Noblett,
Danielle Markle, and
Laura C. Skoczylas*

The bladder has two primary functions: to store urine and to empty at regular intervals. Although simple in concept, these functions involve complex neurologic reflex pathways that allow for coordination of the bladder, urethra, and pelvic floor to achieve effective storage and elimination. Voiding dysfunction affects millions of adults in the United States and can manifest as either an inability to retain urine or an inability to empty the bladder.

Urinary incontinence affects up to 33% of adult women in the United States, with the most common type being stress incontinence. Stress incontinence is generally due to a loss of anatomic support underneath the urethra, a poorly functioning urethral sphincteric mechanism, or a combination of both. The second most common type of incontinence is urge loss. Urge incontinence falls under a broader category of disorders referred to as overactive bladder. The term *overactive bladder* was coined by the pharmaceutical industry as part of an advertising campaign. The term was so favorably accepted by the medical community it was adopted by the International Continence Society (ICS) as part of its official terminology. Two large epidemiologic studies, one in Europe and the second in North America, have estimated that approximately 16% of the adult population has overactive bladder. In the United States this translates into more than 30 million adults, with nearly one third of those actively seeking treatment.

Both stress and urge incontinence increase with age, with some women having both types, a condition termed *mixed incontinence*. Although not life threatening, these conditions have a dramatic impact on all domains of quality of life [1], as well as medical conditions such as infections and depression, and are associated with an increased risk of falls and fractures. We have an aging population, and it is estimated that by 2030 more than 43 million women will be older than 65 years, with another 20 million older than 45 years. This translates into a large number of women at risk of developing these disorders who will actively be seeking treatment to alleviate their symptoms and improve their quality of life [1]. Fortunately, over the past decade awareness of these conditions has increased, and as such, more treatment options are available for both types of incontinence. Having options allows us to work closely with our patients in developing treatment plans that best fit individual patients' lifestyles and meet their goals.

Difficulty in bladder emptying and urinary retention may be due to a myriad of causes, with obstructive causes being much less common in women. The prevalence of retention is not well known due to the lack of strict definitions and to the vague nature of presenting symptoms. Treatment should be tailored to the underlying cause when possible. However, in many cases the cause may be irreversible and treatment options limited. Early recognition and prompt treatment are important in order to avoid associated complications and long-term sequelae.

International Continence Society Classification of Urinary Incontinence

Stress incontinence

Symptom: complaint of involuntary leakage on effort or exertion, or on sneezing or coughing

Sign: observation of involuntary loss of urine through the urethra synchronous with exertion/effort, or sneezing or coughing

Urodynamic stress incontinence: involuntary leakage of urine during increased intra-abdominal pressure, in the absence of a detrusor contraction

Urge incontinence

Overactive bladder

Urgency, with or without urge incontinence, usually with frequency and nocturia, in the absence of pathologic or metabolic factors that would explain these symptoms

Urgency

A sudden, compelling desire to pass urine that is difficult to defer

Frequency

Complaint by the patient that she voids too often by day (generally considered normal to void ≤ 8 times per day)

Nocturia

Complaint that individual has to wake up ≥ I time per night to void

Urge incontinence

The complaint of involuntary leakage accompanied by or immediately preceded by urgency

Detrusor overactivity incontinence

Incontinence due to an involuntary detrusor contraction

Mixed incontinence

Complaint of involuntary leakage associated with urgency and also with exertion, effort, sneezing, or coughing

Extraurethral incontinence

Observation of urine leakage through channels other than the urethra (fistula, ectopic ureter)

Figure 6-1. International Continence Society classification of urinary incontinence 2002 [2].

Treatment Options for Incontinence

Stress incontinence

Behavioral

Support devices

Pharmacologic

Ambulatory procedures

Surgical procedures

Urge incontinence

Behavioral

Pharmacologic

Ambulatory procedures

Surgical procedures

Figure 6-2. Treatment options for incontinence.

Behavioral Management of Stress Incontinence

Pelvic floor exercises

Biofeedback

Vaginal cones

Functional electrical stimulation

Figure 6-3. Behavioral management.

Factors to Consider When Offering Pelvic Muscle Floor Exercises as Treatment
Goal: strengthen muscle tone
Pubococcygeus
Urethral striated sphincter
Requires patient education, motivation, and compliance
Intensity is more important than frequency
Contracting and isolating the proper muscles is essential for success
Maintenance principle (exercising for continence is a lifelong endeavor)
Positive predictors of success
Positive motivation
Recent onset of symptoms
Premenopausal presentation
Ability to contract the pelvic floor
Adverse predictors of success
Lack of motivation
Obesity, chronic cough
Previous pelvic surgery
Long duration of symptoms
Severity of leakage

Figure 6-4. Factors to consider when offering pelvic muscle floor exercises as a treatment modality [3]. Arnold Kegel (1894–1981) introduced the idea of pelvic floor exercises in the 1940s, and since that time these exercises have become a mainstay of therapy for women with urinary incontinence and Kegel's name has become synonymous with the exercises.

Outcomes of Pelvic Floor Muscle Exercises
Efficacy for stress incontinence
Kegel [4] reported 84% success rate
Hospital/physiotherapy–based PFME: 51% (25%–75%)
Home-based PFME: 30% (11%–54%)
41% elected no surgery after PFME [5]
Both show improvement compared with controls
Compliance and motivation seem to be the most important variables in success
Problems with conventional PFME
Exercises can be difficult to teach
Patient has no confirmation whether or not she is doing the exercise correctly
Patient has no way to assess improvement in strength unless or until it impacts her urinary incontinence
With verbal instruction only, 51% perform PFME incorrectly [6]
> 30% of women with stress urinary incontinence after verbal instruction cannot perform a PFME [7–9]
59% of incorrect users learned after first palpation instruction [10]

Figure 6-5. Outcomes with pelvic floor muscle exercises (PFME).

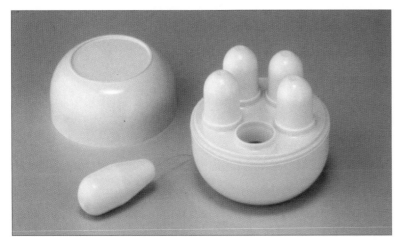

Figure 6-6. Vaginal cones. Weighted vaginal cones can be used to augment strength training in a pelvic floor muscle training program. They are graduated cones with increasing weight from 20 to 100 g that are inserted vaginally and their location is maintained through active contraction of the pelvic floor musculature. A Cochrane review meta-analysis was limited but showed no benefit of vaginal cones over pelvic floor training alone [11]. They may be useful in a select subgroup of patients whose progress has reached a plateau with pelvic floor therapy alone.

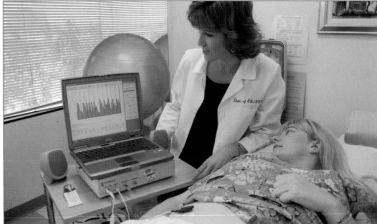

Figure 6-7. Biofeedback using surface electromyography and visual feedback. This is a form of reeducation using visual, auditory, and/or tactile stimuli. This can be in the form of cystometry, electromyography, or perineometry. It generally requires an intelligent and motivated patient. It has been shown to be beneficial for patients with difficulty in performing effective pelvic floor exercises but there has not been statistically significant improvement when used in trials along with pelvic floor muscle training alone.

A randomized trial of 40 patients showed a 55% improvement in stress incontinence with pelvic floor physical therapy with or without biofeedback. This improvement was achieved faster in the biofeedback group [12]. Both groups showed similar improvement of 50% to 69% in a randomized trial of 103 patients with pure stress or mixed incontinence [13].

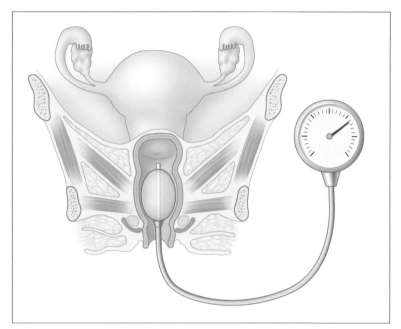

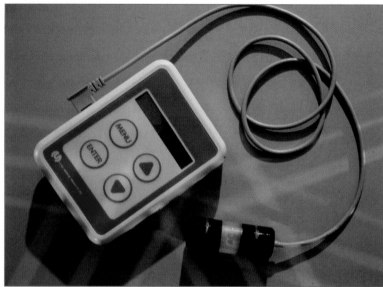

Figure 6-8. Biofeedback using a simple perineometer. Perineometers are the simplest form of biofeedback. Using an intravaginal or intrarectal pressure balloon connected to an external manometer, the pressure in the vagina or rectum can be visualized. This gives the patient confirmation that she is contracting the correct muscles and allows her to follow her progress with the therapy. It is important to instruct the patient on proper use as increases in intra-abdominal pressure may confound the picture.

Figure 6-9. Functional electrical stimulation is used for both stress and urge incontinence. For stress incontinence, this is a "passive" form of pelvic muscle exercise. Electrostimulation delivers a current to the pudendal nerve that causes a pelvic floor contraction. Relapse is common if treatment is stopped.

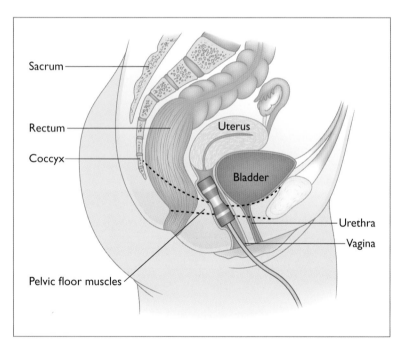

Figure 6-10. Efficacy of functional electrical stimulation. Two hundred women with stress incontinence were assigned to self-help pelvic floor therapy, intensive pelvic floor therapy, or intensive pelvic floor therapy plus electrical stimulation. There was a statistically significant improvement in all groups of 53% to 72%. Intensive pelvic floor therapy showed a benefit over self-help therapy. Electrical stimulation did not add efficacy to intensive pelvic floor training [14].

Fifty-two patients assigned to electrical stimulation versus sham treatment showed statistically significant improvement of at least 50% in 48% to 62% of the active group versus 13% to 19% of the sham group on pad test and voiding diaries [15].

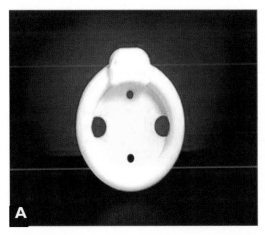
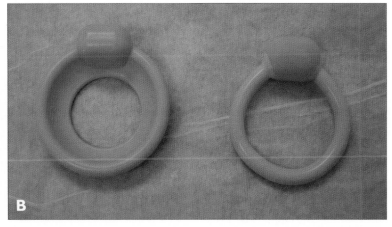

Figure 6-11. **A**, Incontinence pessary ring. **B**, Incontinence pessary dish.

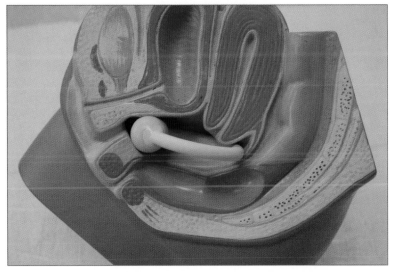

Figure 6-12. Placement of the pessary behind the symphysis provides a backstop of support that theoretically reduces urethral junction hypermobility. Several types are available. The figure illustrates the incontinence dish and ring. Other devices include the Hodge and Regula pessaries with knob and the Gelhorn pessary. In 77 patients who used a continence pessary for 12 weeks, 29% reported complete continence and 51% reported improvement greater than 50%. Minor adverse effects occurred in 26% [16].

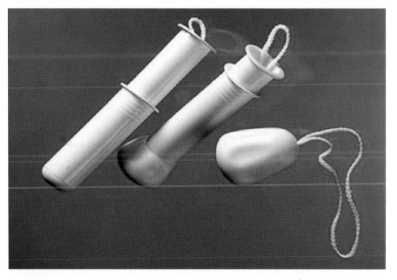

Figure 6-13. Continence tampons. The continence tampons acts to prevent leakage by providing support to the bladder neck. A randomized crossover study with 62 women comparing a Conveen continence guard (no longer marketed) versus a Contrelle continence tampon (Coloplast, Minneapolis, MN) showed a significantly reduced amount of leakage with both devices. The tampon showed significantly greater improvement over the guard. Both were well tolerated, with 63% preferring the tampon versus 26% preferring the guard [17].

A study of 18 women exercising with either a tampon or Hodge pessary showed a significant improvement in urine loss with either device [18]. (*Courtesy of* Coloplast.)

Management of Urinary Incontinence and Retention **115**

Pharmacologic Management of Stress Incontinence

Therapeutic Agent	Pharmacologic Category/Mechanism of Action	Dosing	Comments
PPA	α-Adrenergic agonist acts at α-adrenergic receptors at the bladder neck to cause smooth muscle contraction, increasing MUCP [19]	Most studies use 50 mg PO BID	Often limited by side effects (reported in as many as 33%), including blood pressure elevation, insomnia, headache, tremor, palpitations, cardiac arrhythmia. Use with caution in patients with hypertension, cardiovascular disease, or hyperthyroidism
Imipramine	Has both anticholinergic and α-adrenergic agonist actions. α-Adrenergic activity occurs through blockade of norepinephrine reuptake, increasing MUCP [19]	Typically 25 mg PO TID or QID. Can increase dosage up to 150 mg	Side effects consist of anticholinergic effects. Dose can be started at 25 mg QD and then increased to minimize side effects, especially in the elderly
Duloxetine	Serotonin and norepinephrine reuptake inhibitor increases bladder capacity and striated muscle urethral sphincter activity through central neurologic action [20]	Doses from 20 mg PO QD to 20–40 mg PO BID	Not FDA approved for the treatment of stress incontinence. Up to 23% experience significant nausea. Other significant side effects include fatigue, dry mouth, insomnia, and constipation
Estrogen	Increases UCP, increases urethral blood flow, increases α-adrenergic receptor sensitivity, improves cellular maturation of the urethra and vagina [21–23]	Can be given by oral, transdermal, or vaginal route. Hormone regimen can include conjugated equine estrogens, estriol, estrone, estradiol	Systemic estrogen needs to be given with a progestin to prevent endometrial hyperplasia/carcinoma

Figure 6-14. Pharmacologic therapies for stress incontinence are limited and are not as commonly used as for urge incontinence. Use of estrogen replacement therapy has become controversial. BID—twice daily; FDA—Food and Drug Administration; MUCP—maximal urethral closure pressure; PO—by mouth; QD—daily; QID—four times daily; PPA—phenylpropanolamine; TID—three times daily; UCP—urethral closure pressure.

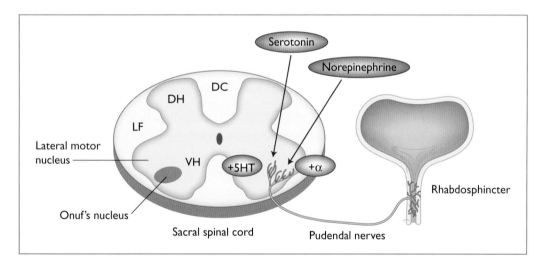

Figure 6-15. Mechanism of action of duloxetine [24]. Duloxetine increases the motor efferent output from Onuf's nucleus (anterior horn cells of S2–4) and thus increases the motor activity at the urethral rhabdosphincter. DC—dorsal column; DH—dorsal horn; 5HT—5-hydroxytryptamine; LF—lateral fasciculus; VH—ventral horn. (*Adapted from* Thor and Katofiasc [24].)

Nurses Health Study

39,436 women were asked two questions in 1996 and 2000:

How often have you leaked urine in the past 12 months?

When you lose your urine, how much usually leaks?

RR of incontinence increased in all current hormone users: 1.45–1.60

Figure 6-16. Use of estrogen is controversial. Table shows outcomes of estrogen trials in the Nurses Health Study [25]. RR—relative risk.

Heart and Estrogen/Progesterone Replacement Study (HERS)

Subanalysis of incidence of incontinence

Based on 2 unvalidated questions

Average age of inclusion was 66.4 years

Compliance rates were 68% in the HRT group, 80% in the placebo group

Outcomes

64% on HRT reported incontinence

49% on placebo reported incontinence (*P* = 0.001)

No effect was seen on women < 60 y

Figure 6-17. Heart and Estrogen/Progesterone Replacement Study (HERS) [26]. HRT—hormone replacement therapy.

Summary of the Women's Health Initiative Study Findings Regarding Urinary Incontinence

	CE and MPA vs Placebo	CE vs Placebo
Amount UI	RR 1.20 (1.06-1.36)	RR 1.59 (1.39–1.82)
Frequency UI	RR 1.38 (1.28–1.49)	RR 1.47 (1.35–1.61)
Bother UI	RR 1.22 (1.13–1.32)	RR 1.50 (1.37–1.65)
Limitations	RR 1.18 (1.06–1.32)	RR 1.29 (1.15–1.45)

Figure 6-18. Summary of the Women's Health Initiative (WHI) study findings regarding urinary incontinence (UI) [27]. The study was designed to evaluate coronary and fracture end points, not incontinence. Groups were not similar in baseline characteristics. Incontinence was diagnosed based on symptoms, and four validated questions were asked, about amount, frequency, limitation, and bother. Medication adherence was 74% in the treatment groups and 81% in the placebo groups at year 1. The overall incidence of incontinence was increased in CE + MPA (conjugated estrogens plus medroxyprogesterone) and in CE alone (relative risk [RR] = 1.39, 1.53), as was the incidence of stress incontinence (RR = 1.87, 2.15) and the incidence of mixed incontinence (RR = 1.49, 1.79). Women younger than 55 years showed no increased incidence of stress incontinence; women younger than 70 years showed no increased incidence of mixed incontinence. The study was not powered to answer study questions in groups less than 60 years of age. Conclusions of the WHI included the following: The relative risk of incontinence is increased in this population, though the original study was not designed to answer incontinence questions. There was no ability to control for vaginal E2 use, which the placebo group was more likely to require. No clear theory was presented on the mechanism; timing of hormone replacement therapy may be critical.

Randomized and Nonrandomized Trials with Oral Estrogen

Nonrandomized clinical trials

	Estrogen Type	Duration	Diagnosis	Outcome Measure	Findings
Góes et al. [28] 2003	Oral CE, 0.625 mg	3 mo	USI	Symptoms UDS	57.9% satisfied 21% dry No Δ UDS
Rud [29] 1980	Oral E2, E3, or intramuscular	3 wk	USI	UDS	E2/E3 increase in MUP and FUL
Sartori et al. [30] 1995	Oral CE, MPA	3 mo	USI	Symptoms UDS	90% improved Increased MUCP
Suzuki et al. [31] 1997	Oral CE, MPA	4 mo	USI	Symptoms UDS	25% improved symptoms 21% improved UDS
Mäkinen et al. [32] 1995	E2 patch, oral MPA	9 mo	USI	Symptoms UDS	76% improvement Increase in FUL

Randomized controlled trials

	Estrogen Type	Duration	Diagnosis	Outcome Measure	Findings
Wilson et al. [33] 1987, n = 36	Oral E1 vs placebo	3 mo	USI	Diary UDS	No significant Δ
Jackson et al. [34] 1999, n = 67	Oral E2 vs placebo	6 mo	USI	Diary UDS SF-36	No significant Δ
Fantl et al. [35] 1996, n = 83	Cyclic CE, MPA	3 mo	MUI	Diary SF-36	No significant Δ
Grady et al. [36] 2001*	Cyclic CE, MPA	4 y	MUI	HERS questions	↑ Incontinence and severity; $P = 0.001$
Hendrix et al. [27] 2005†	CE + MPA and CE alone	1 y	MUI	Incident UI WHI	↑ Incontinence incident RR 1.39

*HERS trial.
†WHI trial.

Figure 6-19. Randomized and nonrandomized trials with oral estrogen. CE—conjugated estrogens; FUL—functional urethral length; HERS—Heart and Estrogen/Progesterone Replacement Study; MPA—medroxyprogesterone; MUCP—maximal urethral closure pressure; MUI—mixed urinary incontinence; MUP—maximal urethral pressure; RR—relative risk; SF-36—Short Form-36; UDS—urodynamic studies; UI—urinary incontinence; USI—urodynamic stress incontinence; WHI—Women's Health Initiative.

Randomized and Nonrandomized Trials with Vaginal Estrogen

Nonrandomized clinical trials

	Estrogen Type	Duration	Diagnosis	Outcome Measure	Findings
Bhatia et al. [37]	Vaginal CE 2 g	6 wk	USI	Symptoms UDS	55% Satisfied Increase in MUCP
Hilton and Stanton [38]	Vaginal CE 2 g	4 wk	USI	Symptoms UDS	Reduced severity of symptoms; increased MUCP
Schmid-Bauer [39]	Vaginal E2	6 wk	MUI	Symptoms Quality of life	69%–82% improved 72% quality of life improved
Schär et al. [40]	Vaginal E2	3 mo	MUI	Symptoms	50% improved
Cardozo et al. [41]	Vaginal E2 vs E3	6 mo	MUI	Symptoms	53%–59% improvement

Randomized controlled trials

	Estrogen Type	Duration	Diagnosis	Outcome Measure	Findings
Dessole et al. [42]	Vaginal E3	6 mo	USI	Symptoms	Significant reduction in incontinence, $P < 0.01$
				UDS	Significant ↑ MUP and MUCP, $P < 0.05$
Sacco et al. [43]	Vaginal E3	2 mo	USI	Symptoms UDS	Clinical improvement ↑ MUCP, FUL, and max capacity*

Not significant.

Figure 6-20. Randomized and nonrandomized trials of vaginal estrogen. CE—conjugated estrogens; FUL—functional urethral length; MUCP—maximal urethral closure pressure; MUI—mixed urinary incontinence; MUP—maximal urethral pressure; UDS—urodynamic studies; USI—urodynamic stress incontinence.

Important Studies on Drug Treatment of Stress Incontinence

Study	Design	Results
PPA		
Lehtonen et al. [44]	Double-blind randomized controlled trial: 43 patients were treated with either placebo or 50 mg PPA	A statistically significant improvement in subjective response with PPA over placebo (15 of 21 treated with PPA vs 8 of 22 treated with placebo); there was a 14% increase in MUCP; rare adverse reactions were noted with no adverse BP effects
Alhasso et al. [45]	Cochrane	Weak evidence to support the use of α-adrenergic agonists over placebo (further, larger studies are needed to fully evaluate)
Imipramine		
Lui et al. [46]	Prospective intervention trial: 40 patients were treated with imipramine 25 mg TID	35% were cured and 25% showed improvement > 50% over baseline analysis for pad test; the success group had a higher pretreatment urethral closure pressure
Duloxetine		
Dmochowski et al. [20]	Double-blind randomized controlled trial: 683 women were randomly assigned to placebo vs 40 mg duloxetine	There was a significant decrease in the incontinence episode frequency with 51% having a 50%–100% improvement vs 34% with placebo; nausea (24%) was the major adverse effect for duloxetine (74% who had nausea completed the trial)
Norton et al. [47]	Double-blind randomized trial: 553 women were randomly assigned to placebo vs 20 mg, 40 mg, or 80 mg of duloxetine	Improvements in median incontinence frequency were seen in a dose-dependent fashion from 20 mg to 40 mg to 80 mg with a nausea frequency that also increased to a maximum of 15%

Figure 6-21. Important studies regarding drug treatment of stress incontinence. BP—blood pressure; MUCP—maximal urethral closure pressure; PPA— phenylpropanolamine; TID—three times daily.

Ambulatory Procedures

Bulking agents

Collagen (Contigen; Bard Urological Products, Covington, GA)

Hydroxyapatite (Coaptite; Bioform Medical, San Mateo, CA)

Hyaluronic acid/dextranomer (Durasphere; Carbon Medical Technologies, St. Paul, MN)

Radiofrequency

Renessa device (Novasys Medical, Newark, CA)

Figure 6-22. Ambulatory procedures.

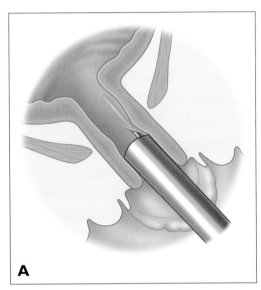 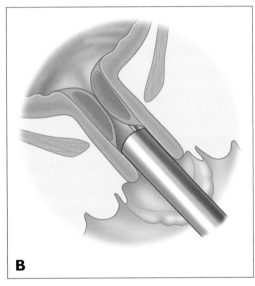

Figure 6-23. Bulking procedures are a minimally invasive option for outpatient treatment of urinary incontinence, including intrinsic sphincter deficiency. **A,** Technique for performing a transurethral bulking procedure. Topical anesthetic is applied transurethrally. A 0° or 12° urethroscope is generally used for the injection. The needle is placed through the mucosa at midurethra and advanced to the bladder neck. **B,** The goal is to achieve coaptation of the urethral mucosa in the midline to provide increased outlet resistance. Generally injections at the 3, 6, and 9 o'clock positions are required to achieve coaptation.

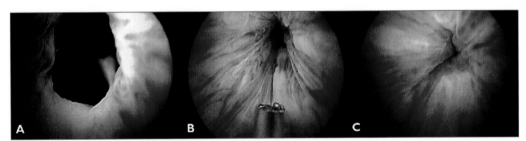

Figure 6-24. Example of a wide open bladder neck prior to bulking (**A**), after injection at 3 and 9 o'clock (**B**), and after injection at 6 o'clock to complete the procedure (**C**). Collagen is the most commonly used agent but is limited by degradation/absorption over time. This can necessitate multiple injections, which can limit the cost effectiveness of the procedure [48].

Corcos and Fournier [49] evaluated 40 patients who had periurethral collagen injections and were evaluated after 4 years. Thirty percent were cured, with four requiring follow-up injection. Forty percent were improved, with five requiring repeat injections.

Hydroxyapatite (Coaptite; Bioform Medical, San Mateo, CA) is a new agent showing promise as a urethral bulking agent. A study of 10 patients followed for 1 year showed a decline of 90% in mean 24-hour pad weight with no significant complications. The injected volume was 3.9 mL and seven of 10 patients required a follow-up injection [50]. Hyaluronic acid/dextranomer gel (Zuidex; Q-Med, Uppsala, Sweden) is a new agent that can be administered blindly using an Implacer device (Q-Med). It is biodegradable and nonimmunogenic. A study of 142 patients (invasive therapy naïve) involving four 0.7-mL injections via the Implacer device showed a 77% response rate after 12 months (as measured by a > 50% reduction in provocation stress test results). The reinjection rate was 43% at 8 months [51].

Renessa Radiofrequency Procedure: Indications and Advantages

Stress incontinence due to hypermobility

Single treatment, 15–20 min total procedure time

Local + oral or conscious sedation

Palpation based (no cystoscopy required)

Excellent safety profile, well tolerated

No incisions, bandages, or dressings

Rapid recovery with minimal limitations

Figure 6-25. Renessa (Novasys Medical, Newark, CA) is a new technology involving radiofrequency (RF) energy delivered to 36 sites from the bladder neck to the midurethra causing focal denaturation of submucosal collagen, which results in reduced wall compliance without narrowing the lumen.

Appell *et al.* [52] randomly assigned 110 of 173 patients to RF microremodeling and 63 to sham treatment. Patients were evaluated up to 12 months after the injection. No statistically significant difference in adverse outcomes was seen between the sham and active groups except for dysuria. Seventy-four percent of patients with moderate to severe stress urinary incontinence had a greater than 10-point improvement in quality of life. Those with mild stress urinary incontinence and placebo had a similar improvement in quality of life. There was a statistically significant increase in mean leak point pressure in the treatment group versus the sham group [52]. No long-term outcome data are available.

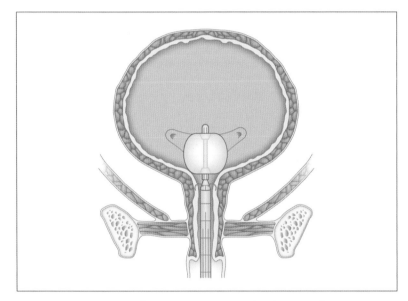

Figure 6-26. Renessa device (Novasys Medical, Newark, CA) demonstrating the prongs embedded in the periurethral tissue.

Historical Surgical Procedures

Anterior colporrhaphy with suburethral plication involves plicating the endopelvic fascia after the vaginal mucosa has been dissected away. One of the first stress incontinence procedures, which has now been abandoned due to poor long-term success rates. Still used frequently for midline anterior vaginal wall prolapse repairs [53]

Marshall-Marchetti-Krantz (MMK) sutures placed at the urethrovesical junction (UVJ) are anchored to the periosteum of the symphysis pubis, elevating and stabilizing the UVJ in the retropubic space. It has been largely replaced by the Burch urethropexy secondary to similar success and the significant complication of osteitis pubis and osteomyelitis in the MMK procedure vs the Burch

Needle bladder neck suspensions: Needle urethropexy has undergone multiple modifications from the initial procedure described by Pereyra in 1959. In general these procedures involve using needles to anchor the vaginal tissue to the rectus fascia, thus stabilizing the bladder neck. They have generally been abandoned secondary to modest success compared with the Burch and suburethral sling procedures [53,54]

In a study by Bergman and Elia [55], 127 patients with stress incontinence were randomly assigned to anterior colporrhaphy, modified Pereyra procedure, or a Burch urethropexy. Burch showed a cure rate of 82%, anterior colporrhaphy 37%, modified Pereyra 43% at 5 years

Figure 6-27. Historical surgical procedures.

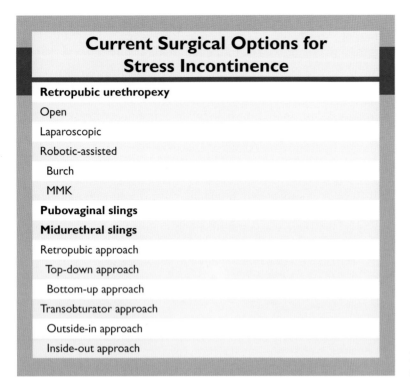

Current Surgical Options for Stress Incontinence

Retropubic urethropexy

Open

Laparoscopic

Robotic-assisted

Burch

MMK

Pubovaginal slings

Midurethral slings

Retropubic approach

Top-down approach

Bottom-up approach

Transobturator approach

Outside-in approach

Inside-out approach

Figure 6-28. Current surgical options for stress incontinence. MMK—Marshall-Marchetti-Krantz.

Advantages and Disadvantages of Current Surgical Options

Surgery	Approach	Success Rates (Follow-up)	Advantages	Disadvantages
Retropubic urethropexy (Burch, MMK)	Abdominal	75%–90% (1–5 y) 69%–90% (10 y)	Longer-term data; low complication rates	More invasive Longer recovery
	Laparoscopic	85% (5 y)		Osteitis pubis, osteomyelitis seen with MMK
Traditional pubovaginal slings	Combined abdominal-vaginal	72%–99% (1 y) 68%–90% (5 y) Meta-analysis at 5 y 86%	Effective for patients with ISD	More invasive Higher morbidity in harvesting autologous tissue Higher rates of postoperative voiding dysfunction
Retropubic midurethral slings	Vaginal Bottom-up Top-down	81%–92% (1–7.6 y) 81%–89% (1–2 y)	Less invasive Quicker Minimal dissection	Potential for bowel/vascular injury Synthetic mesh carries risk for erosion
Transobturator midurethral slings	Vaginal Outside-in Inside-out	84%–94% (1 y) 88%–93% (3–4 mo)	Avoids risk of bowel injury Quicker	Short-term data Risk of groin pain Less effective for patients with ISD

Figure 6-29. Current surgical options for stress incontinence including potential advantages and disadvantages. ISD—intrinsic sphincter deficiency; MMK—Marshall-Marchetti-Krantz.

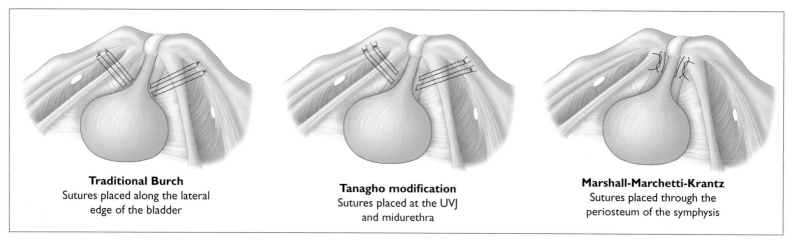

Traditional Burch
Sutures placed along the lateral
edge of the bladder

Tanagho modification
Sutures placed at the UVJ
and midurethra

Marshall-Marchetti-Krantz
Sutures placed through the
periosteum of the symphysis

Figure 6-30. Modifications of Burch retropubic urethropexies.
In the traditional procedure (*left*), sutures (two) are placed bilaterally
in the periurethral endopelvic connective tissue of the anterior vaginal wall at the level of the urethrovesical junction (UVJ) fixing it to
the ipsilateral Cooper's ligament. This provides support to a hyper-
mobile urethra. Success rates have been reported between 70% and
90% at 5 years.

This procedure is not typically used in patients with intrinsic
sphincter deficiency as a high failure rate of greater than 50% was
noted in patients with maximal urethral closure pressures of less than
20 cm H$_2$O [56]. De novo overactive bladder symptoms have been
noted in 5% to 17% of patients, with resolution of symptoms in 50%
to 70% of patients. The Tanagho modification of the procedure (*middle*) involves more lateral placement of the sutures to avoid urethral
injury as well as placement of the second suture at the midurethra
and tying the sutures without excessive elevation and compression of
the urethra by the pubic symphysis [53,54]. The Colpopexy and Urinary Reduction Efforts (CARE) trial showed that addition of the Burch
procedure at the time of abdominal sacrocolpopexy significantly
reduced new stress incontinence postoperatively from 44% to 22%
in women without a history of stress incontinence [57]. The figure on
the *right* shows the Marshall-Marchetti-Krantz procedure.

Pubovaginal Slings

Traditional pubovaginal slings involve harvesting a graft from the rectus fascia or the fascia lata. The graft is then passed up from a vaginal opening
through needles passed under direct contact through the retropubic space. The sling is then positioned at the bladder neck. Other biologic or
synthetic sling materials can be used and are discussed below. Success rates are > 80%.

De novo OAB can be seen in both traditional and synthetic sling procedures at a rate of about 0%–30%.

Newer sling procedures involving synthetic sling materials in either the retropubic or transobturator approach have success rates similar to
those seen with the traditional pubovaginal slings.

Successful in patients with stress incontinence secondary to poor urethral support as well as intrinsic sphincter deficiency [58].

Wadie *et al.* [59] showed a 92%–93% cure rate at 6 mo in both groups in a randomized study of 53 patients assigned to TVT vs rectus fascia sling.

A study involving 142 patients randomly assigned to either Pelvicol pubovaginal sling (Bard Nordic, Helsingborg, Sweden) vs TVT sling showed
similar success rates of > 80% with no difference in complication rates [60].

Figure 6-31. Traditional pubovaginal slings. OAB—overactive bladder; TVT—tension-free tape.

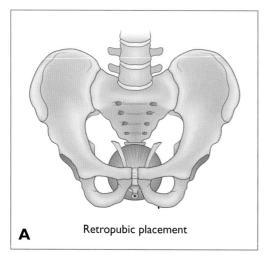

A   Retropubic placement

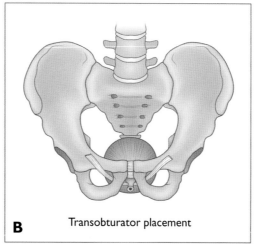

B   Transobturator placement

Figure 6-32. Approaches for midurethral
slings. **A**, Retropubic placement.
B, Transobturator placement.

Bottom-up approach

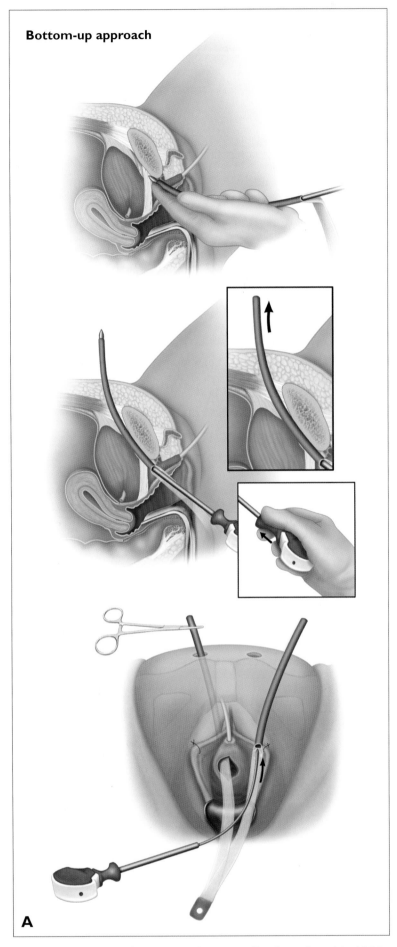

Top-down approach

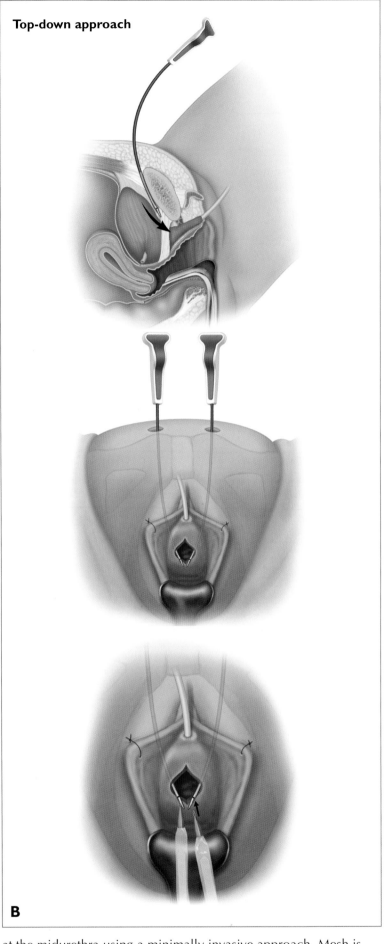

A

B

Figure 6-33. Retropubic approaches were first introduced in 1990 by Petros *et al.* [61] as a minimally invasive surgical alternative for stress incontinence and are marketed by Gynecare (Sommerville, NJ) as the TVT (tension-free vaginal tape). Proline mesh is placed at the midurethra using a minimally invasive approach. Mesh is placed through the retropubic space from either a bottom-up (**A**) or top-down (**B**) approach. Studies show equivalent efficacy with either approach.

Continued on the next page

Figure 6-33. *(Continued)* The procedure is generally performed on an outpatient basis and can be performed with the patient under local anesthesia. Minimal dissection potentially reduces iatrogenic nerve injury. Operative time is short. De novo urge symptoms are seen in 5% to 10% of patients.

Success rates are similar to the Burch retropubic urethropexy and traditional pubovaginal slings with 1- to 7.6-year follow-up. Ninety women with 7.6-year follow-up reported an 81.3% subjective cure rate and 16.3% improvement. Objectively 81.3% were dry by stress test and 24-hour pad test [62]. Multiple variations on the original TVT prototype have been introduced. Early data suggest no significant difference in outcomes regardless of the approach. The treatment is shown to be effective for recurrent incontinence (85%) as well as for those with intrinsic sphincter deficiency (74% cured and 12% improved) [63,64]. Risk factors for failure from one study included a maximal urethral closure pressure of 10 cm H_2O and age greater than 70 years. Other studies have demonstrated that a body mass index of greater than 30 is another risk factor for failure [63].

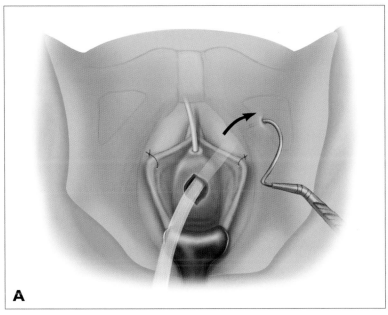
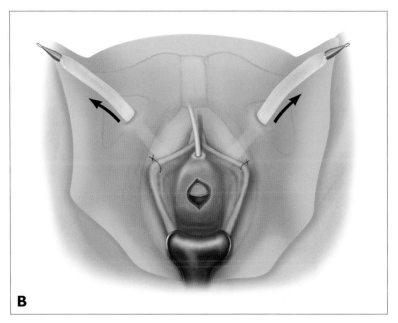

A
B

Figure 6-34. A, Passing of the trocar from an outside-in approach. **B,** Passing of the sling through the transobturator space. The transobturator approach was developed as an alternative to the retropubic sling to avoid the complications associated with that approach, including bladder perforation and vascular or bowel injury. Initially it was thought that cystoscopy was not necessary, but there have been reports of bladder perforation and thus cystoscopy is advised [58]. A small percentage (2.3%) of patients had postoperative groin or perineal pain in one study [65]. Thirty-two patients underwent transobturator sling placement with a success rate of 90.6% at a mean of 17 months with no intraoperative complications. However, five of the 32 had postoperative obstructive symptoms, with one patient requiring intermittent catheterization up to 4 weeks [66].

Meta-analysis of studies comparing retropubic and transobturator slings showed no difference in subjective outcomes at 2 to 12 months of follow-up [67]. There is evidence that the transobturator approach is not as effective for patients with intrinsic sphincter deficiency. In a cohort of 145 patients who underwent either tension-free vaginal tape procedure or Monarc TOT (transobturator tape; American Medical Systems, Minnetonka, MN), those with a maximal urethral closure pressure of less than 42 cm H_2O had a relative risk of 5.89 for failure on objective urodynamic criteria after TOT as compared with tension-free vaginal tape. Differences in subjective reports did not meet statistical significance [68].

Comparative Studies Regarding Surgical Treatment of Stress Incontinence

Surgery	Study	Design	Follow-up	Results
Burch RPU vs modified Pereyra vs anterior repair	Bergman and Elia [55]	RCT	5 y	n = 127; cure rates: Burch 82% Pereyra 43% Anterior repair 37%
Burch vs TVT	Ward and Hilton [69]	RCT	2 y	n = 175 TVT, 169 Burch Cure based on postoperative urodynamics, QOL questionnaires; *Outcomes reported 2 ways:* Intent-to-treat analysis: Burch 51% TVT 63% Group evaluated: Burch 87% TVT 85%
TVT vs TOT	de Tayrac et al. [70]	RCT	1 y	n = 61 Cure rates: TVT (31) 84%, 10% improved TOT (30) 90%, 3% improved
TVT vs SPARC*	Andonian et al. [71]	RCT	1 y	n = 84 (41 SPARC, 43 TVT) Cure based on postoperative urodynamics, pad test, and QOL questionnaires; no difference in objective cure rates: 83% SPARC vs 95% TVT, P = 0.01; no difference in subjective cure rates or complications
TVT vs TOT	Palma et al. [72]	Nonrandomized, prospective clinical trial	16 mo	n = 226 TVT (126), 92% cured, 2.4% improved TOT (100), 94% cured, 2% improved No difference in postoperative voiding dysfunction 10% vs 0% risk of bladder perforation in the TVT vs TOT group

*American Medical Systems, Minnetonka, MN.

Figure 6-35. Important studies comparing surgical treatment of stress incontinence. QOL—quality of life; RCT—randomized controlled trial; RPU—retropubic urethropexy; SPARC—suprapubic arch; TOT—transobturator tape; TVT—tension-free vaginal tape.

Classification of Sling Materials

Biologic

Autologous: rectus fascia or fascia lata

Allograft: cadaveric human fascia lata, dura, or dermis

Xenograft: porcine or bovine dermis and small intestine mucosa

In both allograft and xenograft use, there is a theoretical concern for transmission of prion diseases. The grafts are treated with gamma irradiation or freeze drying and no cases of transmission have been reported. There is concern that this processing weakens the tissue, yet studies have not supported this concern. There is also the risk of graft rejection, but this is rarely reported

Synthetic

Typically used meshes are macroporous (pore size > 75 µm) as opposed to microporous (pore size < 10 µm). Microporous mesh limits tissue ingrowth and macrophage access to bacteria, resulting in poor tissue incorporation and decreased ability to fight infection

Monofilament meshes are preferred over multifilament as multifilament mesh has < 10 µm interstices, which results in the same limitations as seen with the microporous meshes

Experience with polyethylene terephthalate (macroporous multifilament) resulted in erosion rates of 20% to 30% [73,74]

ObTape (Mentor, Santa Barbara, CA), a microporous monofilament mesh, has erosion rates ranging from 4% to 10% [75,76]

Figure 6-36. Classification of sling materials.

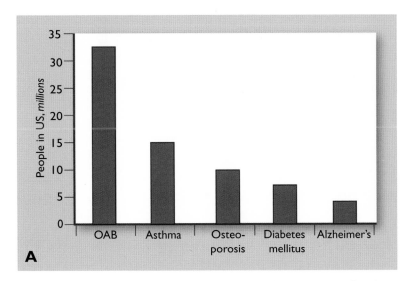

A

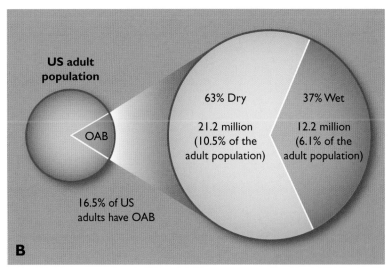

B

Figure 6-37. A, Comparison of overactive bladder (OAB) with other common chronic medical conditions. OAB affects more than 33 million people in the United States, making it more prevalent than many more well-known diseases [77]. Over one third of patients have urge incontinence. Estimated total economic cost of OAB in 2000 was more than $12 billion in the United States. **B**, Breakdown of OAB wet versus OAB dry in the United States. (*Data from* the National Overactive Bladder Evaluation [Noble] Study [77]).

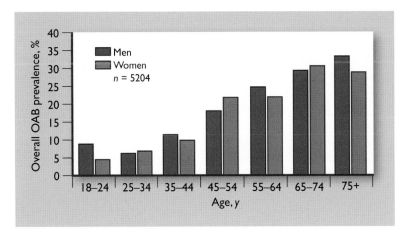

Figure 6-38. The prevalence of overactive bladder (OAB) increases with age in both men and women. The prevalence of OAB with urge incontinence is greater in women, and the prevalence of OAB without incontinence is greater in men. Consequences of OAB include a higher incidence of health problems compared with non-OAB patients [78]; an increase in falls and fractures by 26% and 34%, respectively; a higher rate of urinary tract infections, perineal infections, sleep disturbance, and sexual dysfunction [79]; and a significant reduction in quality of life [80].

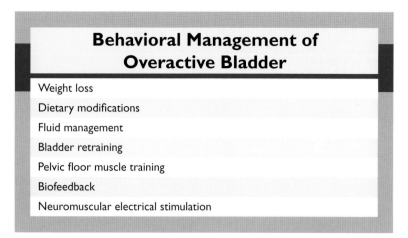

Behavioral Management of Overactive Bladder

Weight loss

Dietary modifications

Fluid management

Bladder retraining

Pelvic floor muscle training

Biofeedback

Neuromuscular electrical stimulation

Figure 6-39. Behavioral management. Lifestyle modifications can be made in an attempt to improve urinary symptoms and incontinence; however, data are limited [81]. Obesity appears to be an independent risk factor for urinary incontinence, and weight loss may be helpful for moderately to morbidly obese women [81]. The benefit of caffeine reduction remains controversial. Although small clinical trials suggest that caffeine reduction improves urinary continence, large cross-sectional studies demonstrate no association [81]. In a large prospective cohort study, coffee, alcohol, and total fluid intake were not found to be independent risk factors for the development of overactive bladder (OAB) [82]. However, most experts recommend limiting daily fluid intake to less than 2 L, and both caffeine and alcohol should be used in moderation.

Bladder retraining is widely used as first-line therapy for patients with overactive bladder and urge incontinence. There is limited evidence demonstrating that bladder training is more effective than no treatment, and insufficient data comparing bladder training with pharmacologic agents. The role of bladder retraining as a supplemental therapy also remains unclear. However, bladder training has no adverse effects and no cost burden and is therefore a safe and easy starting point for patients with OAB [83].

Bladder training focuses on increasing the amount of time between voids, with the goal of increasing bladder capacity and in turn decreasing detrusor overactivity and symptoms of urgency [84]. Bladder training protocols vary. Experts suggest that an outpatient training protocol should include an initial voiding interval of 1 hour during waking hours, which is increased by 15 to 30 minutes per week until a 2- to 3-hour voiding interval is achieved. The voiding schedule is adjusted for tolerance and patients monitor their behavior with bladder diaries. Patients are encouraged to use techniques such as distraction, relaxation, and pelvic floor muscle contraction to suppress urinary urges and to promote bladder control. If no improvement is seen after 3 weeks, it is recommended that other treatment modalities be considered [84].

Physical therapy focuses on teaching patients the ability to suppress the urge to urinate. Pelvic floor muscle training is used primarily for patients with stress urinary incontinence but may also be helpful for those with OAB. By strengthening pelvic floor muscles through Kegel exercises, patients can improve urethral resistance and urinary control. During an episode of urinary urgency, patients are instructed to contract their pelvic floor muscles, relax the rest of the body, and concentrate on suppressing the urge [84].

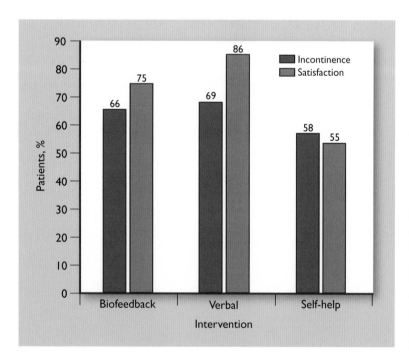

Figure 6-40. Urge incontinence, behavioral training, and biofeedback. Biofeedback can be used to help patients correctly perform pelvic floor muscle exercises and in turn control physiologic responses. Various techniques are used to verify muscle contraction, including vaginal palpation, vaginal cones, the pelvic floor educator, manometry, electromyography, and real-time ultrasound [81].

In a randomized controlled trial of 222 women with urge incontinence aged 55 to 92 years, Burgio *et al.* [85] randomly assigned patients to receive 8 weeks of biofeedback-assisted behavioral training, behavioral training without biofeedback, or self-administered behavioral treatment using a self-help booklet (control condition). Of note, the patients assigned to the "behavioral training without biofeedback" group did receive verbal feedback based on vaginal palpation. No significant difference in reduction of incontinence was seen among the three groups ($P = 0.23$). However, a significant difference was seen with respect to patient satisfaction. Seventy-five percent of the biofeedback group, 85.5% of the verbal feedback group, and 55.7% of the self-help booklet group reported complete satisfaction with treatment ($P = 0.001$).

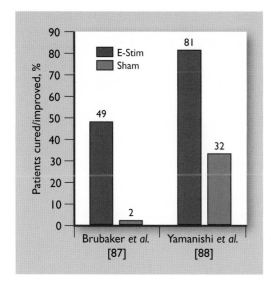

Figure 6-41. Randomized controlled trials (RCTs) of electrical stimulation (E-stim) versus sham device. Neuromuscular electrical stimulation utilizes electrical currents to stimulate pelvic floor muscles and can help patients gain awareness of appropriate muscle contraction. With this technique, patients can make a conscious attempt to join in with the stimulated contraction, with the goal of ultimately initiating a voluntary pelvic floor muscle contraction [86].

Wide variation in E-stim protocols has made it difficult to directly compare studies; however, there appears to be a trend in favor of E-stim over placebo for the treatment of detrusor overactivity [6]. In an RCT of 121 women by Brubaker *et al.* [86], 49% of women with detrusor instability were cured after using a transvaginal electrical device for 8 weeks ($P = 0.0004$). No statistically significant change was seen in the sham device group [12]. In another RCT that involved both men and women with detrusor overactivity, Yamanishi *et al.* [87] found an improvement in 81.3% of patients in the active E-stim group, compared with a 32.1% improvement in the sham group ($P = 0.0001$). More RCTs are needed to fully evaluate this modality.

Pharmacologic Therapy for Overactive Bladder

Therapeutic Agent	Pharmacologic Category	Dosing	Comments
Oxybutynin	Antispasmodic/antimuscarinic Tertiary amine	Immediate release: 5 mg 2–3 times a day; max 20 mg/d	
		Extended release: 5-mg, 10-mg, 15-mg tabs; initial dose 5–10 mg daily, may increase in 5-mg increments; max 30 mg/d	
		Transdermal: 3.9 mg/d; one patch twice weekly (every 3–4 d)	
Tolterodine	Antimuscarinic Tertiary amine	Immediate release: 1-mg, 2-mg tabs; 2 mg twice daily, may decrease to 1 mg twice daily	
		Extended release: 2-mg, 4-mg tabs; 4 mg once daily, may decrease to 2 mg once daily	
Darifenacin	Antimuscarinic Tertiary amine	Extended release: 7.5-mg, 15-mg tabs; 7.5 mg once daily, may increase to 15 mg once daily after 2 wk	Most M_3 selective receptor antagonist
Solifenacin	Antimuscarinic Tertiary amine	5-mg, 10-mg tabs; 5 mg once daily, may increase to 10 mg once daily	50-hour half-life; highest dry rate reported
Trospium chloride	Antispasmodic/antimuscarinic Quaternary amine	20-mg tabs; 20 mg twice daily, may decrease to 20 mg once daily if not well tolerated 60-mg tabs; 60 mg daily	Limited ability to cross the blood-brain barrier, CNS effects should be minimal
Imipramine	Tricyclic antidepressant	25-mg, 50-mg tabs; for children ≥ 6 y, 25 mg daily 1 h before bedtime, after 1 wk can increase to 50 mg for children 6–12 y, up to 75 mg for children for > 12 y	

Figure 6-42. Pharmacologic therapy. Antimuscarinic drugs, such as oxybutynin, tolterodine, darifenacin, and solifenacin, are considered first-line pharmacologic agents in the treatment of overactive bladder with symptoms of urinary frequency, urgency, or urge incontinence. CNS—central nervous system.

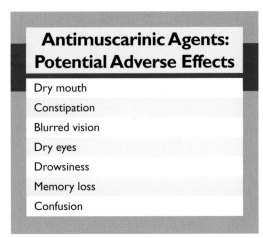

Antimuscarinic Agents: Potential Adverse Effects

Dry mouth

Constipation

Blurred vision

Dry eyes

Drowsiness

Memory loss

Confusion

Figure 6-43. Long-term studies have shown that adverse events such as dry mouth and constipation are most common within the first 3 months of therapy and decrease thereafter [88].

Five Head-to-Head Trials Comparing the Efficacy and Side Effects of Antimuscarinic Agents

Study	Results
The OBJECT Study [89] (Overactive Bladder: Judging Effective Control and Treatment) Compared tolterodine IR 2 mg twice daily to oxybutynin ER 10 mg daily (randomized, double-blind study)	Oxybutynin ER significantly more effective than tolterodine in each of the outcome measures: weekly urge incontinence ($P = 0.03$), total incontinence ($P = 0.02$), and micturition frequency episodes ($P = 0.02$); similar rates of dry mouth and other adverse events for both groups
The OPERA Trial [90] (Overactive Bladder: Performance of Extended Release Agents) Compared tolterodine ER 4 mg daily to oxybutynin ER 10 mg daily (randomized, double-blind study)	Improvements in weekly urge incontinence episodes similar for both groups; oxybutynin significantly more effective in reducing micturition frequency ($P = 0.003$); no episodes of urinary incontinence reported in 23.0% of women in taking oxybutynin, compared with 16.8% in the tolterodine group ($P = 0.03$); dry mouth more common in oxybutynin group; both groups had similar discontinuation rates
The ACET Study [91] (Antimuscarinic Clinical Effectiveness Trial) Compared tolterodine ER 2 or 4 mg to oxybutynin ER 5 or 10 mg (open label study)	The 4-mg group perceived an improved bladder condition compared with approximately 60% in the other groups (all $P < 0.01$); fewer study withdrawals in the tolterodine 4-mg group compared with both oxybutynin groups; less dry mouth reported with tolterodine 4 mg compared with oxybutynin 10 mg
The STAR [92] Trial (Solifenacin OD and Tolterodine ER 4 mg OD as an Active comparator in a Randomized Trial) Compared solifenacin 5 or 10 mg to tolterodine ER 4 mg, patients given option to request a dose increase after 4 wk of treatment (randomized, double-blind study)	Solifenacin, with a flexible dosing regimen, showed greater efficacy than tolterodine with respect to urgency, urge incontinence, and overall incontinence; 74% of patients treated with solifenacin experienced at least a 50% reduction in incontinence episodes, compared with 67% of patients receiving tolterodine ($P = 0.021$); 59% of patients in the solifenacin group become continent, compared with 49% in the tolterodine group ($P = 0.006$); discontinuations for both agents were similar
Chapple and Abrams [93] Three treatment cohorts: darifenacin IR 2.5 mg TID or oxybutynin 2.5 mg TID; darifenacin CR 15 mg once daily or oxybutynin 5 mg TID; darifenacin CR 30 mg daily or oxybutynin 5 mg TID (randomized, double-blind, crossover study)	Improved urodynamic parameters seen for all treatments, with no significant difference between cohorts; both darifenacin CR doses had significantly less effect on salivary flow than IR oxybutynin

Figure 6-44. Five head-to-head trials (four randomized) have compared the efficacy and side effect profiles of the main antimuscarinic agents. CR—controlled release; ER—extended release; IR—immediate release; OD—once daily; TID—three times daily.

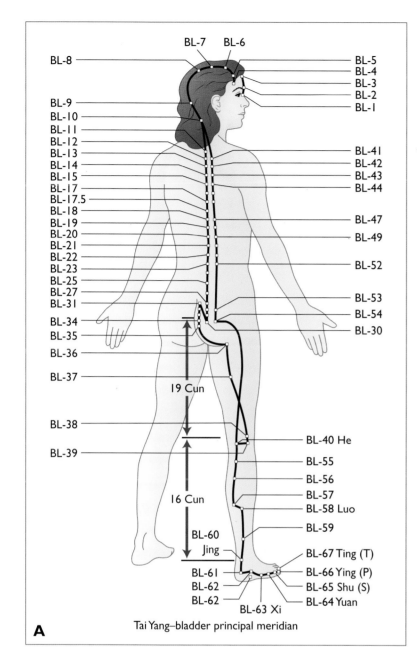

BL-7 BL-6
BL-8
BL-5
BL-4
BL-3
BL-2
BL-1
BL-9
BL-10
BL-11
BL-12
BL-13
BL-14
BL-15
BL-17
BL-17.5
BL-18
BL-19
BL-20
BL-21
BL-22
BL-23
BL-25
BL-27
BL-31
BL-34
BL-35
BL-36
BL-37
19 Cun
BL-38
BL-39
16 Cun
BL-60
Jing
BL-61
BL-62
BL-62
BL-63 Xi
BL-41
BL-42
BL-43
BL-44
BL-47
BL-49
BL-52
BL-53
BL-54
BL-30
BL-40 He
BL-55
BL-56
BL-57
BL-58 Luo
BL-59
BL-67 Ting (T)
BL-66 Ying (P)
BL-65 Shu (S)
BL-64 Yuan

A Tai Yang–bladder principal meridian

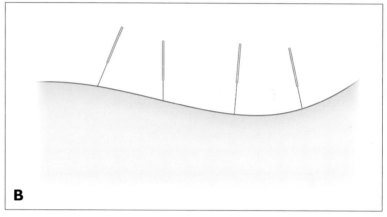

B

Figure 6-45. Acupuncture. **A,** In a randomized placebo-controlled trial of 85 women, patients who received 4 weekly bladder-specific acupuncture treatments had significant improvements in bladder capacity, urgency, frequency, and quality-of-life scores when compared with patients undergoing placebo acupuncture treatments. A significant decrease in the number of incontinent episodes was seen for both groups (59% for treatment and 40% for placebo) with no significant difference in the change between groups [94]. **B,** Acupuncture bladder channel points 32 to 34 are over the S2, 3 foramen.

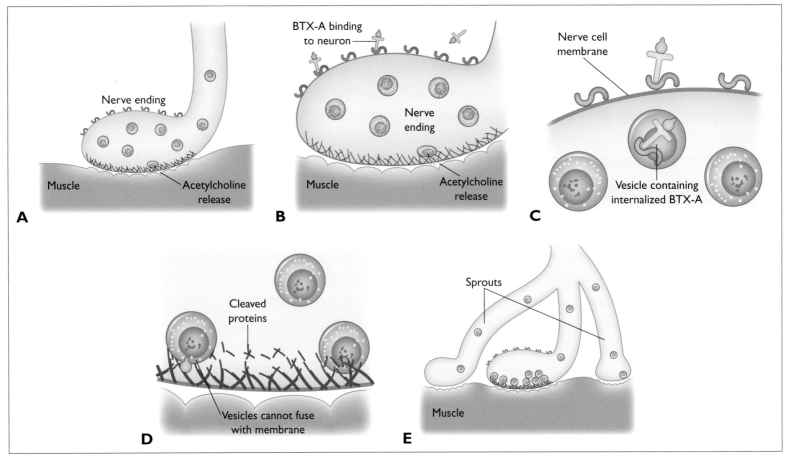

Figure 6-46. Mechanism of action of botulinum toxin type A (BTX-A). BTX-A blocks neuromuscular transmission and inhibits release of acetylcholine. Neurotoxin cleaves SNAP-25 protein, prevents docking and release of acetylcholine, and causes localized reduction in muscle activity. Muscle atrophy leads to axonal sprouting. BTX-A is thought to reduce sensory afferents as well as affecting the sensory feedback loop in the central nervous system [95,96].

A, Endplate sits upon muscle fiber. **B**, Binding: neurotoxin binds to nerve terminal. **C**, Internalization: neurotoxin internalized via receptor-mediated endocytosis. **D**, Blocking: BTX-A blocks fusion of neurotransmitter vesicle with nerve membrane by cleaving SNAP-25. **E**, Sprouting and reestablishment: endplate expands and collateral axonal sprouts emerge.

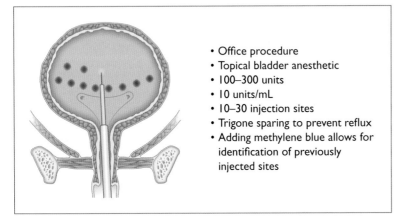

- Office procedure
- Topical bladder anesthetic
- 100–300 units
- 10 units/mL
- 10–30 injection sites
- Trigone sparing to prevent reflux
- Adding methylene blue allows for identification of previously injected sites

Figure 6-47. Technique for intravesical botulinum toxin (BTX) injection. BTX is a highly potent neurotoxin that inhibits acetylcholine release at presynaptic neuromuscular junctions. Serotype A (BTX-A) is commonly used in the treatment of various muscle spasticity disorders and for cosmetic purposes. Although not currently approved by the Food and Drug Administration for this purpose, the use of intradetrusor BTX in humans has shown promising results in the treatment of detrusor overactivity incontinence [97]. Current National Institutes of Health trials are underway to determine efficacy and safety.

Results of Intravesical Botulinum Toxin

Prospective study of 26 women [98]

Refractory nonneurogenic DO

100 units of BTX injected

  14 dry (54%)

  8 improved (30%)

  2 failed (7.6%)

  2 had retention (7.6%)—PVRs 130–230 mL

    Lasted only 1 wk

Most of the effectiveness had worn off by 12 wk

Prospective study of 100 subjects [99]

77 women, 23 men

Refractory nonneurogenic DO and OAB

100 units of BTX injected at 30 sites

Follow-up at 4 and 12 wk

  88% had significant subjective improvement

  Resolution of urgency: 82%

  Resolution of urge incontinence: 86%

  Increased bladder capacity and decreased frequency by 50%, nocturia decreased from 4 to 1.5 micturitions

  No comment on retention rates

Efficacy duration of 6 mo (± 2 mo)

  Based on 20 patients followed out to 36 wk

Figure 6-48. Results of intravesical botulinum toxin (BTX) [98,99]. DO—detrusor overactivity; OAB—overactive bladder; PVR—postvoid residual.

Vanilloids: Capsaicin and Resiniferatoxin

C-fiber afferent neurotoxins that act on the vanilloid receptors

Used primarily to treat neurogenic detrusor overactivity where C-fiber afferentation has become chronically active, such as in spinal cord injuries

Delivered as an intravesical drug therapy. Initially causes depolarization and C-fiber firing, which initially results in pain, but over the long term causes desensitization by ultimately depleting the reservoir of substance P from the C fibers

One installation may last for up to 3 mo

Scoville scale: assigns a heat value to each variety of pepper:

  Bell pepper has a heat value of 1 and is used as the benchmark

  Jalapeno pepper is 1000 times hotter

  Thai pepper is 100,000 times hotter

  Capsaicin is 6 million times hotter

  Resiniferatoxin is 16 billion times hotter (1000 times hotter than capsaicin) but is less pungent and irritating and does not evoke intolerable bladder symptoms during installation

Figure 6-49. Vanilloids: capsaicin and resiniferatoxin.

Results of Intravesical Resiniferatoxin

Prospective study of 20 subjects with chronic spinal cord lesions and refractory detrusor overactivity and detrusor–sphincter dyssynergia [100]

Treated with 30 mL of 10 µmol/L resiniferatoxin for 30 min

Reevaluated at 1 mo after installation

Continence and/or difficulty voiding improved in 12 (60%)

4 Subjects (20%) were dry, and the other 8 were improved

Mean cystometric capacity increased from 102 to 236 mL ($P < 0.001$)

No significant change in the detrusor pressure

There was no relationship seen with the level or completeness of the spinal cord lesion, suggesting that C-fiber sprouting may be similar

Randomized, double-blinded parallel trial comparing capsaicin with resiniferatoxin [101]

39 Subjects with spinal cord injury and neurogenic detrusor overactivity

3-mo follow-up

Clinical improvement was seen in 78% of the capsaicin group and 80% of the resiniferatoxin group at day 30

Urodynamic improvement was seen in 83% of the capsaicin group and 60% of the resiniferatoxin group at day 30

Benefit remained in 2/3 of the 2 groups at 3 mo

No difference in side effects

Figure 6-50. Results of intravesical resiniferatoxin [101,102].

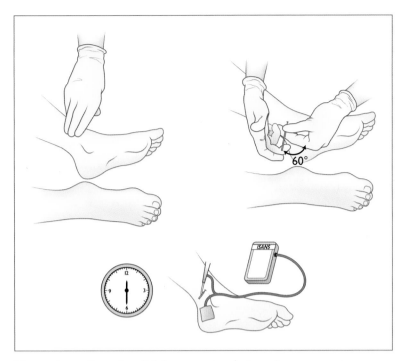

Figure 6-51. Posterior tibial nerve stimulation. An acupuncture needle is placed over the tibial nerve at the level of the medial malleolus and stimulation administered. The procedure is thought to stimulate the inhibitory reflex sacral pathways that control micturition.

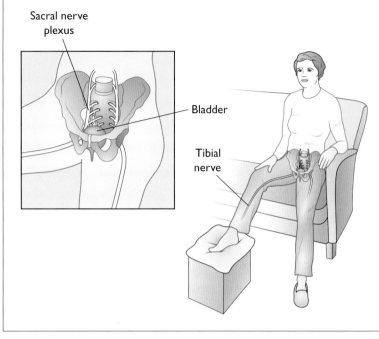

Figure 6-52. Performance of tibial nerve stimulation. The procedure is done in an office-based setting in 30-minute weekly sessions for 12 weeks. The success rate is 92% (37% objective [voiding diaries] and 55% subjective) [102]. Maintenance therapy is necessary [103]. Both subjective and objective deterioration occur if therapy is discontinued. Maintenance therapy is recommended three times weekly.

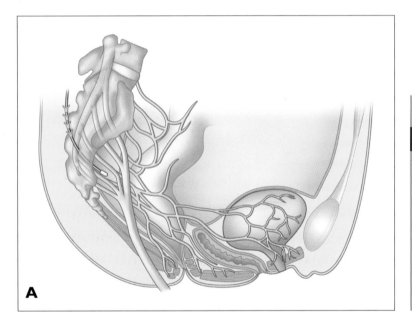

B History of Sacral Nerve Stimulation

1981—Department of Urology, University of California at San Francisco initiated a clinical program

1985 to 1992—Multicenter trial conducted by Urosystems (Sunnyvale, CA)

1994—Medtronic gained approval to market InterStim in Europe for treatment of urge incontinence, retention, and urgency/frequency

1997—FDA approval of InterStim for treatment of urge incontinence

April 1999—FDA approval of the InterStim System for treatment of symptoms of urgency/frequency and urinary retention

Figure 6-53. A, InterStim (Medtronic, Minneapolis, MN) sacral neuromodulation. **B,** History of sacral nerve stimulation. Sacral nerve stimulation involves an implantable, programmable neurostimulation system similar to a pacemaker. An electrode wire is placed adjacent to a sacral nerve root, typically at the S3 level, and attached to a programmable stimulator. Therapy is in two stages, allowing the patient to "trial" the therapy prior to committing to the chronic implant. There is no other surgical procedure that has a similar trial period. The test stimulation phase allows for the patient to make an educated decision to proceed with implant. The implantation phase proceeds if a greater than 50% improvement in symptoms in seen. Indications for InterStim (FDA approved) include urge incontinence, urgency/frequency, nonobstructive retention, and failure of other therapies. FDA—Food and Drug Administration.

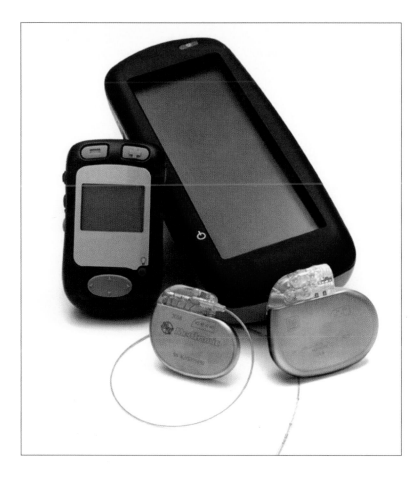

Figure 6-54. InterStim components (Medtronic, Minneapolis, MN). Features include 1) quadripolar tined lead, typically placed parallel to the S3 nerve root; 2) implantable neurostimulator that generates mild electrical pulses that are delivered through the lead electrodes; and 3) clinician and patient programmers that are used to set the parameters of the electrical pulses.

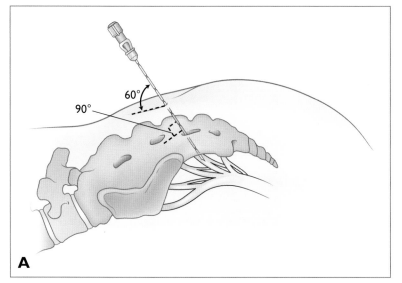

A

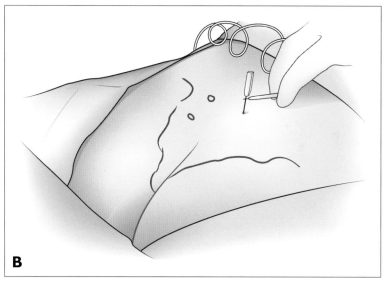

B

Figure 6-55. Placement of the foramen needle. **A,** The needle is placed at a 60° angle in the upper medial quadrant of the S3 foramen. The ideal placement is a parallel line along the nerve to obtain response from all four electrodes. **B,** The procedure is generally performed under fluoroscopic guidance. Proper placement is confirmed using both motor and sensory responses. Motor responses have been shown to be more predictive of a successful implant [104].

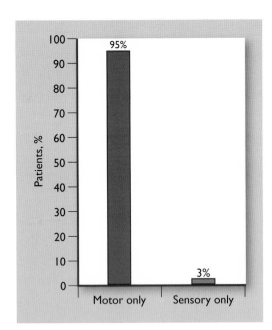

Figure 6-56. Predictors of success for first-stage neuromodulation: motor versus sensory. "Motor only" refers to patients eliciting only a motor response who eventually had an implant. "Sensory only" refers to patients eliciting only a sensory response who eventually had an implant. (*From* Cohen *et al.* [104]; with permission.)

Nerve Innervation	Response		Sensation
	Pelvic floor	**Foot/calf/leg**	
S2 Primary somatic contributor of pudendal nerve for external sphincter, leg, foot	"Clamp"* of anal sphincter	Leg/hip rotation, plantar flexion of entire foot, contraction of calf	Contraction of base of penis, vagina
S3 Virtually all pelvic autonomic functions and striated muscle (levator ani)	"Bellows"† of perineum	Plantar flexion of great toe, occasionally other toes	Pulling in rectum, extending forward to scrotum or labia
S4 Pelvic autonomic and somatic No leg or foot	"Bellows"†	No lower extremity motor stimulation	Pulling in rectum only

* Clamp: contraction of anal sphincter and, in men, retraction of base of penis. Move buttocks and look for anterior/posterior shortening of the perineal structures.
† Bellows: lifting and dropping of pelvic floor. Look for deepening and flattening of buttock groove.

Figure 6-57. Motor and sensory responses. The ideal response is outlined in purple.

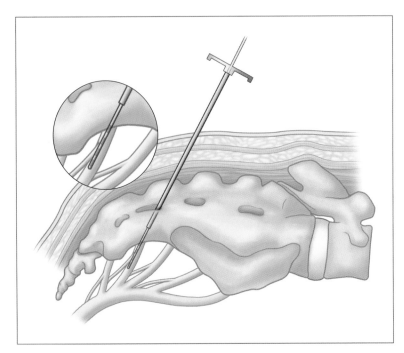

Figure 6-58. Placement of the lead wire: sagittal section of the lead wire with the sheath over the tines but the electrodes exposed. Proper location of the lead is confirmed and adjusted with the protective sheath covering the tines, but exposing the electrodes. This allows for adjusting the position of the lead to ensure the ideal placement.

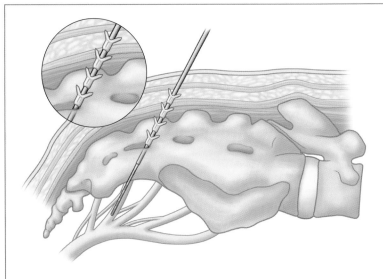

Figure 6-59. Exposure of the tines, securing the lead wire in place. Once proper placement is confirmed, the sheath protecting the tines is removed, thus deploying the tines and securing the lead wire in the proper location. This drawing demonstrates the ideal parallel line along the S3 nerve root. The tines are deployed within the thoracolumbar fascia and paraspinous muscles.

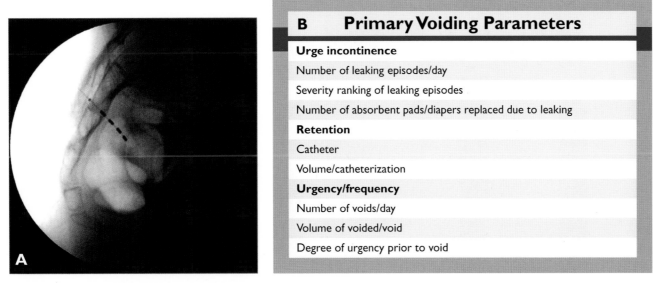

B	Primary Voiding Parameters
Urge incontinence	
Number of leaking episodes/day	
Severity ranking of leaking episodes	
Number of absorbent pads/diapers replaced due to leaking	
Retention	
Catheter	
Volume/catheterization	
Urgency/frequency	
Number of voids/day	
Volume of voided/void	
Degree of urgency prior to void	

Figure 6-60. A, Sagittal view of the quadripolar lead wire in the S3 foramen. **B,** Successful test stimulation is defined as an improvement of 50% or greater in the parameters being measured.

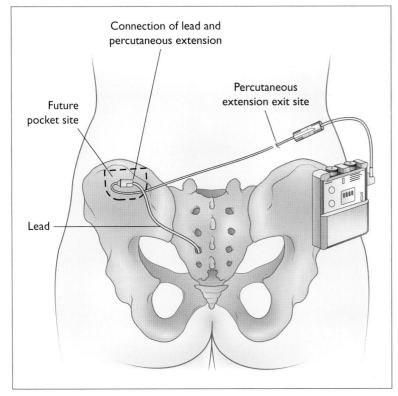

Figure 6-61. Demonstration of the tined lead in place and connected to the temporary extension for the test stimulation phase. Once the tined lead has been secured, the lead wire is tunneled to the ipsilateral posterior hip where a pocket is created in the subcutaneous tissue. The lead is then connected to a temporary extension that is tunneled to the contralateral side and exited through a small stab incision in the skin. This is then attached to the external generator for the test trial.

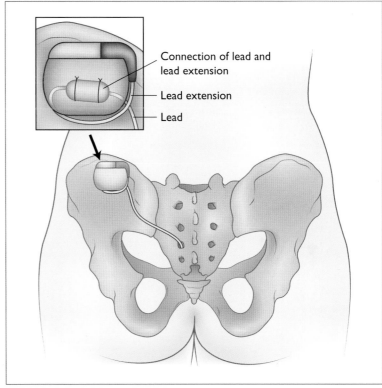

Figure 6-62. Placement of the implantable pulse generator (IPG). If the patient has a greater than 50% response to InterStim therapy (Medtronic, Minneapolis, MN) and elects to proceed, the long-term IPG will be placed into the pocket created in the posterior hip to a depth of 1.5 to 2 cm.

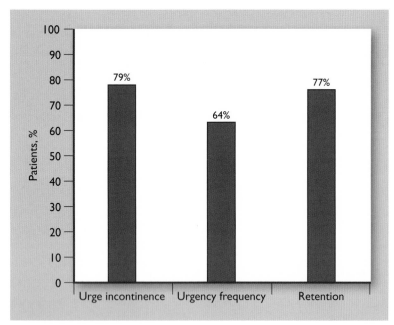 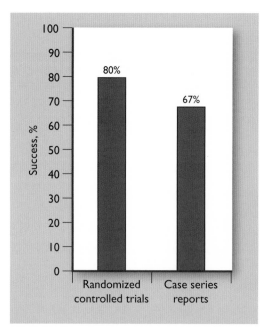

Figure 6-63. Success of InterStim therapy (Medtronic, Minneapolis, MN) for voiding dysfunction in the initial trial. Success was defined as a reduction of 50% or greater in catheterized volumes, an increase of 50% or greater in voided volumes, and a reduction of 50% or more in catheterizations. For urge incontinence, 45% were completely dry; 34% had reduction of 50% or more in leaking episodes. For urgency frequency, 31% had returned to normal voids (four to seven voids/day), and 33% had 50% or greater reduction in voids. For retention, 61% eliminated use of catheters and 16% had 50% or greater reduction in catheter volumes. (MDT-103 study, Medtronic data on file [105].)

Figure 6-64. Current literature on the success rates for urge incontinence. In an independent investigation of 1827 implants from 34 clinical trials, InterStim therapy (Medtronic, Minneapolis, MN) was shown to be an effective option for the treatment of urinary urge incontinence [106].

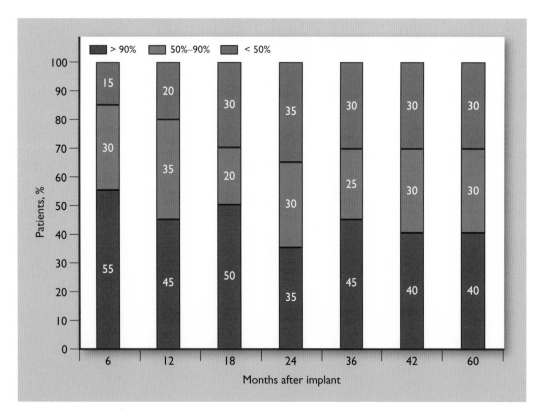

Figure 6-65. Long-term outcome of InterStim therapy (Medtronic, Minneapolis, MN) for urge incontinence. Sustained results of InterStim therapy in patients with urodynamic urge incontinence. Patients were followed for 5 years and were divided into three categories: cured (> 90% improved), improved (< 90% but > 50% improved), and failure (< 50% improved). This study demonstrates the sustained efficacy of InterStim therapy in 70% of patients in whom prior conservative and pharmacologic therapies had failed [107].

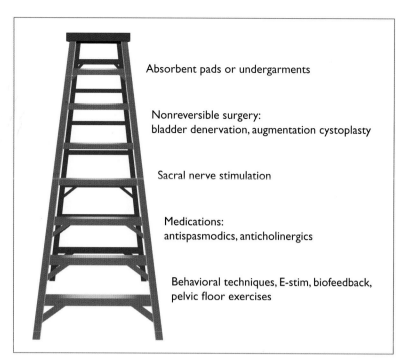

Absorbent pads or undergarments

Nonreversible surgery:
bladder denervation, augmentation cystoplasty

Sacral nerve stimulation

Medications:
antispasmodics, anticholinergics

Behavioral techniques, E-stim, biofeedback,
pelvic floor exercises

Figure 6-66. Treatment ladder for overactive bladder.
E-stim—electrical stimulation.

URINARY RETENTION

Definitions of Urinary Retention

Acute	Chronic
Painful, palpable, or percussable bladder, associated with the inability to pass urine	Nonpainful bladder that remains palpable or percussable after the patient has passed or attempted to pass urine
May be nonpainful under certain conditions (postoperative, postpartum, bulging disk, or after regional anesthesia)	Postvoid residual generally > 300 mL

Figure 6-67. 2002 International Continence Society (ICS) definitions of acute and chronic retention [2]. Patients with chronic retention may be incontinent; however, the ICS no longer recommends the term *overflow incontinence*. Chronic retention excludes transient causes of retention.

Etiologies of Urinary Retention

Pharmacologic	**Neurologic**
Tricyclic antidepressants	Central nervous system lesions
Anticholinergic agents	Multiple sclerosis
α-Adrenergic agents	Cerebrovascular disease
Ganglion blocking agent	Parkinson's disease
Inflammatory	Normal pressure hydrocephalus
Acute urethritis, cystitis, vulvovaginitis	Brain or spinal cord tumor/injury
Acute anogenital infections (herpes simplex)	Cauda equina or conus medullaris lesions
Pelvic floor spasm/tension myalgia	Spinal stenosis
Obstructive	Tabes dorsalis
Intrinsic	Multiple system atrophy (Shy–Drager syndrome)
Stenosis/fibrosis (*ie*, postradiation)	Peripheral nervous system lesions
Acute edema of the urethra (*ie*, postoperative)	Autonomic neuropathy
Foreign body	Herpes zoster
Bladder stone	Radical pelvic surgery
Extrinsic	Pelvic radiation
Pelvic mass	**Idiopathic**
Fibroid (vaginal, urethral, uterine)	Fowler's syndrome
Fecal impaction	Detrusor–sphincter dyssynergia
Entrapped cervix (retroverted uterus, gravid or nongravid)	Hypersensitive female urethra
Anterior vaginal wall prolapse	Pelvic floor hypertonicity
Uterine prolapse	**Iatrogenic**
Female circumcision with subsequent labial fusion	Post–incontinence surgery
Psychogenic	Post–prolapse surgery
Anxiety	Post–botulinum toxin or phenol injection
Depression	Post–radical hysterectomy
Hysteria	
Endocrinologic	
Diabetes	
Hypothyroiditis	

Figure 6-68. Etiologies of urinary retention. Regional anesthesia such as spinal or epidural is the most common pharmacologic cause of acute urinary retention [108]. Current use of antimuscarinics rarely leads to retention because the doses are generally too low to achieve a total blockade of the motor neurons [109]. Vulvovaginal lesions may lead to retention from edema, inflammation, or pain resulting in pelvic floor spasm and subsequent inhibition of pelvic floor relaxation. Obstruction can occur from intrinsic or extrinsic factors, with intrinsic causes being much less common in women. Psychogenic causes are usually a diagnosis of exclusion. Criteria for diagnosis include no obvious neurologic or organic disease, correlation of psychiatric symptoms to the onset of retention, and a positive response to psychotherapy or pharmacotherapy. Psychogenic varieties most commonly occur between the ages of 25 to 45 years and often follow a stressful event. Return to normal voiding occurs in the majority of cases [110,111]. Endocrinologic conditions can lead to a peripheral neuropathy resulting in altered bladder sensation and subsequent retention [112].

Among idiopathic causes, Fowler's syndrome was described in 1998 and is often seen in association with polycystic ovarian disease. Classic urethral electromyographic findings in this condition include the presence of complex repetitive discharges that have a classic "dive bomber" sound [113]. Iatrogenic factors such as postsurgical overcorrection of the bladder neck are one of the most common causes of obstructive voiding in women [114,115]. Regarding neurologic causes, voiding dysfunction manifests differently depending on the neurologic condition and/or level and degree of injury. In general, insults above the sacral micturition center result in detrusor overactivity with simultaneous contraction of the striated urethral sphincter known as detrusor–sphincter dyssynergia. Lesions below the sacral micturition center as well as peripheral lesions result in detrusor areflexia.

Symptoms of Voiding Dysfunction

Hesitancy
Slow or weak stream
Straining to void
Prolonged stream
Postvoid fullness (incomplete void)
Need for positional change to void
Double voiding

Figure 6-69. Symptoms. A detailed medical and surgical history as well as current medications (including nonprescription) should be obtained. Acute retention most often will present with pain and an inability to pass urine.

Signs of Voiding Dysfunction

Pelvic Examination	Neurologic Examination
Prolapse	Mental status
Mass	Motor and sensory of lower limbs
Infection	Reflexes
Pelvic floor spasticity	Deep tendon reflexes
	Proprioception
	Clitoral–anal reflex

Figure 6-70. Signs of voiding dysfunction. A careful neurologic, pelvic, and abdominal examination should be performed to exclude any obvious cause of retention.

Investigations

Voiding diary (frequency–volume chart)
PVR determination
Transurethral catheterization
Bladder ultrasound
Imaging studies
Urodynamics
Cystometry (simple)
Uroflowmetry
Video cystometry
Pressure voiding study
Neurodiagnostic evaluation

Figure 6-71. Investigations should be focused on the primary suspected abnormality and may include a vast array of diagnostic tests. When assessing the postvoid residual (PVR), the total voided volume should be taken into consideration. In general, it is considered normal to empty 80% of the total bladder volume.

Urodynamic Features of Retention

Delayed first sensation
Peak flow consistency < 15 mL/s and/or a postvoid residual of > 50 mL with 150 mL minimum starting bladder volume
Increased bladder capacity (acontractile states)
Detrusor pressure and compliance are generally normal except in association with fibrosis
Low or absent detrusor activity (detrusor failure)
Detrusor pressure > 50 cm H_2O (obstruction)
Upper motor neuron lesions may present with:
Hyperreflexia and reduced bladder capacity
Early first sensation and urgency
Abnormal compliance and end filling detrusor pressures

Figure 6-72. Urodynamic features of retention. For the majority of subjects, cystometry and voiding studies are generally sufficient. Occasionally, video urodynamics may be useful when high-pressure voiding is demonstrated and there is a concern about ureteral reflux. (*Adapted from* Cardozo and Staskin [111].)

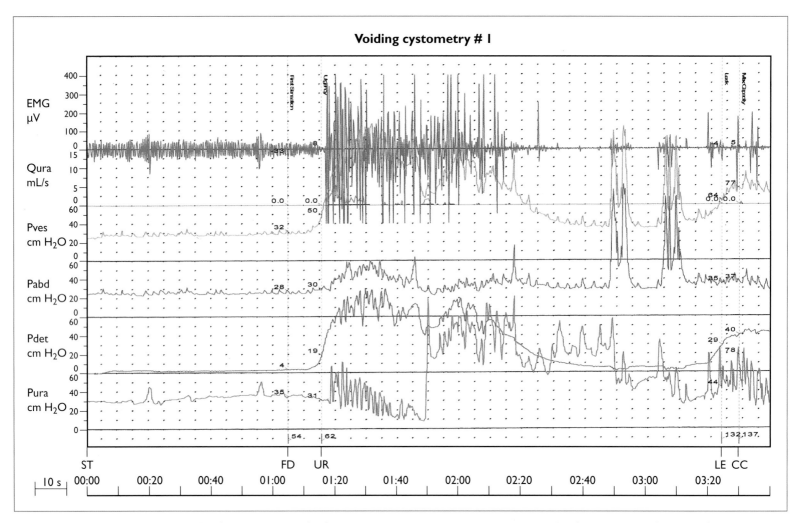

Voiding cystometry # 1

Figure 6-73. Pressure voiding study: demonstrating a high-pressure detrusor contraction during voiding. Most women can empty their bladders with detrusor pressures less than 20 cm H_2O. This detrusor contraction mounted a pressure of more than 60 cm H_2O, which increases suspicion for an obstructive process. CC—maximum cystometric capacity; EMG—electromyography; FD—first desire; LE—leak; Pabd—abdominal pressure; Pdet—detrusor pressure; Pura—urethral pressure; Pves—vesical pressure; Qura—rate of urine loss; ST—start; UR—urge.

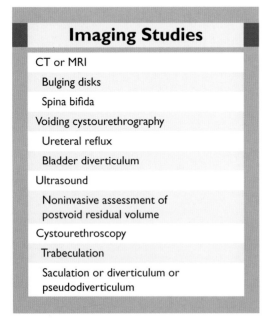

Imaging Studies

CT or MRI
  Bulging disks
  Spina bifida
Voiding cystourethrography
  Ureteral reflux
  Bladder diverticulum
Ultrasound
  Noninvasive assessment of
  postvoid residual volume
Cystourethroscopy
  Trabeculation
  Sacculation or diverticulum or
  pseudodiverticulum

Figure 6-74. Imaging studies.

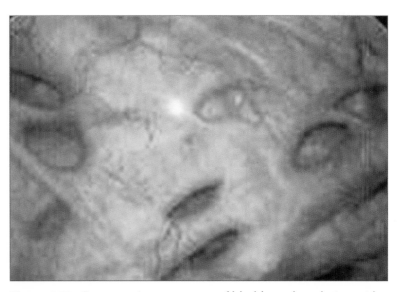

Figure 6-75. Cystoscopic appearance of bladder trabeculation with sacculation.

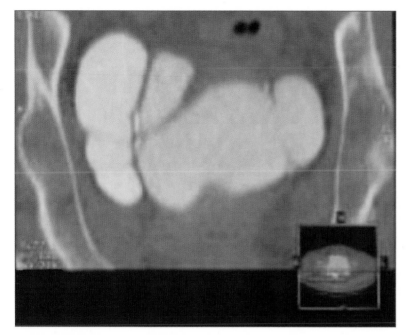

Figure 6-76. CT scan appearance of multiple bladder diverticulum as seen in coronal section. As can be appreciated from the image, bladder diverticulum can commonly be mistaken for complex pelvic masses.

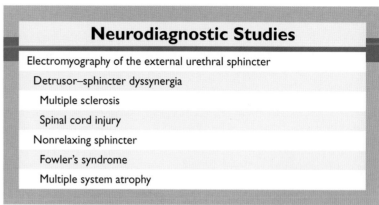

Figure 6-77. Neurodiagnostic studies. Most useful in situations of unexplained acute retention. There are two ways to approach the striated urethral sphincter, either transvaginally or transperineally. The transperineal approach has been shown to provide a higher number of motor unit action potentials versus the transvaginal approach, with equal comfort levels. Topical anesthetic is applied 20 minutes prior to the examination. A 30-gauge needle is placed at the 12 o'clock position 4 to 5 mm anterior to the urethral meatus and advanced approximately 1.5 cm [116]. A common finding in Fowler's syndrome is the presence of pseudomyotonic discharges.

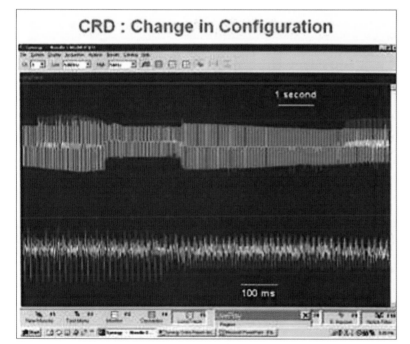

Figure 6-78. Example of an electromyographic tracing of a pseudomyotonic discharge. CRD—complex repetitive discharge.

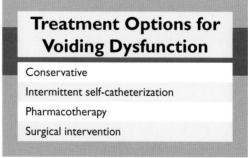

Figure 6-79. Treatment options. Anticipation of postsurgical/ postpartum retention may prevent long-term voiding dysfunction if early intervention is instituted. High-risk situations include surgery for stress incontinence and pelvic organ prolapse, radical pelvic surgery, and use of regional anesthesia [2,109,118].

Conservative Therapies

Prophylactic (acute postprocedural)

  Bladder drainage

Double voiding

Timed voiding (every 3–4 h)

Credé maneuver

  May be contraindicated in patients with evidence of ureteral reflux
  as this may cause high pressures

Pelvic floor physical therapy

  Pelvic floor hypertonic disorders

Figure 6-80. Conservative therapies. Prompt bladder drainage either with a transurethral Foley catheter or use of intermittent catheterization is essential in avoiding bladder overdistension and long-term sequelae including eventual renal compromise [118].

Intermittent Self-Catheterization

Sterile ISC

  Generally reserved for a hospital setting

Clean ISC

  Performed by the individual or caretaker

Frequency varies based on goals

  Avoid incontinence episodes

  Avoid overdistention

Figure 6-81. Introduced in 1966, intermittent self-catheterization (ISC) was used primarily in cases of neurogenic bladder [12]. It has now become the treatment of choice for chronic urinary retention. Although the idea may initially be met with some resistance by the patient, providing support and education and teaching the proper technique will often overcome any barrier [112]. In general, prophylactic antibiotics are not recommended and infections are treated as they occur.

Pharmacotherapy

Cholinergic agents

  Bethanechol

  Distigmine bromide (anticholinesterase)

α-Adrenergic blocking agents

Intravesical prostaglandin E_2 and F_2

Anxiolytic agents (diazepam)

  May be beneficial in postoperative voiding dysfunction

Figure 6-82. Pharmacotherapy. In general the uses of medications in the treatment of female urinary retention have met with disappointing results. Currently there is no evidence to support the use of any of the agents listed in the table [119–123].

Surgical Management

Urethral dilation

  Useful in stenosis (ie, postradiation)

Bladder diverticulectomy

Ureteral bulking agents or reimplantation for reflux conditions

Intraurethral botulinum toxin A injections in for DSD [124]

Chronic indwelling catheter

  Transurethral

  Suprapubic

Urinary diversion

Sacral neuromodulation

Figure 6-83. Surgical management. Surgery for obstruction should be tailored to the underlying causative factor. The role for urethral sphincterotomy is questionable given the overall poor results, high rate of incontinence, and the advent of intrinsic sphincter deficiency (DSD). Treatment of DSD from underlying neurologic disease or spinal cord injury has shown promising results [124].

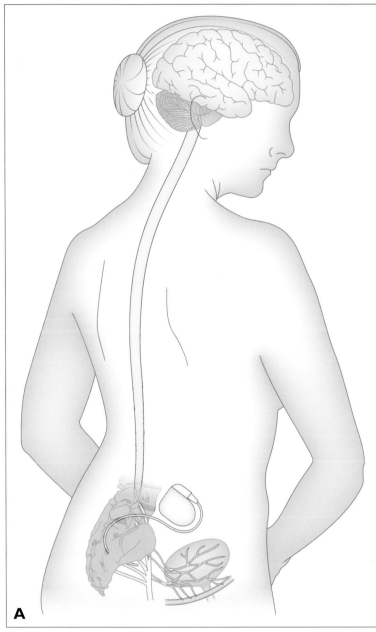

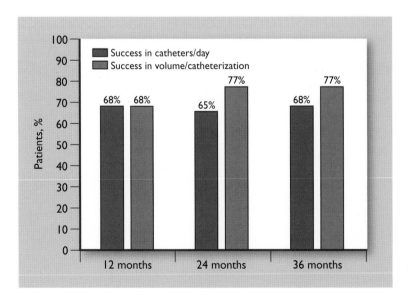

Figure 6-84. A, Sacral neuromodulation was approved by the Food and Drug Administration for the treatment of nonobstructive urinary retention in 1999. The lead is placed via a sacral foramen to lie adjacent to a sacral nerve root. This is done in an identical fashion as for the treatment of urge incontinence described earlier. **B,** Theory of the mechanism of action for facilitating voiding.

B Theory of the Mechanism of Action for Facilitating Voiding

Turn off the sphincter and urethral guarding reflex

Inhibition of the sphincter indirectly facilitates bladder activity

Help patient to relocalize the pelvic floor and regain the capability to relax it and initiate voiding

Figure 6-85. Urinary retention clinical results. This multicenter trial enrolled 177 patients with urinary retention requiring catheterization [125]. In 61% no catheterization was necessary; 16% had greater than 50% improvement in catheterized volumes. In the control group (not implanted yet or off) improvement was only 9%. Benefit was maintained at 18 months [126].

REFERENCES

1. Shull BL: Pelvic organ prolapse: anterior, superior, and posterior vaginal segment defects. *Am J Obstet Gynecol* 1999, 181:1–6.

2. Cardozo L, Staskin D: The standardization of terminology of lower urinary tract function recommended by the International Continence Society 2002. In *Textbook of Female Urology and Urogynecology*, edn 2. London: Informa Healthcare; 2006.

3. Mantle J, Versi E: Physiotherapy for stress urinary incontinence: a national survey. *BMJ* 1991, 302:753–755.

4. Kegel AH: Progressive resistance exercise in the functional restoration of the perineal muscles. *Am J Obstet Gynecol* 1948, 56:238–249.

5. Wells TJ: Pelvic (floor) muscle exercise. *J Am Geriatr Soc* 1990, 38:333–337.

6. Bump RC, Hurt WG, Fantl JA, *et al*.: Assessment of Kegel pelvic muscle exercise performance after brief verbal instruction. *Am J Obstet Gynecol* 1991, 165:322–327; discussion 327.

7. Benvenuti F, Caputo GM, Bandinelli S, *et al*.: Conservative treatment of female genuine stress incontinence. *Am J Phys Med* 1987, 66:155–168.

8. Bo K, Larsen S, Oseid S, *et al*.: Knowledge about and ability to correct pelvic floor exercises in women with urinary stress incontinence. *Neurourol Urodyn* 1988, 7:261–262.

9. Hesse U, Schuessler B, von Obernitz N, Senn E: Effectiveness of a EMG-controlled biofeedback 9 three step pelvic floor reeducation in the treatment of stress urinary incontinence: a clinical assessment. *Neurourol Urodyn* 1990, 9:397–398.

10. Bø K: Pelvic floor muscle exercise for the treatment of stress urinary incontinence: an exercise physiology perspective. *Int Urogynecol J* 1995, 6:282–289.

11. Herbison P, Plevnik S, Mantle J: Weighted vaginal cones for urinary incontinence. *Cochrane Database Syst Rev* 2002, 1:CD002114.

12. Berghmans LC, Frederiks CM, de Bie RA, *et al*.: Efficacy of biofeedback, when included with pelvic floor muscle exercise treatment, for genuine stress incontinence. *Neurourol Urodyn* 1996, 15:37–52.

13. Morkved S, Bø K, Fjortoft T: Effect of adding biofeedback to pelvic floor muscle training to treat urodynamic stress incontinence. *Obstet Gynecol* 2002, 100:730–739.

14. Goode PS, Burgio KL, Locher JL, *et al*.: Effect of behavioral training with or without pelvic floor electrical stimulation on stress incontinence in women: a randomized controlled trial. *JAMA* 2003, 290:345–352.

15. Sand PK, Richardson DA, Staskin DR, *et al*.: Pelvic floor electrical stimulation in the treatment of genuine stress incontinence: a multicenter, placebo-controlled trial. *Am J Obstet Gynecol* 1995, 173:72–79.

16. Kondo A, Yokoyama E, Koshiba K, *et al*.: Bladder neck support prosthesis: a nonoperative treatment for stress or mixed urinary incontinence. *J Urol* 1997, 157:824–827.

17. Thyssen H, Bidmead J, Lose G, *et al*.: A new intravaginal device for stress incontinence in women. *BJU Int* 2001, 88:889–892.

18. Nygaard I: Prevention of exercise incontinence with mechanical devices. *J Reprod Med* 1995, 40:89–94.

19. Cardozo L, Staskin D: Drug treatment of voiding dysfunction in women. In *Textbook of Female Urology and Urogynecology*, edn 2. London: Informa Healthcare; 2006.

20. Dmochowski RR, Miklos JR, Norton PA, *et al*., Duloxetine Urinary Incontinence Study Group: Duloxetine versus placebo for the treatment of North American women with stress urinary incontinence. *J Urol* 2003, 170(4 Pt 1):1259–1263.

21. Waetjen LE, Dwyer PL: Estrogen therapy and urinary incontinence: what is the evidence and what do we tell our patients? *Int Urogynecol J Pelvic Floor Dysfunct* 2006, 17:541–545.

22. Fantl JA, Cardozo L, McClish DK: Estrogen therapy in the management of urinary incontinence in post-menopausal women: a meta-analysis. First report of the Hormones and Urogenital Therapy Committee. *Obstet Gynecol* 1994, 83:12–18.

23. Zullo MA, Oliva C, Falconi G, *et al*.: Efficacy of estrogen therapy in urinary incontinence: a meta-analytic study [in Italian]. *Minerva Ginecol* 1998, 50:199–205.

24. Thor K, Katofiasc MA: Effects of duloxetine, a combined serotonin and norepinephrine reuptake inhibitor, on central neural control of lower urinary tract function in the chloralose-anesthetized female cat. *J Pharmacol Exp Ther* 1995, 274:1014–1024.

25. Danforth KN, Townsend MK, Lifford K, *et al*.: Risk factors for urinary incontinence among middle-aged women. *Am J Obstet Gynecol* 2006, 194:339–345.

26. Steinhauer JE, Waetjen LE, Vittinghoff E, *et al*.: Postmenopausal hormone therapy: does it cause incontinence? *Obstet Gynecol* 2005, 106(5 Pt 1):940–945.

27. Hendrix SL, Cochrane BB, Nygaard IE, *et al*.: Effects of estrogen with and without progestin on urinary incontinence. *JAMA* 2005, 293:935–948.

28. Góes VR, Sartori MG, Baracat EC, *et al*.: Urodynamic and clinical evaluation of postmenopausal women with stress urinary incontinence before and after cyclic estrogen therapy. *Clin Exp Obstet Gynecol* 2003, 30:103–106.

29. Rud T: The effects of estrogens and gestagens on the urethral pressure profile in urinary continent and stress incontinent women. *Acta Obstet Gynecol Scand* 1980, 59:265–270.

30. Sartori MG, Baracat EC, Girão MJ, *et al*.: Menopausal genuine stress urinary incontinence treated with conjugated estrogens plus progestogens. *Int J Gynecol Obstet* 1995, 49:165–169.

31. Suzuki Y, Oishi Y, Yamazaki H, *et al*.: A study of the clinical effect of hormone replacement therapy for patients with stress incontinence [in Japanese]. *Jpn J Urol* 1997, 88:427–433.

32. Mäkinen JI, Pitkänen YA, Salmi TA, *et al*.: Transdermal estrogen for female stress urinary incontinence in postmenopause. *Maturitas* 1995, 22:233–238.

33. Wilson PD, Faragher B, Butler B, *et al*.: Treatment with oral piperazine oestrone sulphate for genuine stress incontinence in postmenopausal women. *Br J Obstet Gynaecol* 1987, 94:568–574.

34. Jackson S, Shepard, A, Brooks S, Abrams P: The effect of oestrogen supplementation on post-menopausal urinary stress incontinence: a double-blind placebo-controlled trial. *Br J Obstet Gynaecol* 1999, 106:711–778.

35. Fantl JA, Bump RC, Robinson D, *et al*.: Efficacy of estrogen supplementation in the treatment of urinary incontinence. The Continence Program for Women Research Group. *Obstet Gynecol* 1996, 88:745–749.

36. Grady D, Brown JS, Vittinghoff E, *et al*.: Postmenopausal hormones and incontinence: the Heart and Estrogen/Progestin Replacement Study. *Obstet Gynecol* 2001, 97:116–120.

37. Bhatia NN, Bergman A, Karram MM: Effects of estrogen on urethral function in women with urinary incontinence. *Am J Obstet Gynecol* 1989, 160:176–181.

38. Hilton P, Stanton SL: The use of intravaginal oestrogen cream in genuine stress incontinence. *Br J Obstet Gynaecol* 1983, 90:940–904.

39. Schmid-Bauer CP: Vaginal estriol administration in treatment of postmenopausal urinary incontinence [in German]. *Urologe A* 1992, 31:384–389.

40. Schär G, Köchli OR, Fritz M, *et al*.: Effect of vaginal estrogen therapy on urinary incontinence in postmenopause [in German]. *Zentralbl Gynakol* 1995, 117:77–80.

41. Cardozo L, Lose G, McClish D, *et al*.: A systematic review of the effects of estrogens for symptoms suggestive of overactive bladder. *Acta Obstet Gynecol Scand* 2004, 83:892–897.

42. Dessole S, Rubbatu G, Ambrosini G, *et al*.: Efficacy of low-dose intravaginal estriol on urogenital aging in postmenopausal women. *Menopause* 2004, 11:49–56.

43. Sacco F, Rigon G, Carbone A, *et al*.: Transvaginal estrogen therapy in urinary stress incontinence [in Italian]. *Minerva Ginecol* 1990, 42:539–544.

44. Lehtonen T, Rannikko S, Lindell O, et al.: The effect of phenylpropanolamine on female stress urinary incontinence. Ann Chir Gynaecol 1986, 75:236–241.

45. Alhasso A, Glazener CM, Pickard R, N'dow J: Adrenergic drugs for urinary incontinence in adults. Cochrane Database Syst Rev 2005, 20:CD001842.

46. Lui HH, Sheu BC, Lo MC, Huang SC: Comparison of treatment outcomes for imipramine for female genuine stress incontinence. Br J Obstet Gynaecol 1999, 106:1089–1092.

47. Norton PA, Zinner NR, Yalcin I, Bump RC, Duloxetine Urinary Incontinence Study Group: Duloxetine versus placebo in the treatment of stress urinary incontinence. Am J Obstet Gynecol 2002, 187:40–48.

48. Cardozo L, Staskin D: Urethral injections for incontinence. In Textbook of Female Urology and Urogynecology, edn 2. London: Informa Healthcare; 2006.

49. Corcos J, Fournier C: Periurethral collagen injection for the treatment of female stress urinary incontinence: 4-year follow-up results. Urology 1999, 54:815–818.

50. Mayer R, Lightfoot M, Jung I: Preliminary evaluation of calcium hydroxylapatite as a transurethral bulking agent for stress urinary incontinence. Urology 2001, 57:434–438.

51. Chapple CR, Haab F, Cervigni M, et al.: An open, multicentre study of NASHA/Dx Gel (Zuidex) for the treatment of stress urinary incontinence. Eur Urol 2005, 48:488–494.

52. Appell RA, Juma S, Wells WG, et al.: Transurethral radiofrequency energy collagen micro-remodeling for the treatment of female stress urinary incontinence. Neurourol Urodyn 2006, 25:331–336.

53. Baggish MS, Karram MM: Atlas of Pelvic Anatomy and Gynecologic Surgery, edn 2. Philadelphia: Elsevier Saunders; 2006.

54. Cardozo L: Abdominal and transvaginal colpourethropexies for stress urinary incontinence. In Textbook of Female Urology and Urogynecology, edn 2. London: Informa Healthcare; 2006.

55. Bergman A, Elia G: Three surgical procedures for genuine stress incontinence: five-year follow-up of a prospective randomized study. Am J Obstet Gynecol 1995, 173:66–71.

56. Sand PK, Bowen LW, Panganiban R, Ostergard DR: The low pressure urethra as a factor in failed retropubic urethropexy. Obstet Gynecol 1987, 69:399–402.

57. Brubaker L, Cundiff GW, Fine P, et al., Pelvic Floor Disorders Network: Abdominal sacrocolpopexy with Burch colposuspension to reduce urinary stress incontinence. N Engl J Med 2006, 354:1557–1566.

58. Cardozo L: An overview of pubovaginal slings: evolution of technology. In Textbook of Female Urology and Urogynecology, edn 2. London: Informa Healthcare; 2006.

59. Wadie BS, Edwan A, Nabeeh AM: Autologous fascial sling vs polypropylene tape at short-term followup: a prospective randomized study. J Urol 2005, 174:990–993.

60. Abdel-Fattah M, Barrington JW, Arunkalaivanan AS: Pelvicol pubovaginal sling versus tension-free vaginal tape for treatment of urodynamic stress incontinence: a prospective randomized three-year follow-up study. Eur Urol 2004, 46:629–635.

61. Petros P, Henriksson L, Johnson P, Varhos G: An ambulatory surgical procedure under local anesthesia for the treatment of female urinary incontinence. Int Urogynecol J 1996, 7:81–86.

62. Nilsson CG, Falconer C, Rezapour M: Seven-year follow-up of the tension-free vaginal tape procedure for treatment of urinary incontinence. Obstet Gynecol 2004, 104:1259–1262.

63. Rezapour M, Falconer C, Ulmsten U: Tension-free vaginal tape (TVT) in stress incontinent women with intrinsic sphincter deficiency (ISD): a long-term follow-up. Int Urogynecol J 2001, 12(Suppl 2):S12–S14.

64. Rardin C, Kohli N, Rosenblatt P, et al.: Tension-free vaginal tape: outcomes among women with primary versus recurrent stress urinary incontinence. Obstet Gynecol 2002, 100:893–897.

65. Krauth JS, Rasoamiaramanana H, Barletta H, et al.: Sub-urethral tape treatment of female urinary incontinence: morbidity assessment of the trans-obturator route and a new tape (I-STOP): a multi-centre experiment involving 604 cases. Eur Urol 2005, 47:102–106.

66. Delorme E, Droupy S, de Tayrac R, Delmas V: Transobturator tape (Uratape): a new minimally-invasive procedure to treat female urinary incontinence. Eur Urol 2004, 45:203–207.

67. Latthe P, Foon R, Toozs-Hobson P: Transobturator and retropubic tape procedures in stress urinary incontinence: a systematic review and meta-analysis of effectiveness and complications. BJOG 2007, 114:522–531.

68. Miller JJ, Botros SM, Akl MN, et al.: Is transobturator tape as effective as tension-free vaginal tape in patients with borderline maximum urethral closure pressure? Am J Obstet Gynecol 2006, 195:1799–1804.

69. Ward KL, Hilton P, UK and Ireland TVT Trial Group: A prospective multi-center randomized trial of tension-free vaginal tape and colposuspension for primary urodynamic stress incontinence: two-year follow-up. Am J Obstet Gynecol 2004, 190:324–331.

70. de Tayrac R, Defieux X, Droupy S, et al.: A prospective randomized trial comparing tension-free vaginal tape and transobturator suburethral tape for surgical treatment of stress urinary incontinence. Am J Obstet Gynecol 2004, 190:602–608. [Retraction in: Am J Obstet Gynecol 2005, 192:339.]

71. Andonian S, Chen T, St.-Denis B, Corcos J: Randomized clinical trial comparing suprapubic arch sling (SPARC) and tension-free vaginal tape (TVT): one-year results. Eur Urol 2005, 47:537–541.

72. Palma PC, Riccetto CL, Dambros M, et al.: SAFYRE: 1 new concept for adjustable minimally invasive sling for female urinary stress incontinence [in Spanish]. Actas Urol Esp 2004, 28:749–755.

73. Roth CC, Holley TD, Winters JC: Synthetic slings: which material, which approach. Curr Opin Urol 2006, 16:234–239.

74. Amrute KV, Badlani GH: Female incontinence: a review of biomaterials and minimally invasive techniques. Curr Opin Urol 2006, 16:54–59.

75. de Tayrac R, Deffieux X, Resten A, et al.: A transvaginal ultrasound study comparing transobturator tape and tension-free vaginal tape after surgical treatment of female stress urinary incontinence. Int Urogynecol J Pelvic Floor Dysfunct 2006, 17:466–471.

76. Bhargava S, Chapple CR: Rising awareness of the complications of synthetic slings. Curr Opin Urol 2004, 14:317–321.

77. Stewart WF, Van Rooyen JB, Cundiff GW, et al.: Prevalence and burden of overactive bladder in the United States. World J Urol 2003, 20:327–336.

78. Brown JS, McGhan WF, Chokroverty S: Comorbidities associated with overactive bladder. Am J Manage Care 2000, 6(11 Suppl):S574–S579.

79. Brown JS, Subak LL, Gras J, et al.: Urge incontinence: the patient's perspective. J Womens Health 1998, 7:1263–1269.

80. Abrams P, Kelleher CJ, Kerr LA, et al.: Overactive bladder significantly affects quality of life. Am J Manage Care 2000, 6(11 Suppl):S580–S590.

81. Cardozo L: Outcomes of conservative treatment. In Textbook of Female Urology and Urogynecology, edn 2. London: Informa Healthcare; 2006.

82. Dallosso HM, McGrother CW, Matthews RJ, Donaldson MM, Leicestershire MRC Incontinence Study Group: The association of diet and other lifestyle factors with overactive bladder and stress incontinence: a longitudinal study in women. BJU Int 2003, 92:69–77.

83. Wallace SA, Roe B, Williams K, Palmer M: Bladder training for urinary incontinence in adults. Cochrane Database Syst Rev 2004, 1:CD001308. DOI: 10.1002/14651858.CD001308.pub2.

84. Garely A: Nondrug therapy options for overactive bladder. Contemp Obstet Gynecol (Suppl) 2005, Sept 1:5–7.

85. Burgio KL, Goode PS, Locher JL, et al.: Behavioral training with and without biofeedback in the treatment of urge incontinence in older women: a randomized controlled trial. JAMA 2002, 288:2293–2299.

86. Brubaker L, Benson JT, Bent A, et al.: Transvaginal electrical stimulation for female urinary incontinence. Am J Obstet Gynecol 1997, 177:536–540.

87. Yamanishi T, Yasuda K, Sakakibara R, et al.: Randomized, double-blind study of electrical stimulation for urinary incontinence due to detrusor overactivity. Urology 2000, 55:353–357.

88. Haab F, Corcos J, Siami P, et al.: Long-term treatment with darifenacin for overactive bladder: results of a 2-year, open-label extension study. BJU Int 2006, 98:1025–1032.

89. Appell RA, Sand P, Dmochowski R, *et al.*, Overactive Bladder: Judging Effective Control and Treatment Study Group: Prospective randomized controlled trial of extended-release oxybutynin chloride and tolterodine tartrate in the treatment of overactive bladder: results of the OBJECT Study. *Mayo Clin Proc* 2001, 76:358–363.

90. Diokno AC, Appell RA, Sand PK, *et al.*, OPERA Study Group: Prospective, randomized, double-blind study of the efficacy and tolerability of the extended-release formulations of oxybutynin and tolterodine for overactive bladder: results of the OPERA trial. *Mayo Clin Proc* 2003, 78:687–695.

91. Sussman D, Garely A: Treatment of overactive bladder with once-daily extended-release tolterodine or oxybutynin: the Antimuscarinic Clinical Effectiveness Trial (ACET). *Curr Med Res Opin* 2002, 18:177–184.

92. Chapple CR, Martinez-Garcia R, Selvaggi L, *et al.*, STAR Study Group: A comparison of the efficacy and tolerability of solifenacin succinate and extended release tolterodine at treating overactive bladder syndrome: results of the STAR trial. *Eur Urol* 2005, 48:464–470.

93. Chapple CR, Abrams P: Comparison of darifenacin and oxybutynin in patients with overactive bladder: assessment of ambulatory urodynamics and impact on salivary flow. *Eur Urol* 2005, 48:102–109.

94. Emmons SL, Otto L: Acupuncture for overactive bladder: a randomized controlled trial. *Obstet Gynecol* 2005, 106:138–143.

95. Rosales RL, Arimura RK, Ikenaga S, *et al.*: Extrafusal and intrafusal muscle effects in experimental botulinum toxin A injection. *Muscle Nerve* 1996, 19:488–496.

96. Filippi GM, Ericco P, SantarelliR, *et al.*: Botulinum A toxin effects on rat jaw muscles spindles. *Acta Otolaryngol* 1993, 113:400–404.

97. Mahajan ST, Brubaker L: Botulinum toxin: from life-threatening disease to novel medical therapy. *Am J Obstet Gynecol* 2007, 196:7–15.

98. Werner M, Schmid DM, Schüssler B: Efficacy of botulinum-A toxin in the treatment of detrusor overactivity incontinence: a prospective nonrandomized study. *Am J Obstet Gynecol* 2005, 192:1735–1740.

99. Schmid DM, Sauermann P, Werner M, *et al.*: Experience with 100 cases treated with botulinum-A toxin injections in the detrusor muscle for idiopathic overactive bladder syndrome refractory to anticholinergics. *J Urol* 2006, 176:177–185.

100. Kuo HC: Effectiveness of intravesical resiniferatoxin in treating detrusor hyper-reflexia and external sphincter dyssynergia in patients with chronic spinal cord lesions. *BJU Int* 2003, 92:597–601.

101. de Seze M, Wiart L, de Seze MP, *et al.*: Intravesical capsaicin versus resiniferatoxin for the treatment of detrusor hyperreflexia in spinal cord injured patients: a double-blind, randomized, controlled trial. *J Urol* 2004, 171:251–255.

102. van Balken MR, Vergunst H, Bemelmans BL: Prognostic factors for successful percutaneous tibial nerve stimulation. *Eur Urol* 2006, 49:360–365.

103. van der Pal F, van Balken MR, Heesakkers JP, *et al.*: Percutaneous tibial nerve stimulation in the treatment of refractory overactive bladder syndrome: is maintenance treatment necessary? *BJU Int* 2006, 97:547–550.

104. Cohen BL, Tunuguntla HS, Gousse A: Predictors of success for first stage neuromodulation: motor versus sensory. *J Urol* 2006, 175:2178–2180.

105. MDT-103 Study, Medtronic data on file.

106. Brazelli M, Murray A, Fraser C: Efficacy and safety of sacral nerve stimulation for the treatment of urinary urge incontinence: a systematic review. *J Urol* 2006, 175:835–841.

107. Bosch J, Groen J: Sacral nerve neuromodulation in the treatment of patients with refractory motor urge incontinence: long-term results of a prospective longitudinal study. *J Urol* 2000, 163:1219–1222.

108. Weiniger CF, Wand S, Nadjari M, *et al.*: Postvoid residual volume in labor: a prospective study comparing parturients with and without epidural anesthesia. *Acta Anaesthesiol Scand* 2006, 50:1297–1303.

109. Andersson KE, Yoshida M: Antimuscarinic and the overactive bladder: which is the main mechanism of action? *Eur Urol* 2003, 1:1–5.

110. Barrett DM: Evaluation of psychogenic urinary retention. *J Urol* 1978, 120:191.

111. Cardozo L, Staskin D: Non-neurogenic voiding difficulty and retention. In *Textbook of Female Urology and Urogynecology*, edn 2. London: Informa Healthcare; 2006.

112. Yu HJ, Chia LW, Ping LS, *et al.*: Unrecognized voiding difficulty in female type 2 diabetic patients in the diabetic clinic: a prospective case control study. *Diabetes Care* 2004, 27:988–989.

113. Fowler CJ, Christmas TJ, Chapple CR, *et al.*: Abnormal electromyographic activity of the urethral sphincter, voiding dysfunction, and polycystic ovaries: a new syndrome? *BMJ* 1998, 297:1436–1438.

114. Smith RW, Cardozo L: Early voiding difficulty after colposuspension. *Br J Urol* 1997, 80:911–914.

115. Kuura N, Nilsson CG: A nationwide analysis of complications associated with the tension-free vaginal tape (TVT) procedure. *Acta Obstet Gynecol Scand* 2002, 81:72–77.

116. Olsen A, Benson JT, McClellan E: Urethral sphincter needle electromyography in women: comparison of periurethral and transvaginal approaches. *Neurourol Urodyn* 1998, 17:531–535.

117. Smith PH, Turnbull GA, Currie DW, Peel KR: The urological complications of Wertheim's hysterectomy. *Br J Urol* 1969, 41:685–688.

118. Gutman L, Frankel H: The value of intermittent self catheterization in the early management of traumatic paraplegia and tetraplegia. *Paraplegia* 1966, 4:63–84.

119. Cameron MD: Distigmine bromide in the prevention of post-operative retention of urine. *J Obstet Gynaecol Br Commonw* 1966, 73:847–848.

120. Delaere KPJ, Thomas CMG, Moorer WA, Debbrycine FMJ: The value of intravesical prostaglandin E2 and F2 alpha in women with abnormalities of bladder emptying. *Br J Urol* 1981, 53:306–309.

121. Tammela T, Kontturi M, Kaar K, Lukkarinen O: Intravesical prostaglandin F2 for promoting bladder emptying after surgery for female stress incontinence. *Br J Urol* 1987, 60:43–46.

122. Barrett DM: The effect of oral bethanechol chloride on voiding in female patients with excessive residual urine: a randomized double blind study. *J Urol* 1981, 126:640–642.

123. Philip NH, Thomas DG, Clarke SJ: Drug effects on the voiding cystometrogram: a comparison of oral bethanecol and carbachol. *Br J Urol* 1980, 52:484–487.

124. Kuo HC: Botulinum A toxin urethral injection for the treatment of lower urinary tract dysfunction. *J Urol* 2003, 170:1908–1912.

125. Jonas U, Fowler CJ, Chancellor MB, *et al.*: Efficacy of sacral nerve stimulation for urinary retention: results 18 months after implantation. *J Urol* 2001, 165:15–19.

126. Medtronic postapproval trial, Medtronic data on file.

7

Evaluation of Fecal Incontinence and Constipation

Dee Fenner and Christina Lewicky-Gaupp

Fecal incontinence is the inability to defer the elimination of stool or gas until there is a socially acceptable time and place to do so. Because maintaining fecal continence is a complex physiologic process that requires a person's ability to perceive the type of fecal bolus, store or retain when necessary, and excrete when desirable, the loss of that ability is equally as complex. Fecal continence requires normal stool consistency and volume, normal colonic transit time, a compliant rectum, innervation of the pelvic floor and the anal sphincters, and the interplay between the puborectalis muscle, rectum, and anal sphincters [1]. Loss of one or more of these abilities can lead to fecal incontinence.

Fecal incontinence can be socially debilitating for the patient. The emotional and psychological impact on the quality of life can be devastating for the patient and her family. In the evaluation of fecal incontinence, the physician and patient must communicate sufficiently to have a clear understanding of the patient's symptoms, including loss of flatus or stool, frequency of incontinence, and impact on the quality of the patient's life. Evaluation and treatment should be based on the severity of the patient's symptoms.

The estimated prevalence of fecal incontinence ranges from 1.3% to 11% in women older than 64 years of age. More than 30% of women reporting urinary incontinence also report fecal incontinence or dual incontinence [2–7].

The most common cause of fecal incontinence in women is damage to the anal sphincters at the time of vaginal delivery with or without neuronal injury. Damage can occur by mechanical disruption or separation of the internal anal sphincter or external anal sphincter or by damage to the muscle innervation by stretching or crushing the pudendal and pelvic nerves. Sultan *et al.* [8] showed that 13% of primiparas and 23% of multiparas developed fecal incontinence or fecal urgency postpartum. By anal ultrasound, all but one woman had evidence of anal sphincter disruption. The chance of muscular injury is increased with midline episiotomy, forceps delivery, and vaginal delivery of larger infants. Not all risk factors are known and not all women are susceptible to pelvic floor damage. Further study is needed to accurately predict which women are at risk.

Evaluation of fecal incontinence should include history, physical examination, prior treatment, and proposed therapy. In addition, certain tests, such as nerve conductance studies, may be helpful in counseling patients before surgical therapy in terms of expected outcomes.

Unlike fecal incontinence, constipation is extremely common in the general population and accounts for 2.5 million physician visits annually in the United States [9]. Estimates of the prevalence of constipation range from 2% to 27% [10,11]. Various risk factors for constipation have been identified and include a history of sexual abuse, depression, and low income [12]. Constipation increases with age [13], and women are more commonly affected than men. Thus it becomes important for obstetricians, gynecologists, and urogynecologists to be familiar with the condition.

The definition of constipation can vary; however, it has recently been redefined by the Rome Foundation (Figure 4-1). Constipation can be classified into three categories: normal-transit, slow-transit, and disorders of defecatory or rectal evacuation. It is important to differentiate the type of constipation a patient has because treatment options can vary. Normal-transit constipation is the most common form of constipation. Patients complain of infrequent and hard stools as well as abdominal bloating and pain. The cause is often related to a poor diet that lacks fiber and is low in fluid intake. The cause of slow-transit constipation, conversely, is likely secondary to colonic inertia, which is demonstrated with delayed passage of radiopaque markers through the colon. These patients also complain of infrequent bowel movements, abdominal bloating, and pain but also demonstrate a blunted response to cholinergic agents [14]. Lastly, patients with disorders of defecatory or rectal evacuation must be considered. Normal defecation involves the coordinated relaxation of the puborectalis muscle and anal sphincter in response to increases in rectal pressure (*eg*, with straining). In patients with this type of constipation, puborectalis dyssynergia can be seen; this is a paradoxical contraction of the puborectalis muscle that occurs with straining, thus blocking the outlet. Also, patients with posterior vaginal wall prolapse and symptoms of obstructed defecation may have trapping of stool within a rectocele pocket and thus present with similar symptoms (complaints of a feeling of incomplete rectal emptying or needing to splint in order to have a bowel movement).

Evaluation of constipation begins with a thorough history and physical examination. If a metabolic cause is suspected, laboratory tests including electrolyte studies, thyroid function tests, and a complete blood count can be helpful. Flexible sigmoidoscopy or colonoscopy or a barium enema are recommended if the screening time is appropriate or symptoms are suggestive of an anatomic lesion or stricture. Other anatomic studies can include defecography if, for example, puborectalis dyssynergia is suspected. If slow-transit constipation is suspected, colonic transit times should be determined (normal transit time < 72 hours) and anorectal manometry performed with a balloon expulsion test [15]. Because treatment options are targeted to the varying pathophysiologies of constipation, it is important to differentiate which type of constipation is present with the above measures.

CAUSES OF FECAL INCONTINENCE

Rome III Criteria for Functional Gastrointestinal Disorders

IBS	At least 3 months, with onset at least 6 months prior to diagnosis of recurrent abdominal pain or discomfort associated with ≥ 2 of the following: 1. Improved with defecation and/or 2. Onset associated with a change in the frequency of stool and/or 3. Onset associated with a change in form (appearance) of stool
Functional constipation	≥ 3 days/month in past 3 months with onset at least 6 months prior to diagnosis with ≥ 2 of the following: 1. Straining ≥ ¼ of defecations 2. Lumpy or hard stools ≥ ¼ defecations 3. Sensation of incomplete evacuation ≥ ¼ defecations 4. Sensation of anorectal obstruction/blockage ≥ ¼ defecations 5. Manual maneuvers to facilitate ≥ ¼ defecations and/or 6. < 3 defecations per week Insufficient criteria for IBS Loose stools rarely present without use of laxatives
Functional diarrhea	At least 3 months, with onset at least 6 months prior to diagnosis of: 1. Loose or watery stools; 2. Present > ¾ time; and 3. No abdominal pain
Functional fecal incontinence	Uncontrolled passage of fecal material for ≥ 3 months, in an individual with a developmental age of ≥ 4 years, associated with: 1. Abnormal functioning of normally innervated and structurally intact muscles 2. Minor abnormalities of sphincter structure and/or innervation and/or 3. Normal or disordered bowel habits (fecal retention or diarrhea) and/or 4. Psychological causes *and* Exclusion of all of the following: abnormal innervation caused by spinal cord lesions, CNS lesions, autonomic neuropathies, anal sphincter abnormalities associated with a multisystem disease, structural or neurologic abnormalities believed to be the major or primary cause of fecal incontinence
Levator ani syndrome	At least 3 months, with onset at least 6 months prior to diagnosis of: 1. Chronic or recurrent rectal pain or aching; and 2. Episodes last ≥ 20 minutes; and 3. Other causes of rectal pain such as inflammatory bowel disease, cryptitis, fissure, hemorrhoids have been excluded 4. Tenderness with posterior traction on puborectalis
Dyssynergic defecation	Patient must satisfy diagnostic criteria for functional constipation During repeated attempts to defecate, must have ≥ 2 of the following: 1. Manometric, EMG, or radiologic evidence for inappropriate contraction of the pelvic floor muscles or < 20% relaxation of basal resting sphincter pressure and/or 2. Inadequate propulsive forces on manometry or imaging and/or 3. Incomplete evacuation based on imaging or balloon expulsion

Figure 7-1. Rome III criteria for functional gastrointestinal disorders [16]. CNS—central nervous system; EMG—electromyography; IBS—irritable bowel syndrome.

Common Causes of Fecal Incontinence

Pathology outside the pelvis

Diarrheal states

  Infectious diarrhea

  Irritable bowel syndrome

  Inflammatory bowel disease

  Short-gut syndrome

  Bacterial overgrowth (common in cases of diabetic gastroparesis)

  Laxative abuse

  Radiation enteritis

  Carcinoid tumor

  Malabsorption

Neurologic diseases

  Congenital anomalies (*eg*, myelomeningocele)

  Multiple sclerosis

  Diabetic neuropathy

  Neoplasms or injury of the brain, spinal cord, or cauda equina

  Scleroderma (reduced rectal compliance)

Pathology inside the pelvis

Obstetric injury

  Disruption of internal anal sphincter

  Disruption of external anal sphincter

  Pelvic floor/anal sphincter denervation

Trauma

  Pelvic fracture

  Anorectal surgery

  Anal intercourse

  Rectovaginal fistula

Rectal neoplasia

Rectal prolapse

Rectocele/perineocele

Hemorrhoids

Overflow

  Impaction

  Encopresis

Figure 7-2. Common causes of fecal incontinence.

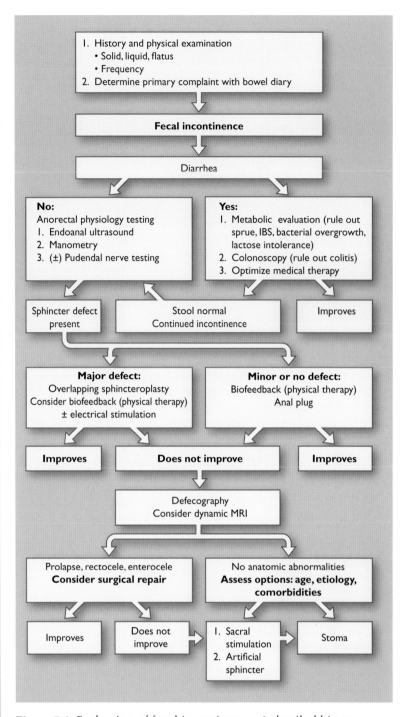

Figure 7-3. Evaluation of fecal incontinence. A detailed history differentiates incontinence of gas, liquid, or solid stool along with frequency, onset, and progression of symptoms. The effect of symptoms on the patient's quality of life should also be examined with a validated questionnaire such as the FIQ-L (Fecal Incontinence Quality of Life) [17]. A history of antecedent anorectal or gynecologic surgery should be obtained as well as a detailed obstetric history including the type of delivery, weight of largest infant, length of second stage of labor, episiotomy, and use of vacuum or forceps. The presence or absence of the sensation of a need to defecate should be elicited to assess for the possibility of neurologic diseases such as multiple sclerosis. Rectal examination should assess resting and squeeze tone, presence of a rectocele or mass, and fecal impaction. Inspection of the rectum and vagina should evaluate for a rectovaginal fistula, prolapsing hemorrhoids, or rectal prolapse. Further evaluation, including radiologic and physiologic tests, has been shown in a prospective study at a tertiary colorectal referral clinic to alter the final diagnosis of the cause of fecal incontinence in 19% of cases [18]. IBS—irritable bowel syndrome.

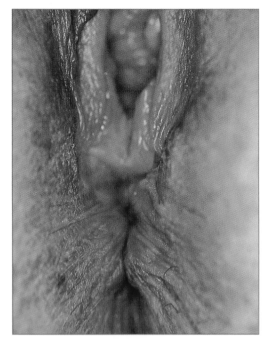

Figure 7-4. Perineum with chronic laceration of external anal sphincter (EAS). Inspection of the perineum shows the classic "dovetail" sign with loss of the anal skin creases anteriorly due to a chronic third-degree laceration of the EAS. Normally, with an intact sphincter, the skin creases are arranged radially around the anus.

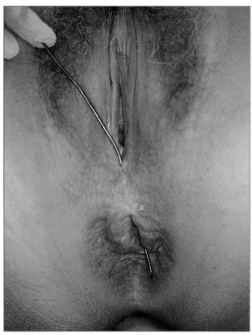

Figure 7-5. Rectovaginal fistula. A rectovaginal fistula should be considered in a patient who has had a recent vaginal delivery with or without known lacerations, a recent pelvic surgery, or a history of inflammatory bowel disease. Patients generally report a constant stool drainage or vaginal discharge. Anal sphincter injuries are commonly found in conjunction with fistulas, so the entire sphincter mechanism should be fully evaluated before a surgical repair is attempted.

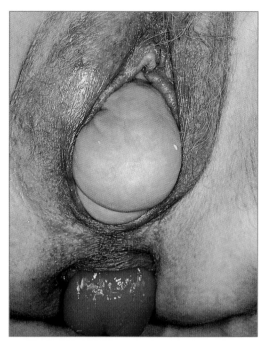

Figure 7-6. Rectal prolapse. Rectal prolapse is accompanied by fecal incontinence in 40% to 60% of patients and may be due to stretching of either the internal anal sphincter by the prolapse or the pudendal nerves as a consequence of chronic straining and perineal descent. Following prolapse repair, continence improves in about 50% of patients [19]. This patient also has vaginal vault prolapse, commonly seen in conjunction with rectal prolapse due to straining and loss of pelvic floor function.

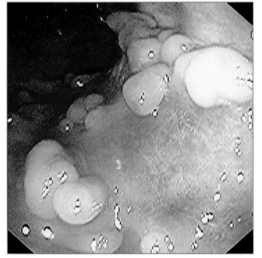

Figure 7-7. Crohn's disease. Crohn's disease on colonoscopy shows areas of normal bowel with pseudopolyps from chronic inflammation. The severity of incontinence from chronic diarrhea resulting from inflammatory bowel disease or irritable bowel syndrome is dependent on anal sphincter function and rectal compliance. If the rectum is diseased from Crohn's proctitis, rectal compliance and storage capability are reduced, causing fecal urgency, soilage, and incontinence. Prior anal surgery and fistulas can also impair sphincter function.

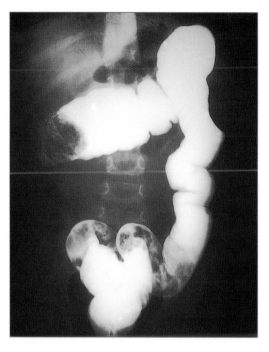

Figure 7-8. Intussusception of the proximal transverse colon on barium enema. This patient presented with intermittent abdominal pain, diarrhea, and fecal incontinence. Fecal incontinence is secondary to the bowel spasm and liquid stool that "overcomes" the anal sphincter. Patients with a weakened or shortened anal sphincter may become incontinent only to liquid stool.

DIAGNOSTIC METHODS

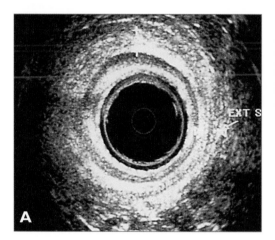
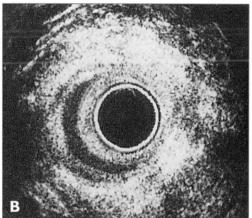
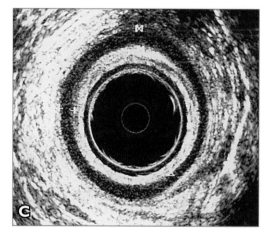

Figure 7-9. Anal ultrasound. **A**, Anal ultrasound has significantly enhanced the ability to delineate defects of both the internal and external anal sphincters. The internal anal sphincter is visible as a hypoechoic circle and the external anal sphincter is seen as a hyperechoic circle. Scarred areas have a homogeneous, gray appearance. **B**, With the patient lying on her left side, a defect in both the internal and external anal sphincters is seen at the 3 o'clock position. This injury is the result of a difficult vaginal delivery. **C**, With the vagina again at the 3 o'clock position, there is an intact internal anal sphincter and a defect in the external anal sphincter.

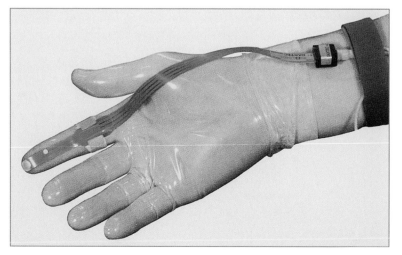

Figure 7-10. St. Mark's electrode. Neurophysiologic testing for evaluation of fecal incontinence can include pudendal nerve terminal motor latencies (PNTMLs) and needle electromyography. Pictured is a St. Mark's electrode used to stimulate the pudendal nerve at the level of the ischial spine, transrectally or transvaginally, and to record the response at the anal sphincter. This test evaluates the neuromuscular function of the anal sphincter. Prolonged PNTML can be found in patients with idiopathic fecal incontinence and after vaginal delivery or pelvic surgery. Pudendal neuropathy may predict continence after surgeries for rectal prolapse and sphincter lacerations. Laurberg *et al*. [20] noted that eight of 10 patients with normal PNTML findings had excellent or good results after a sphincteroplasty and only one of nine patients with abnormal PNTML findings had good results after a sphincteroplasty for obstetric trauma.

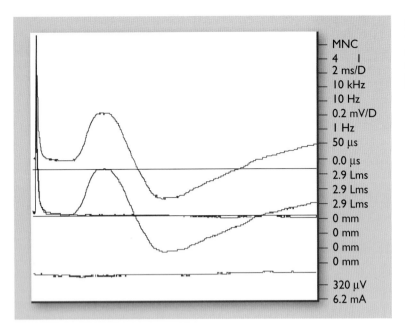

MNC
4   I
2 ms/D
10 kHz
10 Hz
0.2 mV/D
1 Hz
50 μs
0.0 μs
2.9 Lms
2.9 Lms
2.9 Lms
0 mm
0 mm
0 mm
0 mm

320 μV
6.2 mA

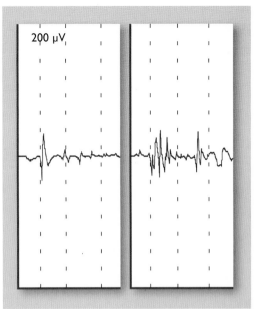

200 μV

Figure 7-11. Pudendal nerve terminal motor latencies (PNTMLs). Normal bilateral PNTMLs have been shown to be 2.0 ± 0.2 ms. The latency response is measured from the onset of the stimulus to the onset of the response in the external anal sphincter. Normal PNTML is the measurement of the fastest response of the pudendal nerve and does not necessarily mean the entire nerve is normal. Neither does an abnormal latency indicate abnormal muscle function. A damaged nerve can heal and reinnervate the muscle, and although the PNTML may be slightly prolonged, the muscle functions normally. Lms—latency milliseconds; MNC—motor nerve conduction.

Figure 7-12. Sphincter electromyography (EMG). Single-fiber EMG may be used to investigate the external anal sphincter. On the left half of the diagram is a normal single-fiber EMG tracing of a single muscle fiber, firing in a time-locked manner as a constituent of a motor unit. A motor unit consists of the anterior horn cell, its axon and branches, and the muscle fibers it supplies. Each motor unit potential will have a characteristic amplitude, duration, and characteristic shape of electrical response. The waveform on the right reflects several muscle fiber action potentials as a result of "grouping" from reinnervation resulting in several fibers belonging to a motor unit. Counting several fields estimates the fiber density that is increased in neurogenic and myopathic conditions. EMG mapping of the sphincter requires multiple insertions around the anal sphincter to detect areas of scarring or gaps in the muscle.

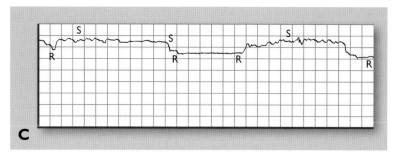

A — Manometry

Test	Sphincter Characteristics
Longitudinal resting pullout	Length
	Maximum average pressure
	Pressure volume
	Cross-sectional asymmetry
Station squeeze	Voluntary augmentation
	Fatigue
	Rest vs squeeze cross-section
Motility	Slow wave
	Ultraslow wave
Balloon reflex	Rectal–anal inhibitory reflex
	Rectal–anal excitatory reflex

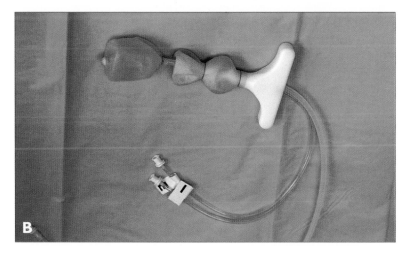

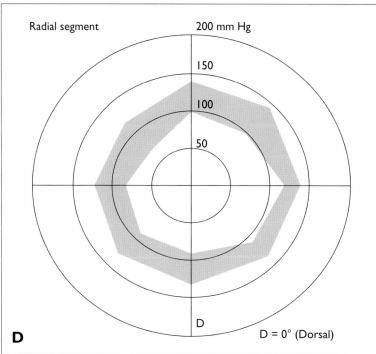

Figure 7-13. Anal manometry. **A,** There are many different types and methods for performing anal manometry. Essentially a balloon or probe is inserted into the rectum and a pressure transducer relays information to a recorder or computer. Important manometric parameters include sphincter length, resting and squeeze pressures, anal canal sensation, compliance, and the presence of the anorectal inhibitory reflex. **B,** A double-balloon manometry device with third distention balloon in the rectum. The top balloon is inserted to the level of the rectum. Filling of the top balloon assesses rectal compliance, sensation, and the rectoanal inhibitory reflex. The middle balloon records the pressures in the internal anal sphincter, and the outer balloon records those in the external anal sphincter. **C,** Anal manometry can determine the baseline resting pressure of the anal canal (R) and the squeeze pressure (S). The internal anal sphincter contributes 80% of the resting pressure. Voluntary contraction or squeezing of the external anal sphincter should double the resting pressures [21]. **D,** Perfusion anal manometry. A radial cross-section of the resting or squeeze pressures can be obtained using an eight-channel water profusion probe that records pressures radially around the anal canal. The pressures are sent to a computer that analyzes the data and develops the model. A sphincter defect at the 12 o'clock position would cause a loss of pressure in that position and asymmetry of the diagram.

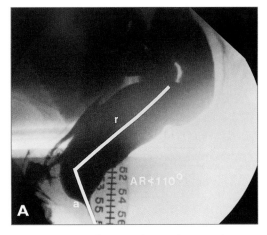 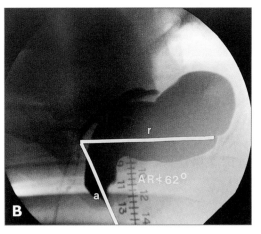 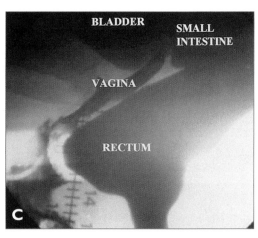

Figure 7-14. Defecography. Defecography is used in the evaluation of defecation disorders, including constipation and fecal incontinence, as well as in the evaluation of pelvic organ prolapse. Barium paste is inserted into the rectum, the small bowel is opacified by oral contrast agent, and the vagina and bladder may also be highlighted using barium paste and liquid contrast. The patient sits on a radiolucent commode and is asked to squeeze her pelvic floor, to relax her pelvic floor, and to evacuate her bowels. Fluoroscopy is used to record the dynamic activity of the bowel and pelvic organs. Defecography is used to identify rectal prolapse, internal rectal intussusception, or rectocele. In general, it is not a first-line test in evaluating fecal incontinence. **A** and **B**, The anorectal angle, as measured on these defecographies, was once thought to be predictive of pelvic floor function and useful in evaluating fecal incontinence. Although some studies show that incontinent patients have a more obtuse angle at rest, during straining, and during voluntary contraction of the sphincter, the overlap with results from normal control patients is too great for diagnostic significance. **C**, Defecography showing a large rectocele. Rectoceles can trap stool at the time of defecation that occasionally evacuates without sensation, causing fecal soiling. Fecal impaction can work similarly from chronic distention of the rectum, leading to relaxation of the internal anal sphincter, loss of resting tone, and stool leakage.

Common Causes of Constipation

Pathology outside the pelvis	Pathology inside the pelvis
Metabolic states	Obstruction
Hypothyroidism	Colon
Diabetes mellitus	Stricture
Hypercalcemia	Neoplasm
Hypokalemia	Diverticula
Uremia	Rectum
Anorexia nervosa	Fissure
Panhypopituitarism	Stenosis
Pregnancy	Rectal prolapse
Neurologic states	Rectocele/perineocele
Congenital	Paradoxical puborectalis contraction
Hirschprung's disease	Impaction
Acquired	
Chagas' disease	
CNS or spinal cord tumor	
Parkinson's disease	
Multiple sclerosis	
Autonomic neuropathy	
Diabetes mellitus	
Medications	
Antidepressants	
Mineral supplementations (eg, iron, calcium)	
Anticholinergics	
Narcotics	
Pychiatric	

Figure 7-15. Common causes of constipation. CNS—central nervous system.

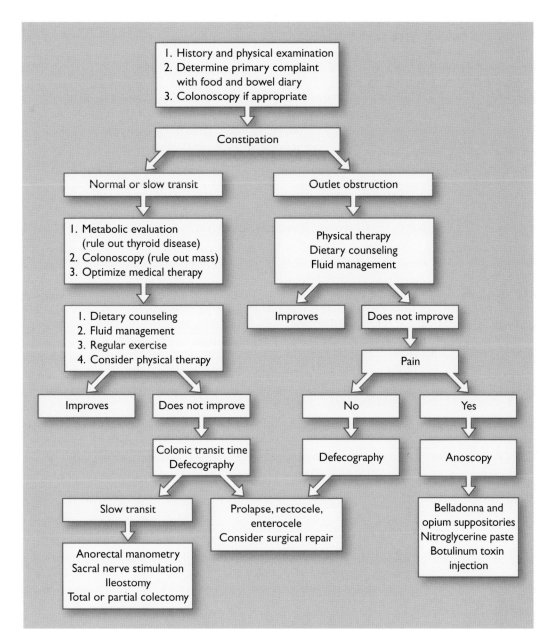

Figure 7-16. Evaluation of constipation. A detailed history should include the number of stools per week, pain with defecation, and need to splint or manually disimpact stool from the rectum in order to have a bowel movement. The patient's daily intake of fluids and fiber should also be assessed. The effect of symptoms on the patient's quality of life should also be elicited with a validated questionnaire such as the PAC-QOL (Patient Assessment of Constipation Quality of Life) [22]. A thorough medical history including use of medications (including chronic laxative abuse) and antecedent anorectal or gynecologic surgery is important as well. Recent lifestyle modifications should be considered including quitting smoking and significant decreases in caffeine intake. On physical examination, the abdomen should be palpated to note distension and the presence of bowel sounds. Examination of the vagina should be performed to note the presence of a rectocele or pelvic/rectal mass as well as any fissures or fistulas. The presence or absence of stool in the rectum or impaction should be noted. Flexible sigmoidoscopy or colonoscopy should be considered [23].

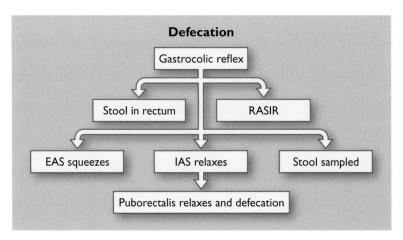

Figure 7-17. Normal defecation. When a bolus of stool or gas is sensed in the rectum, the rectoanal sphincteric inhibitory reflex (RASIR) is activated. While the external anal sphincter (EAS) squeezes, the internal anal sphincter (IAS) has a reflex relaxation that allows for colonic contents to be sampled by the anal canal. This sampling allows for differentiation of solid, liquid, and gas forms of the material. If the time is appropriate, after sampling, the IAS, puborectalis, and EAS should all relax and allow for defecation. If the time is not appropriate for defecation, the IAS contracts and allows fecal material to be pushed back into the rectum.

REFERENCES

1. Lee RA, Madoff RD, Pemberton J, Fleshman J: Panel presentation: current understanding of anal continence/incontinence. *J Pelvic Surg* 1998, 4:115–125.

2. Madoff RD, Williams JG, Caushau PF: Fecal incontinence. *N Engl J Med* 1992, 326:1002–1007.

3. Kamm MA: Obstetric damage and fecal incontinence. *Lancet* 1994, 344:730–733.

4. Jackson SI, Weber AM, Hull TL, *et al.*: Fecal incontinence in women with urinary incontinence and pelvic organ prolapse. *Obstet Gynecol* 1997, 89:423–427.

5. Melville JL, Fan MY, Newton K, Fenner D: Fecal incontinence in US women: a population based study. *Am J Obstet Gynecol* 2005, 193:2071–2076.

6. Pretlove SJ, Radley S, Toozs-Hobson PM, *et al.*: Prevalence of anal incontinence according to age and gender: a systematic review and meta-regression analysis. *Int Urogynecol J* 2006, 17:407–417.

7. Nirhira MA, Cundiff GW. Fecal incontinence. In *Ostergard's Urogynecology and Pelvic Floor Dysfunction*, edn 5. Philadelphia: Lippincott & Wilkins; 2003:41–353.

8. Sultan AH, Kamm MA, Hudson CN, *et al.*: Anal-sphincter disruption during vaginal delivery. *N Engl J Med* 1993, 329:1905–1911.

9. Sonnenberg A, Koch TR: Physician visits in the United States for constipation: 1958-1986. *Dig Dis Sci* 1989, 34:606.

10. Stewart WF, Liberman JN, Sandler RS, *et al.*: Epidemiology of Constipation (EPOC) study in the United States: relation of clinical subtypes to socio-demographic features. *Am J Gastroenterol* 1999, 94:3530–3540.

11. Pare P, Ferrazzi S, Thompson WG, Irvine EJ, *et al.*: An epidemiological survey of constipation in Canada: definitions, rates, demographics, and predictors of health care seeking. *Am J Gastroenterol* 2001, 96:3130–3137.

12. Everhart JE, Go VL, Johannes RS, *et al.*: A longitudinal survey of self-reported bowel habits in the United States. *Dig Dis Sci* 1989, 34:1153–1162.

13. Higgins PD, Johanson JF: Epidemiology of constipation in North America: a systematic review. *Am J Gastroenterol* 2004, 99:750–759.

14. Bassotti G, Chiationi G, Imbibo BP, *et al.*: Impaired colonic motor response to cholinergic stimulation in patients with severe chronic idiopathic (slow transit type) constipation. *Dig Dis Sci* 1993, 38:1040–1045.

15. Lembo A, Camilleri C: Chronic constipation. *N Engl J Med* 2003, 349:1360–1368.

16. Rome Foundation: Guidelines: Rome III diagnostic criteria for functional gastrointestinal disorders. *J Gastrointest Liver Dis* 2006, 15:307–312.

17. Rockwood TH, Church JM, Fleshman JW, *et al.*: Fecal incontinence quality of life scale: quality of life instrument for patients with fecal incontinence. *Dis Colon Rectum* 2000, 43:9–17.

18. Keating JP, Stewert PJ, Eyers AA, *et al.*: Are special investigations of value in the management of patients with fecal incontinence? *Dis Colon Rectum* 1997, 40:896–901.

19. Snooks SJ, Henry MM, Swash M: Anorectal incontinence and rectal prolapse: differential assessment of the innervation of the puborectalis and external anal sphincter muscles. *Gut* 1985, 26:470–476.

20. Laurberg S, Swash SJ, Henry MM: Delayed external sphincter repair for obstetric tear. *Br J Surg* 1988, 75:786–788.

21. Pemberton JH, Kelly KA: Achieving enteric continence: principles and applications. *Mayo Clin Proc* 1986, 61:586–599.

22. Marquis R, De La Loge C, Bubois D, *et al.*: Development and validation of the Patient Assessment of Constipation Quality of Life questionnaire. *Scand J Gastroenterol* 2005, 40:540–551.

23. Hull T: Constipation. In *Urogynecology and Pelvic Reconstructive Pelvic Surgery*, edn 2. St. Louis: Mosby; 1999:269–276.

8

Treatment of Fecal Incontinence and Constipation

Dee Fenner and
Christina Lewicky-Gaupp

The hope for successful management of fecal incontinence depends on the clinician's thorough understanding of normal pelvic anatomy and function. This understanding will guide the clinician in obtaining the appropriate diagnostic tests to identify the cause of symptoms and thus treat the problem appropriately. Continence is not fully understood but depends on bowel consistency and frequency; intact myenteric reflexes and autonomic, sensory, and motor nerves; and pelvic anatomy. If only one of these factors is abnormal, compensation can occur so that there may be no noticeable or significant symptoms. If one or more of the factors is sufficiently compromised, the person can become incontinent. Incontinence may be very mild and hardly noticeable or it may be severe and lead to a confined lifestyle. A detailed history is necessary to determine the degree of incontinence. This is important because the severity of symptoms dictates the aggressiveness of management. If a patient has a major sphincter abnormality, but no fecal incontinence, then treatment is not warranted. If a patient has very severe symptoms that significantly affect her lifestyle and mental state, then even risky or experimental surgery may be in order. A detailed history is also necessary to help identify the causative factors (eg, childbirth). This will guide the physical examination or ancillary testing to help identify a specific anatomic or functional abnormality (eg, sphincter defect) resulting in optimal treatment (eg, sphincteroplasty) and continence. The options for treatment of fecal incontinence are the focus of discussion.

Similarly, the clinician's understanding of the various pathophysiologies of constipation allows for directed treatments and optimization for success and patient satisfaction. Increasing fiber intake, good hydration, and regular exercise should be recommended for all patients. However, three types of constipation have been identified and include normal-transit, slow-transit, and disorders of defecatory or rectal evacuation; targeted therapy for each subgroup is important as well.

The mainstay therapy for normal-transit constipation includes dietary fiber with addition of osmotic laxatives. Patients with slow-transit constipation, however, have less of a response to dietary fiber and laxatives [1]. Thus, treatment may require the addition of a prokinetic agent after a neurologic cause such as Hirschsprung's disease has been excluded as the cause. For patients with evacuation difficulty secondary to obstruction, therapy is varied. For example, if puborectalis dyssynergia is seen, therapy is targeted to biofeedback. Because relaxation of the muscles involves central nervous inhibition of the spinal defecatory reflex, biofeedback employs the use of visual and digital feedback in order to learn techniques of pelvic floor and anal sphincter muscle relaxation when straining. Conversely, in patients with posterior vaginal wall prolapse and symptoms of obstructed defecation with trapping of stool within a rectocele pocket, surgical intervention may be indicated. The options for treatment of constipation are also the focus of this discussion.

Factors Contributing to Fecal Incontinence

Functional	Neurologic (ie, diabetes, trauma, spinal defects, multiple sclerosis)
Irritable bowel syndrome	Pelvic defects
Diarrhea (ie, malabsorption, endocrine disorder, upper intestinal disease, food intolerance)	Enterocele
Constipation, impaction	Rectocele
Diet	Enterogenital fistula
Medications (ie, laxatives)	Rectal intussusception/prolapse
Proctitis/colitis	Anal outlet defects
Infectious	Birth defects (ie, anal atresia, imperforate anus)
Idiopathic (ulcerative colitis, Crohn's disease)	Traumatic delivery
Polyp/cancer	Iatrogenic (fistulotomy, sphincterotomy, hemorrhoidectomy, mucosal ectropion)
Diverticulitis/volvulus	

Figure 8-1. Factors contributing to fecal incontinence. Multiple factors may contribute to fecal incontinence. A thorough history and physical examination will often identify these factors and lead to an appropriate diagnosis and treatment plan.

Figure 8-2. Nonsurgical treatment of fecal incontinence. Functional fecal incontinence, when the patient has no history of sphincter trauma and no major sphincter deformity, can be treated very successfully by nonsurgical means, even in severe cases. The first line of management is to encourage and educate the patient to eat a high-fiber diet with plenty of fluids and fiber supplements as needed. This is helpful and sometimes all that is required. The fiber with the fluids tends to make the bowels more consistent, regular, and predictable, allowing for an easier and more complete fecal evacuation. In patients who tend to have loose or frequent bowel movements, the addition of loperamide or diphenoxylate with atropine as indicated can decrease the bowel frequency to a more manageable level. Kegel sphincter strengthening exercises are also recommended as a first-line treatment. Patients are instructed to practice contracting the anal sphincter and holding it in that state for a count to 10, for a series of 10 times, several times per day. They are encouraged to do this routinely whether it is while sitting down for meals or while driving to and from regular activities, such as work. The more often a person performs that exercise, the more successful it will be. It may take several weeks to accomplish noticeable improvement. A bowel training regimen may be beneficial when the initial measures are unsuccessful. Initially, daily suppositories, glycerin or bisacodyl, or enemas are given at the same hour every morning. Ideally, these measures are administered 15 to 20 minutes after breakfast to take advantage of the gastrocolic reflex. Lower abdominal massage can be performed at the same time. As the bowels become more predictable, the frequency of this type of stimulation can be decreased.

In patients with spinal cord injuries, digital stimulation is performed to accomplish the same purpose by stimulating a rectocolic evacuation reflex. If these measures are unsuccessful or if the patient is not a candidate for a sphincteroplasty, or if a sphincteroplasty has failed, then different types of biofeedback have about a 70% success rate [2]. Sensory biofeedback can be accomplished with an electromyographic electrode or a distal rectal balloon by applying either increasing electrical current or increasing the volume of water, respectively, to train the patient to

Nonsurgical Treatment of Fecal Incontinence

Manipulation of stool consistency

   Diet—high fiber, fiber supplements, fluids

   Medication—loperamide hydrochloride or diphenoxylate hydrochloride with atropine sulfate

Kegel exercises

Bowel training regimen

   Regular periodic suppositories or enemas

   Digital stimulation

Biofeedback

   Electromyography—sensory, topical, stimulatory

   Manometry—sensory, pressure

Anal plug

recognize these stimuli at lower levels of current or water volume. Biofeedback trains the patient to recognize the presence of rectal contents at a lower threshold. This allows the patient more time to voluntarily contract the sphincter or head toward the bathroom and avoid an episode of incontinence. Sphincter motor function can be trained electrically or manometrically by placing topical electrical leads in the anal region or a manometry catheter in the anal canal to pick up electrical activity or pressure responses to sphincter contraction. The electrical activity reading or pressure measurement is the feedback that the patient sees to gauge success. These measures have been successful, but not as successful in patients with a pudendal neuropathy. In those patients with no or minimal sphincter activity, electrical stimulation to the muscle at gradually increasing levels to accomplish a tetanizing stimulus to the sphincter has also led to improved symptoms [3]. The anal plug has been reported to be successful in some patients, but that device has not been widely used [4].

Antidiarrheal Medications	
Drug	**Mechanism of Action**
Loperamide	Inhibits circular and longitudinal muscle contraction
Diphenoxylate with atropine	Direct action on circular smooth muscle to decrease peristalsis
Hyoscyamine sulfate	Anticholinergic
Cholestyramine	Binds bile acids after cholecystectomy (helpful for patients who develop diarrhea after cholecystectomy)

Figure 8-3. Antidiarrheal medications. In every patient, maintaining normal stool consistency and frequency is imperative. Soft, mushy stools can be very difficult for patients to control and evacuate completely. This, in turn, can lead to constant seepage and the inability to wipe clean. If the patient is having several bowel movements throughout the day, this implies rapid colonic motility or an enhanced gastrocolic reflex, both of which can create symptoms of fecal urgency and incontinence. The medications listed here often successfully slow the gastrointestinal tract, and titration of the selected medication over the course of a month can achieve the desired result of a single bowel movement in the morning.

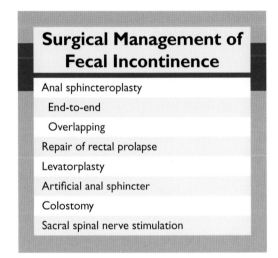

Surgical Management of
Fecal Incontinence

Anal sphincteroplasty

End-to-end

Overlapping

Repair of rectal prolapse

Levatorplasty

Artificial anal sphincter

Colostomy

Sacral spinal nerve stimulation

Figure 8-4. Surgical management of fecal incontinence. With the exception of colostomy, the goal of surgical management is to improve the function of the anal sphincter. Anal sphincteroplasty has proven to be the most successful approach to date; however, as discussed later in the chapter, it is still suboptimal in achieving complete continence. Both overlapping and end-to-end techniques of the anal sphincteroplasty have shown similar success rates [5–7]. Biofeedback has also been shown to improve on the success rates after sphincteroplasty as well [8].

Another development has been the application of electrostimulation to the sacral spinal nerves. So far, with limited experience, there has been some success [9,10].

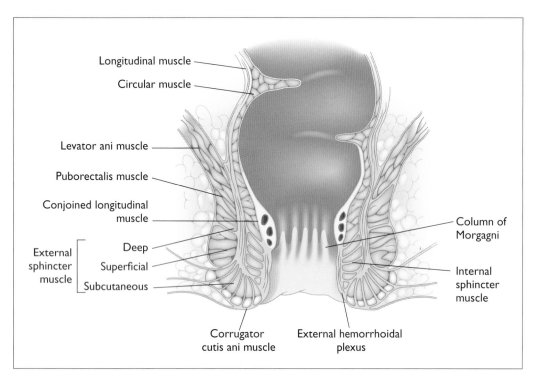

Longitudinal muscle

Circular muscle

Levator ani muscle

Puborectalis muscle

Conjoined longitudinal muscle

External sphincter muscle

Deep

Superficial

Subcutaneous

Corrugator cutis ani muscle

External hemorrhoidal plexus

Column of Morgagni

Internal sphincter muscle

Figure 8-5. Anal anatomy. An understanding of sphincter anatomy is important in accomplishing a good repair and result. The internal sphincter, an involuntary smooth muscle, has the major role of maintaining the resting sphincter tone. It is a continuation of the inner muscular layer of the rectum, which is thickened, and resides in the inner upper two thirds of the anal canal. A problem with this portion of the sphincter can lead to problems with fine tuning of bowel control. The voluntary sphincter mechanism consists of the medial-most portion of the levator contribution, the puborectalis muscle, which is a sling wrapped posteriorly and laterally on the rectum and inserted bilaterally on the pubis. The distal two thirds of the anal canal is the circumferential external sphincter, which extends about 1.5 cm distal to the lower extent of the internal sphincter. The external anal sphincter is innervated by the pudendal nerve from below. The puborectalis is innervated most likely by the direct bundles of the pelvic plexus from above. The internal anal sphincter is innervated by sacral parasympathetics and visceral (prevertebral) sympathetics. The external sphincter and puborectalis are responsible for the voluntary contraction squeeze pressure that closes the anus. Minor defects may be asymptomatic. Major defects in this mechanism may (though not necessarily) lead to significant symptoms of incontinence. It is critical to repair both the voluntary and involuntary sphincter mechanism to its full length to obtain optimal results. The repair must be such that from the baseline tonic state it would allow both relaxation with opening of the canal and contraction with tight closing. The result must be as close to normal anatomy as possible; otherwise patulence or stenosis can occur.

A   Operative Techniques for Anal Sphincteroplasty

1) Preoperative bowel preparation with either enemas or an oral laxative (eg, polyethylene glycol) is recommended.

2) The patient should be placed in dorsal lithotomy position under general anesthesia. Paralysis should be avoided in order to allow for muscle identification and stimulation with a nerve stimulator intraoperatively.

3) Using a no. 15 blade scalpel, a hemicircumferential incision along the perineum just cephalad to the anal sphincter is made. The incision should be as near to the posterior fourchette as possible, with enough room to allow for dissection of the scarred muscle ends.

4) This incision should be extended down to the ischioanal fat on either side of the anus, and the vagina should be separated from the scar tissue.

5) Any perineal scar tissue should then be transected in its entire length.

6) With one finger in the rectum, using sharp, meticulous dissection, the external anal sphincter muscles should then be separated from the anal canal. A nerve stimulator can be utilized to aid in the identification of the external anal sphincter.

7) The internal anal sphincter should be visible at this point. If it is separated from the external sphincter, it should be reapproximated in the midline using monofilament, delayed-absorbable sutures such as 3-0 PDS in an interrupted or mattress fashion.

8) The divided external anal sphincter muscles should then be grasped with Allis tissue forceps bilaterally for retraction and exposure.

9) Interrupted, monofilament, delayed-absorbable sutures such as 2-0 or 3-0 PDS should be placed into the separated external sphincter muscles to allow for their reapproximation in an overlapping or end-to-end fashion. The repair of the sphincter should continue to a level about 1 to 1.5 cm distal to the lower end of the internal anal sphincter.

10) For a large sphincter tear, an overlapping technique using mattress sutures is preferred. In order to successfully overlap the muscles, it is necessary to sharply dissect laterally into the ischioanal fossa; this allows the full length of the muscles to be mobilized from the ischioanal fat. The overlapping technique results in a greater surface area or contact between the muscles.

11) If the sphincter is only partially torn, an end-to-end approach can be performed. In this case, it is not necessary to expose the full length of the torn sphincter. Mattress or interrupted sutures are placed in the exposed sphincter in a standard fashion.

12) The perineal body should then be imbricated over the repaired external anal sphincter using 3-0 polyglactin 910 vertical mattress sutures, thus reconstructing the perineal body.

13) The bulbocavernosus muscles should be sutured to the perineal body.

14) The vaginal epithelium and perineal skin are then closed in a running fashion with a rapidly absorbable suture such as 3-0 polyglactin 910 after copious irrigation of the surgical site.

15) A rectovaginal examination should be performed at the end of the procedure to ensure that the repair is complete.

B   Operative Techniques for Episiotomy Repair

1) When performing an episiotomy repair that involves the anal sphincter as well as the rectal mucosa, it is imperative to optimize the patient's comfort with regional anesthesia and to maximize exposure of the perineum. Regional anesthesia with either a spinal or an epidural facilitates relaxation and identification of the anal sphincter, which often retracts into its capsule.

2) The full extent of the injury should be determined.

3) Attention should first be focused on the anorectal mucosa. This should be repaired with interrupted or running absorbable sutures such as 3-0 polyglactin 910. The knots should be tied in the anal lumen.

4) The internal anal sphincter should be identified. If it is torn, the ends should be grasped with Allis tissue forceps and reapproximated with interrupted or mattress sutures using a monofilament, delayed-absorbable suture such as 3-0 PDS.

5) The external anal sphincter muscles should then be grasped bilaterally with Allis tissue forceps. Using sharp dissection, they should be mobilized laterally. Then, using a monofilament, delayed-absorbable suture such as 3-0 PDS, the torn ends should be reapproximated in an overlapping fashion.

6) Once the sphincter is repaired, the bulbocavernosus muscles should be sutured together in order to reconstruct the perineal body, thus adding support to the repaired sphincter. This lengthening of the perineal body makes it less vulnerable to tearing during a subsequent vaginal delivery.

7) The vaginal epithelium is then repaired using an absorbable suture such as 3-0 polyglactin 910 in a subcuticular fashion.

8) A rectovaginal examination should be performed to ensure that the repair is complete and no residual defects exist.

Figure 8-6. Operative technique for anal sphincteroplasty (**A**) and episiotomy repair (**B**). PDS—polydioxanone. (*Adapted from* Sultan *et al.* [11].)

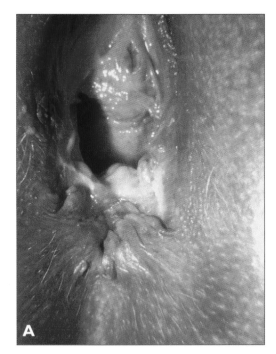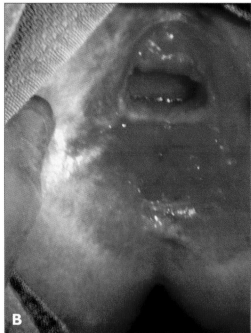

Figure 8-7. Childbirth trauma. **A**, This major, easily identified sphincter defect was caused by trauma from childbirth. There is complete absence of the perineal body and anterior sphincter with major patulence of the anal canal. **B**, This is another example of a major sphincter defect from childbirth injury. There is retraction of both the internal and external sphincter musculature to about the 3 and 9 o'clock positions, with anterior being 12 o'clock.

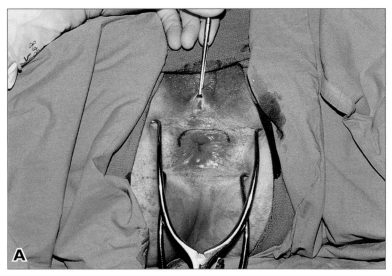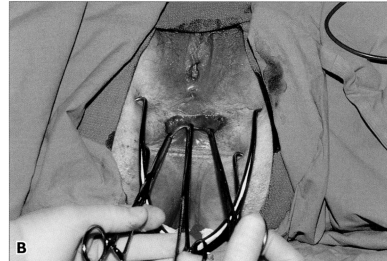

Figure 8-8. Technique. This series of figures gives a detailed description and visualization of the location of the incision, technique of exposure, technique of instrument placement, and the steps to ensure adequate dissection of the sphincter. **A**, The initial incision is a "sad" incision (concentric curved) with an inverted Y-closure as the sphincter ends are brought together and the anal canal is closed. This illustration shows a lithotomy position with a povidone-iodine preparation. The defect in this patient is a minor defect that was easily identified on physical examination. **B**, The skin incision is performed with a no. 15 blade and clamps are placed on the skin flap as the perianal skin is dissected up into the anal canal. The internal sphincter is beginning to be exposed and a space developed to bring the sphincters together. Gelpi retractors are used for exposure. In a case with significant loss of perineal length, a "sad" incision is made anterior to the anus combined with a "smile" incision posterior to the vagina, with the incisions meeting in the middle. This allows for better exposure, wide dissection, and a greater area in the midline to reconstruct the perineum (not shown).

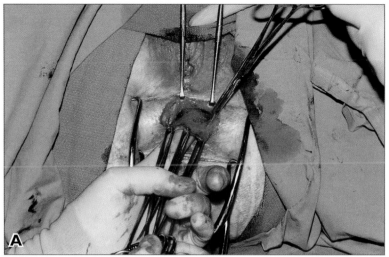

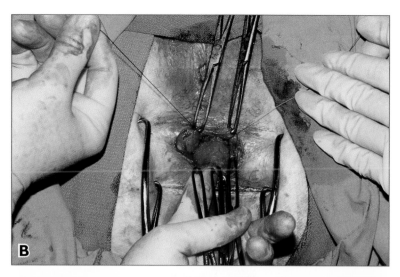

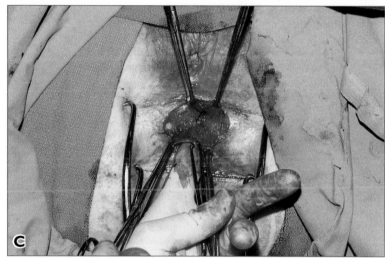

Figure 8-9. Internal sphincter. **A,** With a gloved hand in the anal canal holding the inferior skin flap, retractor clamps are placed on the midline perineal scar tissue and a portion of the retracted external sphincter. The dissection is extended superiorly at least to the same level as the puborectalis, which is superior and lateral. This depth of dissection is important so that a satisfactory length on the internal sphincter repair will be accomplished. Next, the right lateral clamp is placed on the sphincter in the 2 o'clock position and retracted anteriorly while the anal canal digit is palpating the location of the internal sphincter. As the clamp is gently and repeatedly tugged, the location of the internal sphincter is identified. **B,** This exposure allows for the complete identification of the internal sphincter superiorly to lead to a satisfactory length to the internal sphincter repair. This illustration shows the first suture being placed in the internal sphincter at the superior extent of the anal canal at the level of the puborectalis. Sutures with 2-0 polyglactin 910 are placed, and ideally the assistant would tie them so that the surgeon could leave the anal canal digit in place, therefore avoiding the need to continually change gloves to tie knots. After each layer of dissection and closure is done, the wound is irrigated with saline or povidone-iodine. **C,** These interrupted sutures are continued to the same inferior position as the posterior internal sphincter, which can be palpated with the anal canal digit.

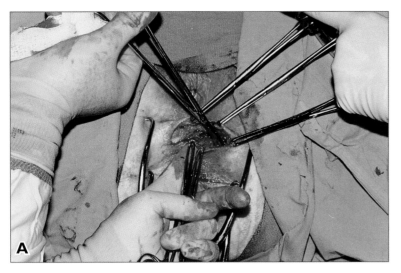

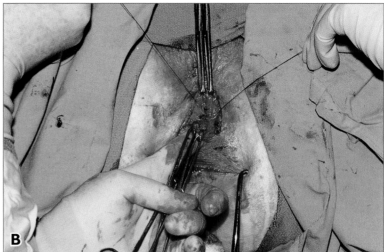

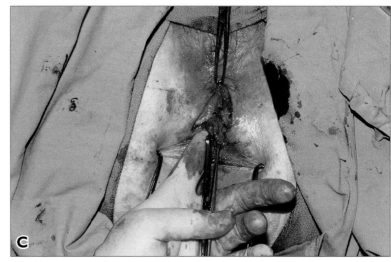

Figure 8-10. External sphincter. **A**, The external sphincter is then elevated from the scar tissue and the perianal skin laterally and posteriorly bilaterally. This is only done at the skin level, as illustrated, and not dissected lateral to the sphincter in the ischial rectal space. Limiting the lateral dissection will help to avoid injury to the anal branch of the pudendal nerve. The sphincter only needs to be dissected so that it can be brought to the midline without excessive tension. Sharp dissection is necessary to allow freeing of this muscle and to avoid skin dimpling. **B**, The external sphincter is exposed with clamps and retracted superiorly; apical superior sutures are placed in the external sphincter with the goal of providing a satisfactory length to the external sphincter. The first suture is placed in the external sphincter near the level of the puborectalis, which can be felt posteriorly and laterally. Sutures of 2-0 polyglactin 910 are used for each layer, except for the skin where 3-0 or 4-0 polyglactin 910 sutures are used. It should be noted that the scar tissue is not excised at any time during the sphincter dissection. In fact, it is used to anchor and secure the sutures. **C**, The repair is then continued externally so that the external sphincter is repaired to a level about 1.0 to 1.5 cm distal to the lower extent of the internal sphincter.

The external sphincter should be repaired to the same level as the palpable external sphincter posteriorly. Some degree of imbrication occurs at this distal point. The sphincter should be snug, but the examining index finger should be able to be inserted fairly easily.

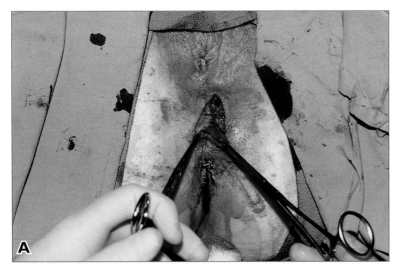

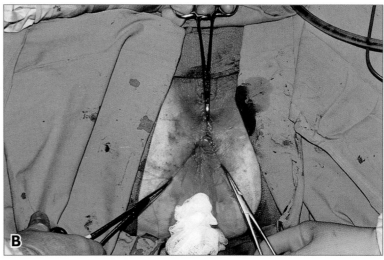

Figure 8-11. Perineal body. **A**, Sutures are also placed in the perineal body and, at this point, it can be seen that the perineal body is lengthened, especially in cases where there are major sphincter injuries. The wound is then irrigated and closed. Some surgeons do a sphincterotomy at the 5 o'clock position to decrease tension on the suture line and prevent stenosis [12]. **B**, This closure has an inverted Y appearance. It is helpful not to trim off any skin if possible to help decrease the risk of anal stenosis. The clamps are on the tails of the knots on the Y limb. This patient had an excellent result.

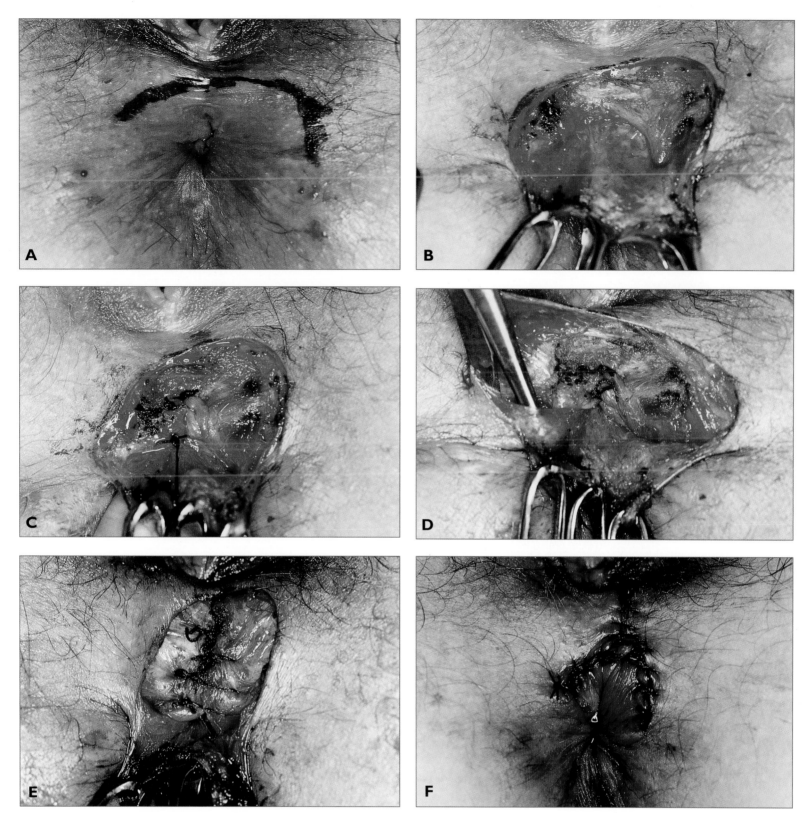

Figure 8-12. Minor sphincter defect. **A,** A closer view of an obvious minor sphincter defect on physical examination is seen, again with a "sad" incision from the 10 o'clock to 3 o'clock position. The incision is extended just past the edge of the palpable retracted external sphincter. Again, anterior is up. **B,** The anoderm is elevated off of the scar tissue superiorly to the level of the puborectalis, which could be palpated posteriorly. Care is taken to avoid a hole in this flap because this may result in an abscess or fistula. The scar is left intact and used to secure the suture material. **C,** The interrupted sutures are placed in the internal sphincter. The finger in the anal canal is used to identify the internal sphincter so that it can be repaired to the appropriate proximal and distal extent. **D,** The external sphincter is then freed from the scar in the skin using sharp dissection with Metzenbaum's scissors. **E,** Interrupted sutures are used to close this external sphincter and imbricate it to the appropriate tension as previously mentioned. **F,** A Y-closure can be accomplished with a running polyglactin 910 suture.

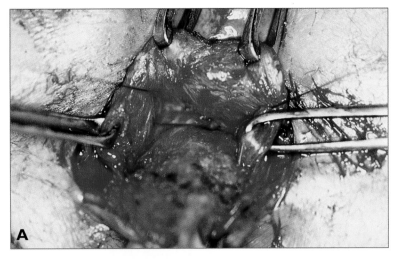

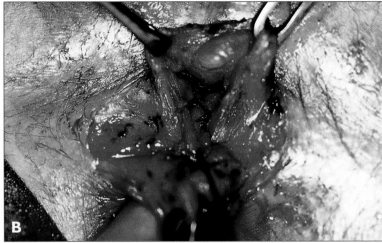

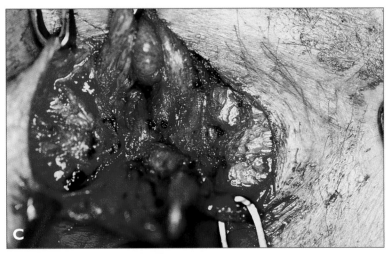

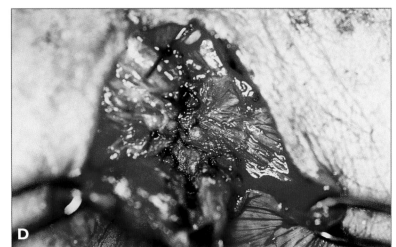

Figure 8-13. Depth of dissection of anal flap. **A**, These photographs illustrate the significant depth of dissection of the anal flap. Clamps are placed laterally on the most inferior internal sphincter. The first interrupted suture is being placed in the proximal internal sphincter. Anterior clamps are placed on the skin and perineal scar for exposure. **B**, The internal sphincter repair leaves a small cavity to allow closure of the external sphincter and perineal body. This is done with interrupted sutures. **C**, The skin flaps are then dissected, giving better exposure to the external sphincter. **D**, Finally, this is closed with some degree of imbrication in the midline. The anal canal finger should be fairly easily insertable with slight resistance as an indication of the tension of the repair.

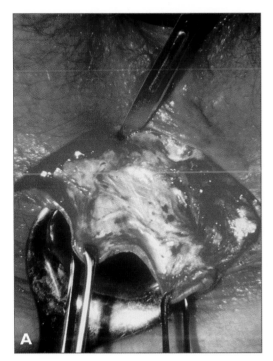 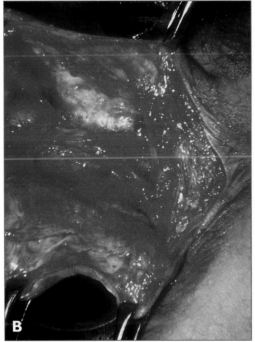 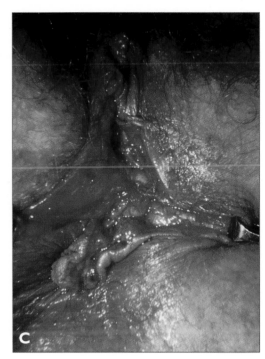

Figure 8-14. Dissection in major sphincter defect. **A,** This case illustrates the amount of dissection necessary in the repair of a major sphincter defect. A large incision is necessary with major anoderm elevation superiorly and laterally to identify the internal and external sphincter. **B,** Once these flaps are elevated in all directions, exposing the muscles, there is a large midline space, giving room to bring these muscles into the midline. Again, the scar tissue is left intact to allow secure suture placement. **C,** Multiple layers of sutures are placed in the internal and external sphincter, as well as the perineal muscles, to reconstruct the perineum. What was once a "sad"-shaped incision is now a vertical incision in the midline radiating between the anus and the vagina. Excessive skin may be trimmed if necessary.

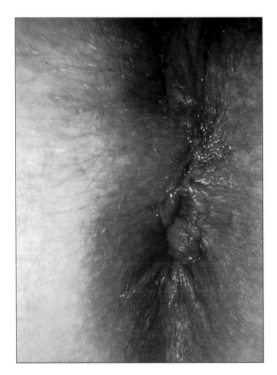

Figure 8-15. Mobilization. In this case, so much mobilization was necessary that a linear skin closure was accomplished. Ideally, a good repair should be performed at the time of the initial sphincter damage using excellent lighting and sphincter exposure and identification of the same anatomic elements as discussed in this chapter. However, delayed sphincter repairs lead to good to excellent resolution of symptoms in 60% to 90% of cases. Complications are uncommon but include infection, fistula, and stenosis. This procedure can generally be performed on an outpatient basis and the postoperative care includes the use of a high-fiber diet, fiber supplements, plenty of fluids, laxatives until the first bowel movement occurs, and sitz baths. Some surgeons use constipating agents, such as codeine, to try to delay bowel movements in their patients. We have not found that necessary and are concerned about the risk of impaction and resultant damage to the repair.

Long-Term Outcomes for Anal Sphincteroplasty

Study	Follow-Up, y	Outcomes
'Karoui et al. [13], 2000 (France)	3.3	28% continent 23% incontinent flatus only 49% incontinent of stool
Halverson et al. [14], 2002 (US)	5.8	14% continent 32% incontinent flatus only 54% incontinent of stool
Malouf et al. [15], 2000 (UK)	6.4	0% continent 10% incontinent flatus only 63% incontinent of stool
Bravo Gutierrez et al. [16], 2004 (US)	10.3	6% continent 18% incontinent flatus only 60% incontinent of stool
Trowbridge et al. [17] 2006 (US)	5.6	10% continent 15% incontinent to flatus only 75% incontinent of solid stool

Figure 8-16. Long-term outcomes for anal sphincteroplasty [13–17]. This table shows a comparison of outcomes from five different studies on anal sphincteroplasty [18]. Unfortunately, the reports of long-term results for a mean follow-up of 3 to 10 years are less than promising, with cure rates ranging from 0% to 28% after overlapping repair. (*Adapted from* Rogers et al. [19].)

Recommended High-Fiber Diet

	Insoluble Fiber	Soluble Fiber
Functions	Move bulk through intestines Control and balance pH in intestines	Bind with fatty acids Prolong gastric emptying to allow slower release and absorption of sugars
Benefits	Promote regular bowel movements Prevent colon cancer by keeping optimal pH	Lower total cholesterol and LDL Regulate blood sugars (especially in diabetic patients)
Food sources	Vegetables (green beans) Fruit skins and root vegetable skins Whole wheat products Wheat oat Corn bran Seeds and nuts	Oats/oat bran Dried beans and peas Nuts Barley Flax seed Fruits (oranges and apples) Vegetables (carrots) Psyllium husk

Figure 8-17. Recommended high-fiber diet. The functions and benefits of both insoluble and soluble fiber are listed along with various food sources. Patients who are reluctant to use bulking laxatives may find benefit from increasing their consumption of these foods. Increasing fiber intake is vital in the treatment of any kind of constipation. In the United States, the Department of Agriculture recommends that adults consume from 20 to 35 g of fiber a day. Fiber intake promotes stool evacuation by increasing not only its bulk but also its water content. Insoluble fiber alone increases stool bulk as well. LDL—low-density lipoprotein.

Medical Therapies for Constipation

Type of Laxative	Examples	Description
Bulking agents	Psyllium Methylcellulose	Absorbs liquid in intestines and swells to form a soft, bulky stool
Stool softeners	Docusate	Helps liquids mix into stools (eases straining rather than causing a bowel movement)
Osmotic laxatives	Polyethylene glycol Saline laxatives: magnesium hydroxide, magnesium citrate Poorly absorbed sugars: lactulose, mannitol, sorbitol, glycerin suppositories	Lactulose and PEG have been shown to increase stool frequency and improve consistency
Stimulant laxatives	Diphenylmethane derivatives: bisacodyl, sodium picosulfate, castor oil, mineral oil Anthraquinones: senna, cascara sagrada, aloe	Insufficient data to make a recommendation regarding use (no placebo-controlled trials)
5-HT$_4$ agonists	Tegaserod	Improves stool frequency, consistency, and straining

Figure 8-18. Medical therapies for constipation. For constipated patients, bulking agents, stool softeners, and osmotic laxatives are generally first-line therapy. Stool softeners have both a hydrophilic and hydrophobic component that together work to degrade stool, thus allowing water and other substrates to enter it. This causes stool softening and increases stool bulk. Osmotic laxatives contain insoluble or poorly absorbed substances that draw water into the lumen of the colon. This works to increase stool volume, which in turn, stimulates intestinal peristalsis to facilitate a bowel movement. Stimulant laxatives are generally not recommended for long-term use. Most are readily available anthraquinone derivatives whose action results from direct stimulation of the smooth muscle of the colon. Long-term use may lead to melanosis coli (dark colonic pigmentation), cathartic colon syndrome (extremely dilated, atonic colon), and neuronal desensitization. Tegaserod has been studied in patients with constipation-dependent irritable bowel syndrome and is not yet approved for long-term use [20].

Functional Outcome of Rectocele Repairs

Study	Patients, n	Follow-up, mo	Type of Repair	Symptom	Preoperative, %	Postoperative, %
Kahn and Stanton [22]	171	42	Levator ani plication	Subjective prolapse Obstructed defecation Constipation Dyspareunia	64 — 22 18	31 33 33 27
Cundiff et al. [23]	69	12	Discrete fascial repair	Subjective prolapse Obstructed defecation Constipation Dyspareunia	62 39 46 29	12 25 13 19
Kenton et al. [24]	55	12	Discrete fascial repair	Subjective prolapse Obstructed defecation Constipation Dyspareunia	86 30 41 28	5 15 20 24
Porter et al. [25]	125	18	Discrete fascial repair	Subjective prolapse Obstructed defecation Constipation Dyspareunia	100 30 60 67	18 14 50 46

Figure 8-19. Functional outcome of rectocele repairs [21–25]. Large studies have been done to address the issue of whether a posterior colporrhaphy is beneficial in treating a woman with constipation and a rectocele; still no clear-cut answer is available. Four of these studies are illustrated here [21]. Both discrete fascial repair and plication of the rectovaginal muscularis are routinely performed, and although anatomic outcomes (such as subjective prolapse) do improve significantly, some patients have less successful functional outcomes (such as continued constipation and new-onset dyspareunia). Most experts advocate the maximization of medical and behavioral therapy prior to surgical correction of an anatomic defect, because the majority of patients can achieve satisfactory results with conservative interventions. Surgical intervention for posterior compartment defects should be considered only when all stool motility and consistency abnormalities have been addressed in order to optimize surgical success and patient satisfaction.

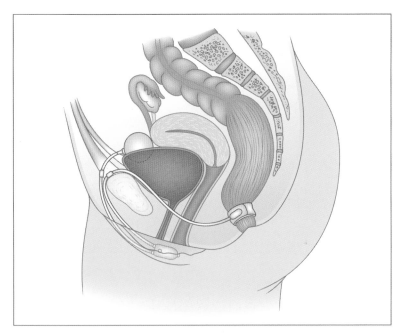

Figure 8-20. Artificial sphincter. The use of the artificial sphincter has indications similar to those of the muscle transpositions and can be used when those muscles are not available. The procedure does not bear the risks involved with muscle harvest such as a defunctionalizing injury to the nerves. The device has three parts: an inflatable cuff placed around the anus, the control pump implanted in the scrotum or labia, and the pressure-regulating balloon placed in the abdomen. Deflation of the cuff allows for fecal evacuation. The artificial sphincter carries the risks of mechanical failure and infection. Despite this, the artificial sphincter has had reasonable success: 75% success and 33% complication rates, similar to the muscle transpositions but with greater ease of placement [26]. Another experimental artificial sphincter technique is being engineered to be placed transabdominally, deep into the pelvis, along the rectum, just above the levators. Theoretically, this works by kinking/folding the bowel under low pressure. The drawbacks to this technique would be significant, including the risks of major abdominal surgery [27].

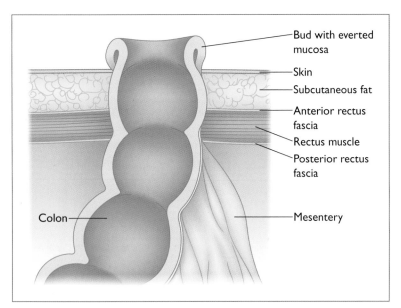

Bud with everted mucosa

Skin

Subcutaneous fat

Anterior rectus fascia

Rectus muscle

Posterior rectus fascia

Colon

Mesentery

Figure 8-21. Colostomy. When the other appropriate medical and surgical measures are unsuccessful in managing fecal incontinence, colostomy placement, usually at the level of the left colon, is a good option. Although this is a major operation, the technique is very familiar to colon and rectal surgeons and is successful in controlling anal incontinence. A laparoscopic approach may decrease operative morbidity. Colostomy placement can be difficult in obese patients or in those with a history of multiple abdominal operations. It is important to make sure that there is an adequate length to allow an everted bud external to the skin. This ensures a better fit of the ostomy collection device and thus prevents leakage and skin excoriation. The most common long-term complication is a peristomal hernia. This is usually repairable but may require a repeat laparotomy. It is important that the physician and the enterostomal therapist work together to provide education, appropriate equipment, and emotional and technical support. This will help the patient to accept the stoma and pursue a normal lifestyle with few, if any, limitations.

REFERENCES

1. Rieger NA, Wattchow DA, Sarre RG, et al.: Prospective trial of pelvic floor retraining in patients with fecal incontinence. Dis Colon Rectum 1997, 40:821–826.

2. Pescatori M, Pavesio R, Anastasio G, Daini S: Transanal electrostimulation for fecal incontinence: clinical, psychologic, and manometric prospective study. Dis Colon Rectum 1991, 34:540–545.

3. Mortensen N, Humphreys MS: The anal continence plug: a disposable device for patients with anorectal incontinence. Lancet 1991, 338:295.

4. Matzel KE, Stadelmaier U, Hohenfellner M: Electrical stimulation of sacral spinal nerves for treatment of fecal incontinence. Lancet 1995, 346:1124–1127.

5. Engel AF, Kamm MA, Sultan AH, et al.: Anterior anal sphincter repair in patients with obstetric trauma. Br J Surg 1994, 81:1231–1234.

6. Jensen LL, Lowry AC: Biofeedback improves functional outcome after sphincteroplasty. Dis Colon Rectum 1997, 40:197–200.

7. Ternent CA, Shashidharan M, Blatchford GJ, et al.: Transanal ultrasound and anorectal physiology findings affecting continence after sphincteroplasty. Dis Colon Rectum 1997, 40:462–467.

8. Sentovich SM, Wong WD, Blatchford GJ: Accuracy and reliability of transanal ultrasound for anterior and sphincter injury. Dis Colon Rectum 1998, 41:1000–1004.

9. VanTets WF, Kuijpers JHC: Pelvic floor procedures produce no consistent changes in anatomy or physiology. Dis Colon Rectum 1998, 41:365–369.

10. Geerdes BP, Heineman E, Konsten J, et al.: Dynamic graciloplasty. Dis Colon Rectum 1996, 39:8, 912–917.

11. Sultan AH, Thakar R, Fenner DE, eds: Perineal and Anal Sphincter Trauma. London: Springer; 2007.

12. Tancer ML, Lasser D, Rosenblum N: Rectovaginal fistula or perineal and anal sphincter disruption, or both, after vaginal delivery. Surg Gynecol Obstet 1990, 171:43-46.

13. Karoui S, Leroi AM, Koning E, et al.: Results of sphincteroplasty in 86 patients with anal incontinence. Dis Colon Rectum 2000, 43:813–820.

14. Halverson AL, Hull TL: Long-term outcome of overlapping anal sphincter repair. Dis Colon Rectum 2002, 45:345–348.

15. Malouf AJ, Norton CS, Engel AF, et al.: Long-term results of overlapping anterior anal-sphincter repair for obstetric trauma. Lancet 2000, 355:260–265.

16. Bravo Gutierrez A, Madoff RD, Lowry AC, et al.: Long-term results of anterior sphincteroplasty. Dis Colon Rectum 2004, 47:727–731.

17. Trowbridge E, Morgan D, Trowbridge MJ, et al.: Sexual function, quality of life, and severity of anal incontinence after anal sphincteroplasty. Am J Obstet Gynecol 2006, 195:1753–1757.

18. Wexner SD, Gonzalez-Padron A, Rius J, et al.: Stimulated gracilis neosphincter operation. Dis Colon Rectum 1996, 39:957–964.

19. Rogers GR, Husam A, Fenner DE: Current diagnosis and treatment algorithms for anal incontinence. BJU Int 2006, 98(Suppl 1):97–106; discussion 107–109.

20. Devesa JM, Fernandez Madrid JM, Rodriguez Gallego B, et al.: Bilateral gluteoplasty for fecal incontinence. Dis Colon Rectum 1997, 40:957–964.

21. Christiansen J, Ronholt Hansen C, Rasmussen O: Bilateral gluteus maximus transposition for anal incontinence. Br J Surg 1995, 82:883–888.

22. Kahn MA, Stanton SL: Posterior colporrhaphy: its effects on bowel and sexual function. Br J Obstet Gynaecol 1997, 104:82–86.

23. Cundiff GW, Weidner AC, Visco AG, et al.: An anatomic and functional assessment of the discrete defect rectocele repair. Am J Obstet Gynecol 1998, 179:1451–1457.

24. Kenton K, Shott S, Brubaker L: Outcome after rectovaginal fascia reattachment for rectocele repair. Am J Obstet Gynecol 1999, 181:1360–1364.

25. Porter WE, Steele A, Walsh P, et al.: The anatomic and functional outcomes of defect-specific rectocele repairs. Am J Obstet Gynecol 1999, 181:1353–1359.

26. Wong WD, Jensen LL, Bartolo DC, Rothenberger DA: Artificial anal sphincter. Dis Colon Rectum 1996, 39:1345–1351.

27. Hajivassiliou CA, Carter KB, Finlay IG: Assessment of a novel implantable artificial anal sphincter. Dis Colon Rectum 1997, 40:711–717.

9

Diagnostic Evaluation of Pelvic Organ Prolapse

Linda Brubaker

More than a decade has passed since the Pelvic Organ Prolapse Quantification system for quantitatively describing prolapse was accepted by the relevant professional societies. Since that time, several important studies have clarified other aspects of the diagnostic evaluation of pelvic organ prolapse (POP), especially with regard to concomitant conditions such as urinary incontinence and defecatory dysfunction. This chapter will update the reader regarding best practices for the physical examination of POP. In addition, ancillary material for surgical testing is reviewed.

As more research on POP emerges, the issue of population screening has become more important. The focus of this chapter is on symptomatic women. However, there is new information about the poor correlation of specific symptoms that are commonly attributable to POP. The symptom of a vaginal bulge that can be felt or seen is highly specific for POP. Urinary incontinence and defecatory dysfunction are nonspecific symptoms and should not be assumed to indicate the presence of POP.

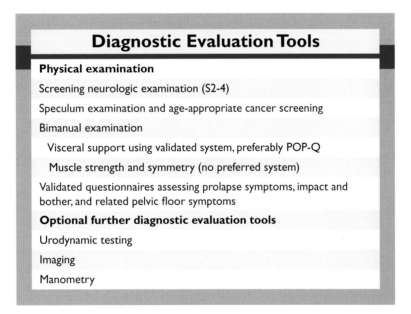

Diagnostic Evaluation Tools

Physical examination

Screening neurologic examination (S2-4)

Speculum examination and age-appropriate cancer screening

Bimanual examination

  Visceral support using validated system, preferably POP-Q

  Muscle strength and symmetry (no preferred system)

Validated questionnaires assessing prolapse symptoms, impact and bother, and related pelvic floor symptoms

Optional further diagnostic evaluation tools

Urodynamic testing

Imaging

Manometry

Figure 9-1. Diagnostic evaluation tools: assessment of vaginal support. The physical examination is the most essential evaluation tool for assessment of vaginal support. Unfortunately, there is no clear dichotomy between "normal" and "pelvic organ prolapse." Moreover, it is clear that normal, asymptomatic, vaginally parous women have different vaginal support than nulliparous women. POP-Q—Pelvic Organ Prolapse Quantification system.

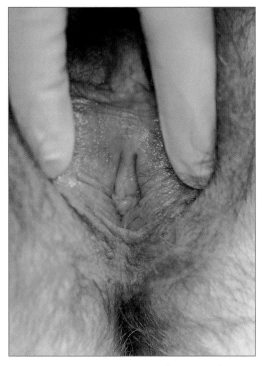

Figure 9-2. The typical vaginal support for nulliparous women is categorized as either stage 0 or I using the Pelvic Organ Prolapse Quantification system. The vaginal wall is rugous, with lateral attachments to the pelvic sidewall at the arcus tendinous fasciae pelvic. The corresponding vaginal topography of this attachment is the lateral sulci at 10 and 2 o'clock (with the patient in the dorsal lithotomy position). The distal rectovaginal septum is attached broadly to the perineal body.

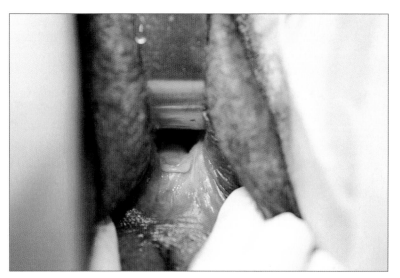

Figure 9-3. The external urethral meatus and urethrovesical junction are typically well supported both at rest and during strain. The urethrovesical junction is approximately 3 cm proximal to the hymen and corresponds roughly with point Aa in the Pelvic Organ Prolapse Quantification (POP-Q) system [1]. The introital opening is held closed, with small POP-Q genital hiatus measurements. The perineal body is well developed. The distance between the external urethral meatus and the midanal opening is significantly smaller than in vaginally parous women [2].

PAROUS WOMEN

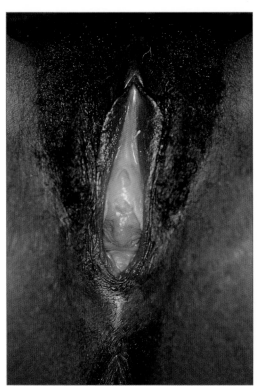

Figure 9-4. After at least one vaginal delivery, the vaginal topography is altered. Common support changes may result in the Ba (anterior) or Bp (posterior) wall being located at the hymen according to the Pelvic Organ Prolapse Quantification (POP-Q) system (point = 0). Using the POP-Q system, such women are categorized in POP-Q stage 2 although many do not have clear symptoms of pelvic organ prolapse (POP). Such women do not require further evaluation or treatment. The natural history of these parity-related topography changes is not known.

There are few data to guide physicians in evaluating the uterine support loss that remains within the vagina. Clearly, there is a threshold at which the uterine (apical) support loss becomes symptomatic but, similar to POP overall, there is no dichotomy between "normal" and "abnormal" uterine support.

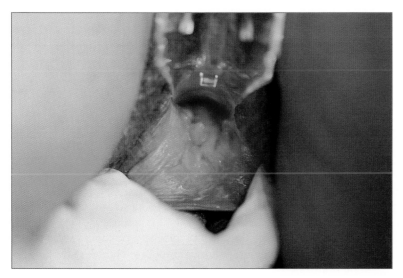

Figure 9-5. Physical examination of the integrity of the connection of the rectovaginal septum to the perineal body is commonly recommended. However, the validity of the examiner's interpretation of "laxity" has not been tested. Multiple emerging studies report that the severity of defecatory symptoms is not related to the severity of prolapse [3,4]. In addition, limited data question the utility of a concomitant posterior wall support procedure at the time of sacrocolpopexy. In an ancillary analysis of the colpopexy and urinary reduction efforts study, women who underwent concomitant posterior vaginal support procedures were no more likely to experience relief for the majority of defecatory symptoms, but were more likely to report postoperative dyspareunia [3,5–7].

ABNORMAL

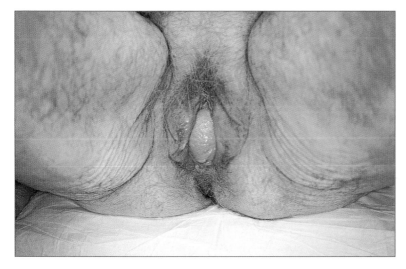

Figure 9-6. Although the posterior cul-de-sac Pelvic Organ Prolapse Quantification (POP-Q) system measurement is not present in women with prior hysterectomy, support abnormalities occur and should be quantified in the presence or absence of the uterus. Support abnormalities that protrude beyond the hymen are more likely to be associated with symptomatic pelvic organ prolapse (POP). Using the POP-Q system, once any aspect of the prolapse extends more than 1 cm beyond the hymen, the woman's support is quantified as stage 3 or 4, depending on her specific support abnormalities.

It is critically important to assess apical support. Nearly all women with symptomatic POP have apical support loss. Support of the apex can secondarily support the anterior and posterior walls. Although it may be difficult to identify the specific abnormalities involved in a given woman's prolapse, it is prudent to assume that apical support is lost and to work hard to disprove that belief. Recent studies have reported that when the anterior wall has lost support, the apex support is also lost. There is a mathematical relationship that describes this finding [8,9].

The importance of apical support is greatest in uterovaginal prolapse. A surgical treatment that removes the uterus, but does not support the apex well, is unlikely to resolve POP.

AREAS OF CONTROVERSY IN SUPPORT ASSESSMENT

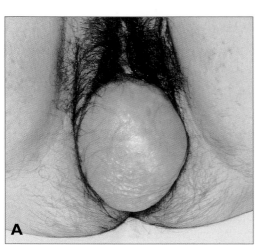

A

Figure 9-7. Examination position. A, Posthysterctomy. B, Uterus in place. Expert opinion and one National Institutes of Health Pelvic Floor Disorders Network study suggest that it is important for the physician examining affected women to visualize the maximum extent of the prolapse [10]. In women with complete anatomic loss, this can often be accomplished with the patient in the supine position. However, in the majority of women seeking evaluation for pelvic organ prolapse (POP), the standing, straining examination is more revealing.

Vaginal rugosity. The presence or absence of vaginal rugosity is interpreted in different ways by different expert surgeons. The majority expert opinion suggests that loss of rugosity indicates significant loss of underlying fibromuscular tissue [11,12].

Continued on the next page

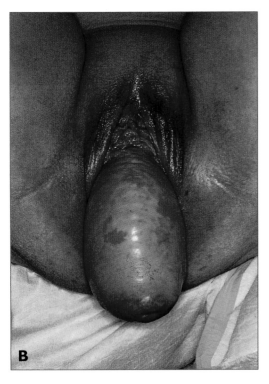

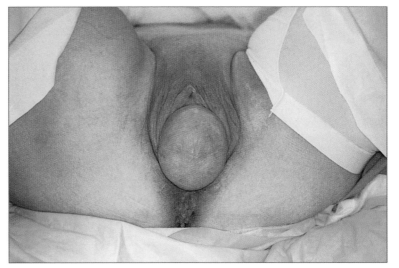

Figure 9-7. *(Continued)* Urethral hypermobility. Similar to POP overall, there is no clear dichotomy between "normal" and "abnormal" urethral support. In the Pelvic Organ Prolapse Quantification (POP-Q) system, point Aa is approximately equivalent to the urethrovesical junction. Recent studies suggest that there is adequate correlation between this physical examination finding and traditional Q-tip measures of urethral support [13]. The Q-tip assessment is not a recommended evaluation for clinical care and has a questionable role even in research settings. The relationship of fluoroscopy during urodynamics has suggested that fluoroscopy is superior to physical examination techniques, including the Q-tip [14]. Some investigators have demonstrated that urethral support can be reliably measured in the research setting using MRI [15].

Routine imaging. Some investigators have recommended that the complete support assessment requires some form of imaging, usually MRI. The routine use of fluoroscopy, such as defecography, is not recommended. Although these tools may be useful for women with special circumstances or unusual findings on physical examination, there is no evidence to support routine imaging in the diagnostic assessment for women with POP.

DISCUSSION OF OTHER POP CASES

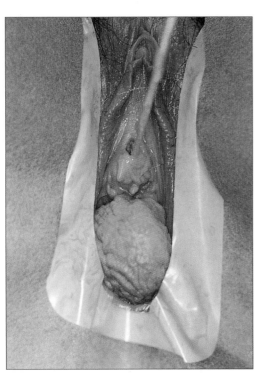

Figure 9-8. Stage 3 pelvic organ prolapse. The posterior vaginal wall may lose its support superiorly (at the upper vagina) and demonstrate prolapse beyond the hymen. The normal rugosity of this posterior wall is generally believed to represent the presence of the rectovaginal fascia, which is composed of smooth muscle and modified connective tissue.

Figure 9-9. Stage 4 pelvic organ prolapse (POP). The anatomic support of the entire posterior vaginal wall may be lost, resulting in complete eversion of the posterior vaginal wall, which commonly exists with a complete vaginal vault prolapse. Beginning at the hymen, the entire posterior wall is everted. Although a rectocele may be present, approximately 30% of patients with this topography do not have fluoroscopic evidence for rectocele formation. It is desirable to consider apical prolapse as the primary problem because the uterus is essentially an innocent passenger in the process of support loss. Removal of the uterus without restoring apical support may achieve a suboptimal surgical outcome. The normal apical structures (*see* Chapter 1) are no longer effective.

Continued on the next page

Figure 9-9. *(Continued)* The evaluation of apical support must distinguish whether or not there is cervical elongation. In cases of cervical elongation, the initial finding of cervical protrusion may be mistaken for uterine prolapse. This is best assessed with the patient in the standing, straining position.

Apical evaluation: abnormal support 1 year after vaginal hysterectomy for prolapse (stage 4 pelvic organ prolapse). In complete support loss, support for the entire anterior and posterior walls is lost, usually secondarily to apical loss. During the physical examination in the office setting, replacement of the apex may be useful to plan surgical repair. However, this does not always guide the need for separate anterior or posterior wall placation. There is little evidence to guide surgical decisions based on this aspect of physical examination.

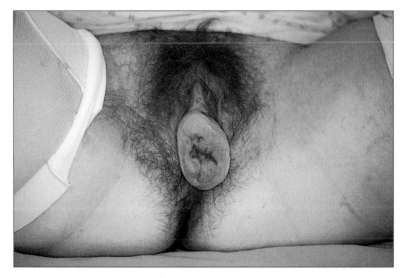

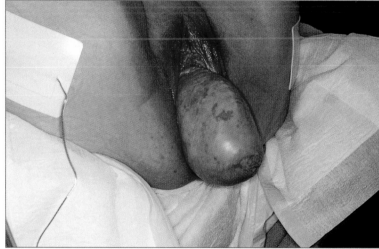

Figure 9-10. Stage 3 uterovaginal pelvic organ prolapse. The normal-sized uterus is present. Due to a loss of uterosacral integrity, the uterus has descended several centimeters below the hymen. Standing, straining evaluation is essential to demonstrate additional components of this prolapse. Although the primary support loss is apical, the clinician must assess the anterior and posterior walls as well. Hysterectomy must be accompanied by adequate apical support measures beyond simple attachment of elongated uterosacral ligament pedicles to the cuff. As discussed in the subsequent treatment chapters, the use of uterosacral ligaments for apical support requires shortening and reinforcement of these structures. If these ligaments are surgically inadequate, alternative apical support procedures must be performed.

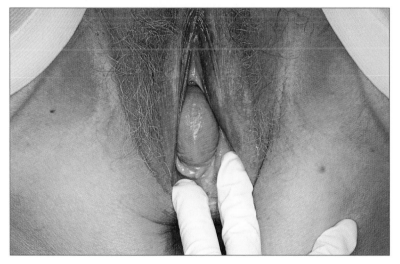

Figure 9-11. Stage 3 pelvic organ prolapse. This posterior vaginal prolapse is secondary to apical prolapse following vaginal hysterectomy and became apparent shortly following prior vaginal hysterectomy without specific apical support. This apical support loss can be suspected given the time course of recurrent prolapse shortly after a primary prolapse operation that included hysterectomy. This apical support loss can be visualized during a straining, half-speculum examination as the blade is slowly withdrawn from the upper third of the vagina.

Figure 9-12. Stage 4 uterovaginal pelvic organ prolapse. This postmenopausal woman presents with complete lack of vaginal support. The 40-g uterus has descended well outside the body because the normal support structures of the vagina failed completely. When complete eversion is present in the supine position, it is not necessary to examine the patient in the standing, straining position because all vaginal points are maximally everted at rest.

Diagnostic Evaluation of Pelvic Organ Prolapse

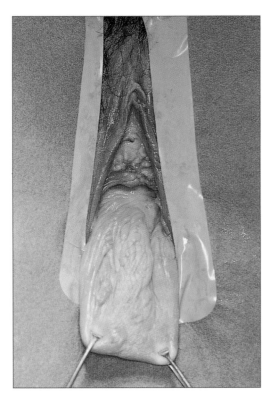

Figure 9-13. Stage 4 pelvic organ prolapse (POP) following hysterectomy. Hysterectomy for stage 4 POP without effective treatment of the apical loss will result in persistent prolapse, as demonstrated in this patient. Anatomically, it is important to recognize that the patient in Figure 9-12 and this patient both have apical failures. The major difference is the presence or absence of the uterus.

EVALUATION OF THE PERINEAL BODY AND GENITAL HIATUS

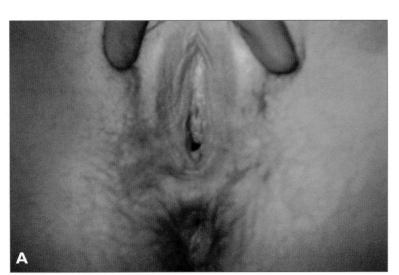

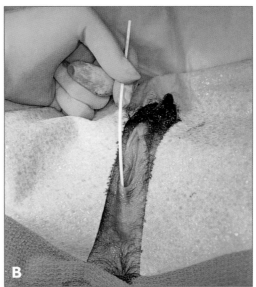

Figure 9-14. Once a decision for surgery has been made, the surgeon must counsel the patient regarding specific surgical procedures, including potential reconstruction of the perineal body. These images are illustrative of issues in this regard.

A, Perineal body/genital hiatus. Closure of the genital hiatus is facilitated by the levator ani muscle complex. When this muscle group is poorly functioning, a widened vaginal opening may be apparent. This may or may not coexist with a small perineal body of poor integrity. Many nulliparous women have perineal body lengths of 2 to 3 cm. The function of the muscle group is certain-

ly more important than the length of the perineal body. However, the importance of rectovaginal fascial attachment to the perineal body is critical for optimal defecation. **B,** A surgically lengthened perineal body is often a surgeon's goal during reconstruction. Preoperatively, the perineal body must be palpated carefully for strength and integrity. A surgically created bridge of skin may mask recurrent or persistent pelvic organ prolapse. This patient reported postoperative dyspareunia and a pelvic pressure consistent with the prolapsing viscera, which was held in by this band of perineal skin.

POP: Methods of Recording

System of Grading	Advantages	Disadvantages
Recommended		
POP-Q [1]	Most quantitative	Not widely adopted
	Demonstrated reproducibility	Not intuitive for many clinicians
	Suited for research and outcome measures	Limited in descriptions of the anatomic site
		Limited in the ability to describe anterior and posterior walls
Baden-Walker halfway system [2]	Used clinically	Pools data into four categorical groups
	Describes apical loss well	Limited usefulness for research
	Easy to use and understand	Reproducibility not known
Not recommended (of historical interest only)		
Grades (0/1–3/4) [3]	Most well known	Poorly described
	Easy	Reproducibility poor
		Inadequate for outcomes research
Stages (0/1–4) [3]	Easy	Poorly described
		Reproducibility poor
		Inadequate for outcomes research

Figure 9-15. Multiple methods have been reported for describing the severity of pelvic organ prolapse (POP). Each system has its aspects of clinical utility and limitations and each physician must select and adhere to his or her preferred system. Objective outcomes of surgical results are best achieved with a quantified system such as the Pelvic Organ Prolapse Quantification (POP-Q) system [1].

Multiple methods for describing the severity of POP have been promulgated. Each system has advantages and disadvantages. The POP-Q system is the most detailed and useful for research settings. The Baden-Walker halfway system is also useful for research, although there are fewer inter- and intraobserver reliability studies on this system. The use of other systems is not recommended for clinical or research description.

Sites of POP-Q

Description	Range of Possible Values
Anterior wall	
Aa: Single point 3 cm from the hymen	-3 to +3
Ab: Using a segment from 3 cm (Aa) to the apex, which describes the position of the most distal point of the anterior wall	-3 to +3 total vaginal length
Posterior wall	
Pa: Single point 3 cm from the hymen	-3 to +3
Pb: Using a segment from 3 in (Pa) to the apex, which describes the position of the most distal point of the posterior wall	-3 to +3 total vaginal length
Apex	
C: Position of the apex when prolapse is at the maximum protrusion	
D: If the uterus is present, position of the posterior fornix, which is helpful in determining the extent of cervical elongation	
Total vaginal length (to cuff or cervix)	

Figure 9-16. Sites of the Pelvic Organ Prolapse Quantification (POP-Q) system. The specific sites of the POP-Q examination become more familiar with frequent use. These points are particularly helpful in recording the surgical outcomes in an objective manner. The conditions of the examination (patient position, use of strain, recording instrument) should be identical before and after surgery to obtain a meaningful comparison of any change. For a diagram of the POP-Q system sites, *see* Figure 4-18.

Point Aa anterior wall	Point Ba anterior wall	Point C cervix or cuff
Gh genital hiatus	Pb perineal body	tvl total vaginal length
Point Ap posterior wall	Point Bp posterior wall	Point D posterior fornix

Figure 9-17. Recording the Pelvic Organ Prolapse Quantification (POP-Q) system—numeric form. This figure shows a simple method of recording the POP-Q values in an office chart. Although this method is convenient, each clinician may develop a method most suited to his or her situation.

OTHER CLINICAL CONDITIONS MIMICKING OR RELATED TO POP

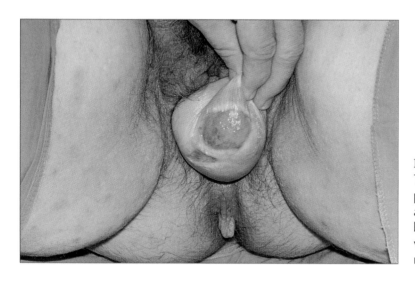

Figure 9-18. Chronic ulceration of long-standing vaginal prolapse. This patient was told that she did not require surgical repair of her posthysterectomy prolapse because she was no longer sexually active. She sought care when she experienced increasing vaginal bleeding. The chronic ulceration should prompt evaluation for vaginal neoplasia. Experts consider these patients to be at increased risk for vaginal evisceration.

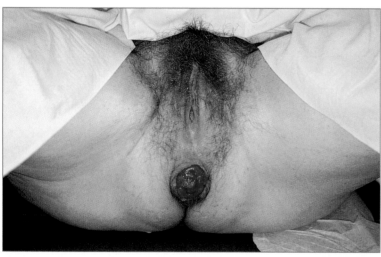

Figure 9-19. Rectal prolapse. The report of hemorrhoids should prompt evaluation of defecation habits and careful anorectal examination. This patient believed her rectal prolapse was severe hemorrhoids. Although she did have hemorrhoids in the typical locations, they were very small. The rectal prolapse extended about 4 cm outside her anal skin and became increasingly difficult to replace, prompting her to consult a physician.

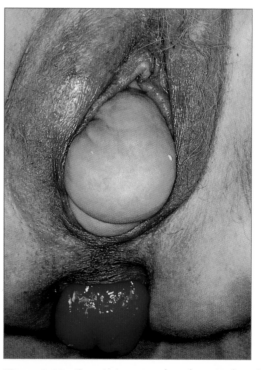

Figure 9-20. Coexisting rectal and vaginal prolapse. Rectal and vaginal prolapse can coexist, albeit uncommonly. Simultaneous repair procedures can be accomplished, relieving the patient of both conditions with an adequate surgical outcome.

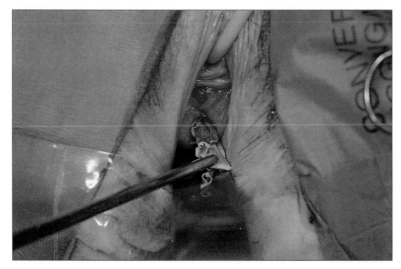

Figure 9-21. Foreign body complications. The use of synthetic materials to treat pelvic organ prolapse (POP) is increasing, especially in women with recurrent prolapse. Although there is no evidence supporting the routine use of synthetic materials for primary POP repairs, this clinical situation is also becoming more common. Thus, surgeons who treat POP will encounter foreign body complications. The typical presenting symptoms of vaginal erosion of synthetic materials include persistent, abnormal vaginal discharge, spotting, and a foul odor. The optimal synthetic material for POP repair is not known, although certain materials are more prone to erosion and should be avoided in prolapse repair.

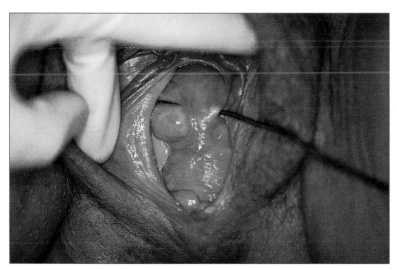

Figure 9-22. Loss of vaginal length after colporrhaphy. This patient had recurrent pelvic organ prolapse that was treated with a series of three anterior and posterior colporrhaphies. Her chief complaint of pelvic pressure persisted. The vaginal length had been reduced to 4 cm with a markedly reduced caliber and pliability.

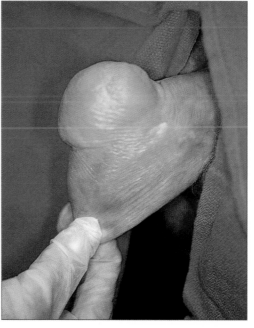

Figure 9-23. Recurrent prolapse. This patient presented with pelvic organ prolapse after a transvaginal paravaginal with sacrospinous ligament suspension performed for posthysterectomy vaginal vault prolapse. The unusual midline defect may have resulted from an undetected preoperative midline defect, which was exacerbated by lateral attachments.

Urodynamic testing. Women with pelvic organ prolapse (POP) commonly have symptoms of urinary tract dysfunction, including stress urinary incontinence (SUI). The current nomenclature describing incontinence is not adequate for describing the clinical situations in women with POP. In a recent study of women undergoing sacrocolpopexy, only 3% demonstrated urodynamic stress incontinence without prolapse reduction.

For women with overt symptoms of SUI, reduction testing will demonstrate the urodynamic finding of urodynamic stress incontinence (USI) in the majority of women. The optimal technique for POP reduction (POP replacement) is not known. The colpopexy and urinary reduction efforts data suggested that reduction with swabs most closely approximates the untreated postoperative stress incontinence outcome

[16]. There are no evidence-based guidelines for selection of concomitant stress incontinence procedures based on any measure of sphincteric integrity.

The colpopexy and urinary reduction efforts trial also demonstrated the protective benefit of Burch colposuspension at the time of sacrocolpopexy in stress-continent women [6]. Women who demonstrated USI during urodynamic testing were more likely to leak than those who did not demonstrate USI. However, based on the overall protective role of the Burch colposuspension at the time of sacrocolpopexy, this procedure should be offered at the time of sacrocolpopexy. An ongoing study will provide information about stress-continent women selecting vaginal POP repairs. Generalizations to other continence procedures or other routes of surgery should be made with caution.

MANOMETRY

Bowel symptoms are common in women, especially in women with prolapse. In an ancillary study of the colpopexy and urinary reduction efforts sacrocolpopexy population, bowel symptoms were common and did not reliably improve with anatomical correction following surgery [3]. Manometry is not recommended as a routine test for the diagnostic evaluation of pelvic organ prolapse

(POP). However, women with concomitant anal incontinence or severe defecatory symptoms may benefit from this additional evaluation.

Pelvic floor fluoroscopy can be used selectively to clarify the visceral abnormalities associated with recurrent or unusual forms of POP. This technique is not recommended as a routine evaluation for POP.

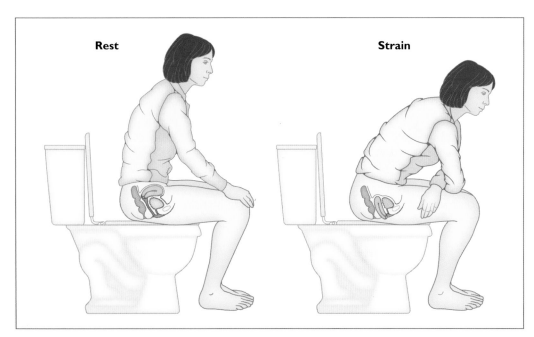

Figure 9-24. Defecating cystoproctography is one of the terms used for fluoroscopic, dynamic imaging of the pelvic viscera. This technique can be performed using opacification of a single viscera or all four of the relevant pelvic viscera (bladder, vaginal, small bowel, and large bowel). This adjunct to physical examination provides additional information about visceral function and support. Technical aspects have been described elsewhere [17]. The pelvis is imaged in the lateral, seated position. Simulated defecation efforts promote maximal protrusion of the prolapsed structures. The patient is seated on a radiolucent commode. After contrast administration, defecation of the rectal contrast occurs. Serial lateral images are obtained throughout the defecation process. This degree of strain maximizes the prolapse, frequently beyond what was visible during a standard physical examination.

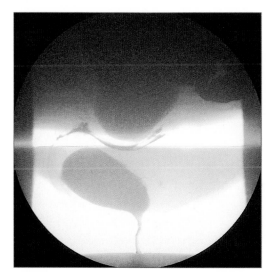 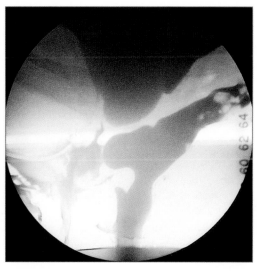 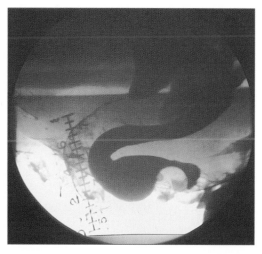

Figure 9-25. Retaining rectocele. This image demonstrates a large rectal protrusion that persists and appears to trap contrast at the end of spontaneous defecation. This distal abnormality is the most common appearance of a rectocele on fluoroscopy. The distal location is typical for the initial presentation of a rectocele, whereas previously operated rectoceles may be located more proximally.

Figure 9-26. Abnormal position of rectocele (postcolporrhaphy). This image demonstrates the more proximal position of a recurrent rectocele after posterior colporrhaphy. The plication of the levator complex can be seen distally. Proximal to this plication, the area of lesser strength protrudes over the plicated muscles. The patient reported persistently difficult defecation with the need to manually assist her defecation.

Figure 9-27. Sigmoidocele. Less commonly, a posterior wall or apical prolapse can be caused by redundant rectosigmoid. The optimal surgical management of this finding remains under study.

Most MRI sequences are completed with the patient in the supine position. However, some anatomic associations with pelvic organ prolapse may be seen using this technique, including abnormalities of muscular attachment or gross integrity [18–20]. Given the limitations and cost of this examination, MRI imaging is reserved for highly selected situations or the research setting.

REFERENCES

1. Bump RC, Mattiasson A, Bo K, *et al.*: The standardization of terminology of female pelvic organ prolapse and pelvic floor dysfunction. *Am J Obstet Gynecol* 1996, 175:10–17.

2. Delancey JO, Hurd WW: Size of the urogenital hiatus in the levator ani muscles in normal women and women with pelvic organ prolapse. *Obstet Gynecol* 1998, 91:364–368.

3. Bradley CS, Brown MB, Cundiff GW, *et al.*: Bowel symptoms in women planning surgery for pelvic organ prolapse. *Am J Obstet Gynecol* 2006, 195:1814–1819.

4. Dooley Y, West K, Kenton K, *et al.*: Bowel symptoms and POP-Q stage are poorly correlated. *Am J Obstet Gynecol* 2006, 12:263–266.

5. Brubaker L, Cundiff G, Fine P, *et al.*: A randomized trial of colpopexy and urinary reduction efforts (CARE): design and methods. *Control Clin Trials* 2003, 24:629–642.

6. Brubaker L, Cundiff GW, Fine P, *et al.*: Abdominal sacrocolpopexy with Burch colposuspension to reduce urinary stress incontinence. *N Engl J Med* 2006, 13:1557–1566.

7. Brubaker L, Nygaard I, Richter H, *et al.*: Two-year outcomes after sacrocolpopexy with and without Burch to prevent stress urinary incontinence: a randomized controlled trial. *Obstet Gynecol* 2008, 112.

8. Rooney K, Kenton K, Mueller ER, *et al.*: Advanced anterior vaginal wall prolapse is highly correlated with apical prolapse. *Am J Obstet Gynecol* 2006, 195:1837–1840.

9. Chen L, Ashton-Miller J, DeLancey J: Do pubococcygeus muscle and the cardinal uterosacral ligament complex impairments interact to affect anterior vaginal wall descent? *J Pelvic Med Surg* 2005, 11(suppl 1):S2.

10. Visco AG, Wei JT, McClure LA, *et al.*: Effects of examination technique modifications on pelvic organ prolapse quantification (POP-Q) results. *Int Urogynecol J Pelvic Floor Dysfunct* 2003, 14:136–140.

11. Delancey JO: Fascial and muscular abnormalities in women with urethral hypermobility and anterior vaginal wall prolapse. *Am J Obstet Gynecol* 2002, 187:93–98.

12. Hsu Y, Chen L, Delancey JO, Ashton-Miller JA: Vaginal thickness, cross-sectional area, and perimeter in women with and those without prolapse. *Obstet Gynecol* 2005, 105:1012–1017.

13. Zyzynski H, Lloyd K, Kenton K, *et al.*: Correlation of Q-tip values and point Aa in stress incontinent women. *Obstet Gynecol* 2007, 110:39–43.

14. Zimmern P, Nager CW, Albo M, *et al.*: Urinary incontinence treatment network interrater reliability of filling cystometrogram interpretation in a multicenter study. *J Urol* 2006, 175:2174–2177.

15. Chou Q, DeLancey JO: A structured system to evaluate urethral support anatomy in magnetic resonance images. *Am J Obstet Gynecol* 2001, 185:44–50.

16. Visco AG for the Pelvic Floor Disorders Network: *The Role of Pre-Operative Urodynamic Testing in Stress Continent Women Undergoing Sacrocolpopexy: The Colpopexy and Urinary Reduction Efforts (CARE) Randomized Surgical Trial.* Tucson, AZ: Society for Gynecologic Surgeons (SGS); 2006.

17. Brubaker L, Retzky S, Smith C, Saclarides T: Pelvic floor evaluation with dynamic fluoroscopy. *Obstet Gynecol* 1993, 82:863–868.

18. Hsu Y, Chen L, Huebner M, *et al.*: Quantification of levator ani cross-sectional area differences between women with and those without prolapse. *Obstet Gynecol* 2006, 108:879–883.

19. Hsu Y, Summers A, Hussain HK, *et al.*: Levator plate angle in women with pelvic organ prolapse compared to women with normal support using dynamic MR imaging. *Am J Obstet Gynecol* 2006, 194:1427–1433.

20. Margulies RU, Hsu Y, Kearney R, *et al.*: Appearance of the levator ani muscle subdivisions in magnetic resonance images. *Obstet Gynecol* 2006, 107:1064–1069.

10

Nonsurgical Management of Pelvic Organ Prolapse

Stephen B. Young

Many women with pelvic organ prolapse (POP) are best served or prefer to have nonsurgical therapy as a first-line treatment. This chapter details the use of pessaries, the most common and definitive nonsurgical therapy for POP. Other nonsurgical therapy revolves around a variety of approaches to increase levator ani control and strength, the use of vaginal estrogen, and lifestyle changes. Increasing levator ani strength and control, meant to combat POP progression, can be accomplished by the proper performance of Kegel exercises [1] or other modalities to achieve effective levator ani muscle tone. These include physical therapy, biofeedback, functional electric stimulation, and the use of vaginal weighted cones.

Bo [2] hypothesizes two mechanisms for how pelvic floor muscle training may be effective in the treatment of POP: 1) women learn to consciously contract before and with increases in abdominal pressure and continue to perform such contractions as a behavioral modification to prevent descent of the pelvic floor. 2) Women are taught to perform regular strength training over time in order to build-up "stiffness" and structural support of the pelvic floor. Improving the strength of the pelvic musculature may have a beneficial effect both on pessary retention and prevention of POP progression. Preoperative physiotherapy may improve the outcomes of reconstructive pelvic surgery for POP [3]. There are specially trained physical therapists and nurse specialists who have a clinical interest in pelvic floor rehabilitation. Kegel exercises must be continued over the course of many years if their beneficial effect is to be maintained. However, long-term adherence to training is low [4].

Pessaries are excellent devices to prepare for, postpone, or prevent surgical intervention. Many postmenopausal women with exteriorized prolapse (stages III and IV) present with atrophic, dry, thin, cracked, and frequently ulcerated vaginal skin outside the vulva. To prepare for optimal surgical intervention, a minimum of 2 months of topical intravaginal estrogen cream should be applied or inserted. A pessary will keep the exteriorized bulge in situ, allowing for improvement in the local environment by relieving vascular kinking, air drying, and decreasing friction from contact with clothing. The now replaced vagina can maintain prolonged contact with the estrogen cream, which is inserted each night. This will encourage thickening, increased vascularity, and perhaps even improvement in the dissection planes to permit optimized surgical technique. Other patients with prolapse want to wait a period of months before surgery. The schoolteacher, the "snowbird," and the caregiver of a sick husband may need to postpone definitive correction to a more appropriate time. Many older women have multiple significant medical conditions that render them poor candidates for lengthy pelvic reconstruction or even obliteration. They may be treated effectively with long-term pessary use.

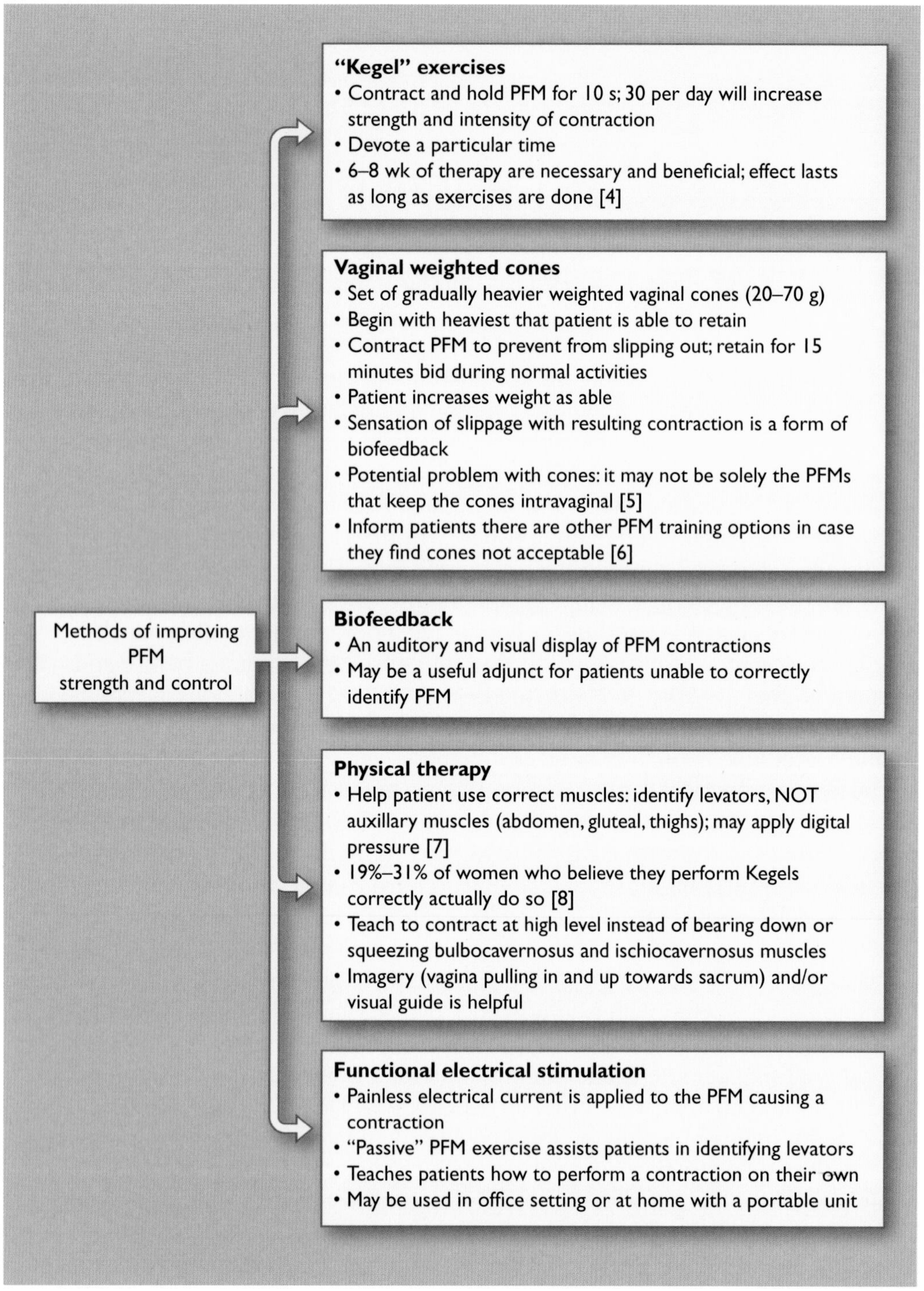

"Kegel" exercises
- Contract and hold PFM for 10 s; 30 per day will increase strength and intensity of contraction
- Devote a particular time
- 6–8 wk of therapy are necessary and beneficial; effect lasts as long as exercises are done [4]

Vaginal weighted cones
- Set of gradually heavier weighted vaginal cones (20–70 g)
- Begin with heaviest that patient is able to retain
- Contract PFM to prevent from slipping out; retain for 15 minutes bid during normal activities
- Patient increases weight as able
- Sensation of slippage with resulting contraction is a form of biofeedback
- Potential problem with cones: it may not be solely the PFMs that keep the cones intravaginal [5]
- Inform patients there are other PFM training options in case they find cones not acceptable [6]

Methods of improving PFM strength and control

Biofeedback
- An auditory and visual display of PFM contractions
- May be a useful adjunct for patients unable to correctly identify PFM

Physical therapy
- Help patient use correct muscles: identify levators, NOT auxillary muscles (abdomen, gluteal, thighs); may apply digital pressure [7]
- 19%–31% of women who believe they perform Kegels correctly actually do so [8]
- Teach to contract at high level instead of bearing down or squeezing bulbocavernosus and ischiocavernosus muscles
- Imagery (vagina pulling in and up towards sacrum) and/or visual guide is helpful

Functional electrical stimulation
- Painless electrical current is applied to the PFM causing a contraction
- "Passive" PFM exercise assists patients in identifying levators
- Teaches patients how to perform a contraction on their own
- May be used in office setting or at home with a portable unit

Figure 10-1. Pelvic floor muscle (PFM) training. Physical therapy using PFM should be used to treat patients with pelvic organ prolapse. PFM training has no known side effects and has shown to be effective in clinical trials and systematic reviews on the treatment of stress urinary incontinence and mixed incontinence. Many women present with both pelvic organ prolapse and stress urinary incontinence [9]. bid—twice daily.

Effects of Estrogen Therapy

Estrogen positively affects much of the pelvic floor

Serum estrogen levels and estrogen receptor values are lower in the uterosacral and cardinal ligaments of premenopausal women with POP [10]

Estrogen receptor values correlate positively with years postmenopausal [10]

Systemic effects

Estrogen can be administered systemically via oral, transdermal, or (secondarily) transvaginal absorption from local creams, rings, or tablets

Estrogen's role in pelvic support is not fully understood and there is no evidence currently to support use of estrogen to prevent or treat prolapse [11]

Selective estrogen receptor modulators have been associated with worsening POP in a systematic review [12]

Intravaginal effects

Urogenital symptoms that clearly respond to estrogen therapy include atrophic vaginitis, dryness, and accompanying dyspareunia [13]

It is a long held belief that vaginal estrogen cream, when used regularly for at least 2 months, will contribute to vaginal thickening, increased vasculature, and facilitated postoperative healing

The estrogen in topical cream preparations is of low potency

Even the lowest-dose estrogen shows evidence of systemic absorption and therefore should be intermittently opposed with progestins in women with uteri [13]

However, in the recent NAMS position statement [14], an alternative position is taken: progestogen is generally not indicated when low-dose estrogen is administered locally

Figure 10-2. Vaginal estrogen. Estrogen positively affects much of the pelvic floor. NAMS—North American Menopausal Society; POP—pelvic organ prolapse.

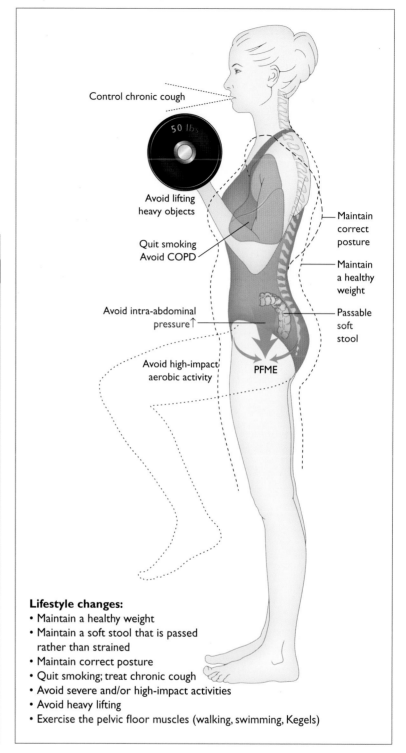

Lifestyle changes:
- Maintain a healthy weight
- Maintain a soft stool that is passed rather than strained
- Maintain correct posture
- Quit smoking; treat chronic cough
- Avoid severe and/or high-impact activities
- Avoid heavy lifting
- Exercise the pelvic floor muscles (walking, swimming, Kegels)

Figure 10-3. Lifestyle changes. Simple modifications in a patient's lifestyle may limit the progression of pelvic organ prolapse and ease its symptoms. These include preventing or treating obesity, instituting pelvic floor muscles exercises (PFME) (walking and swimming), achieving physiologic bowel habits (work-up and treat constipation/straining), quitting smoking and treating chronic cough, and maintaining correct posture. Handa *et al.* [15] found prolapse to be associated with increasing parity and waist circumference. COPD—chronic obstructive pulmonary disease.

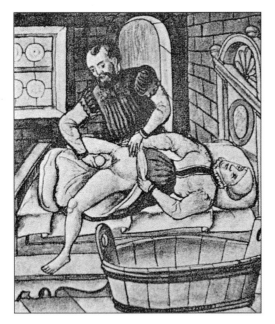

Figure 10-4. The history of pessaries dates back to the Greek and Roman eras and is rich and fascinating in the varieties of organic and inorganic materials used for replacement of vaginal contents. Famous medical names through ancient and medieval times are associated with the development of pessaries. Hippocrates and later Soranus and Diocles used half of a pomegranate sometimes soaked in vinegar. Near the end of the Roman era, emollient, astringent, and aperient drug-soaked pledgets tied with string were used. In the Middle Ages, around 1050 AD, Trotula, the first recorded female gynecologist, made a ball pessary of linen strips, which she held in place with a T-binder. In 1559, Caspar Stromayr (pictured in the woodcut) used a tightly rolled sponge, bound with string, dipped in wax and covered with oil or butter. The great physician Ambrose Paré invented an oval pessary of hammered brass and waxed cork as well as pear-shaped and ring pessaries. The anatomist William Harvey also used pessaries. The first surgical gynecology textbook, by Hendrik Van Roonhuyse in 1663, described a cork with a hole dipped in wax [16]. When complications from pessary use, including discharge and viscus perforation, were discovered, the field evolved. In 1783, Jean Juville invented a soft rubber pessary that could be self-inserted.

Over the past 200 years, pessaries have been used for a variety of uncertain conditions including uterine inflammation, displacement, or retroversion. Over the past 150 years, the invention and development of rubber vulcanization, plastics, and more recently, silicone-based materials have facilitated the evolution of better materials for manufacture. Most pessaries currently in use for the treatment of pelvic organ prolapse are simple, soft, flexible, inert devices made of silicone and supplied in various shapes and sizes. (*From* Miller [16]; with permission.)

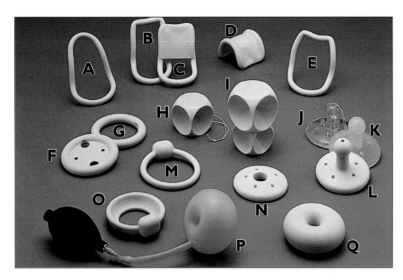

Figure 10-5. Milex pessaries. Milex Products (Chicago, IL) distributes a wide selection of largely silicone-flexible pessaries. **Bold** indicates the pessaries most frequently used and detailed in this chapter.

A. Smith (silicone, folding)
B. Hodge without support (silicone, folding)
C. Hodge with support (silicone, folding)
D. **Gehrung with support (silicone, folding)**
E. Risser (silicone, folding)
F. **Ring with support (silicone, folding)**
G. **Ring without support (silicone, folding)**
H. **Cube (silicone, flexible)**
I. Tandem-Cube (silicone, flexible)

J. Rigid Gellhorn (acrylic, multiple drain)
K. 95% Rigid Gellhorn (silicone, multiple drain)
L. **Flexible Gellhorn (silicone, multiple drain)**
M. Ring incontinence (silicone)
N. Shaatz (silicone, folding)
O. Incontinence dish (silicone, folding)
P. Inflato Ball (latex)
Q. **Donut (silicone)**

In choosing a particular pessary for an individual patient's needs, we try to use the least invasive device that will remain in the vagina, hold the pelvic organs in situ, cause the least number of local symptoms, and require the gentlest and most infrequent change. A properly sized and positioned pessary will sit obliquely behind the symphysis and will just barely appear, if at all, proximal to the levators, on lithotomy Valsalva with the labia separated. A device that is too small will fall out with any activity. A device that is too large may not sit properly behind the symphysis and will cause discomfort and pressure. It may also interfere with micturition and defecation. When possible, we instruct the patient in self-removal, cleaning, and reinsertion. This allows her to change her own pessary in the privacy of her home, taking it out at night and reinserting in the morning so that the vagina can be free of the foreign body while she is at rest. This markedly decreases pessary-related vaginitis and local erosions, by far the most frequent complications of pessary use. It also allows her independence, requiring far fewer pessary follow-up visits. (*From* Milex Products, Chicago, IL.)

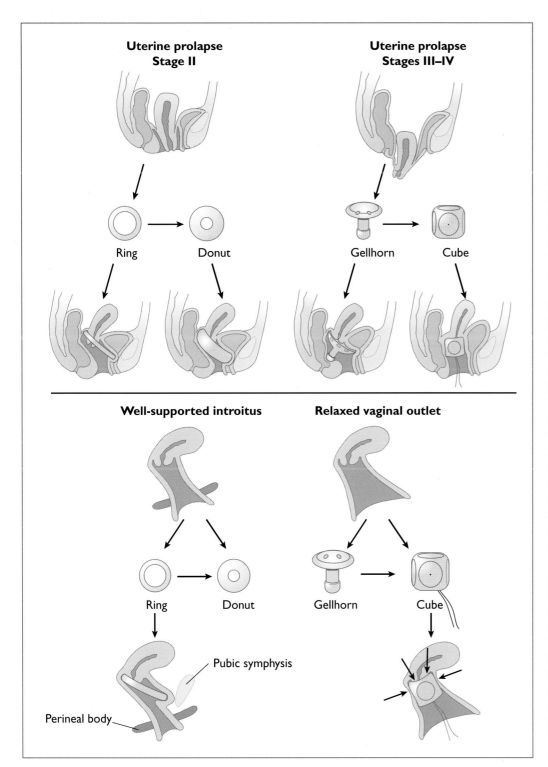

Figure 10-6. Two factors determining pessary choice are the degree of pelvic organ prolapse (*top*) and the integrity of the pelvic outlet (*bottom*). Lesser degrees of pelvic organ prolapse are usually managed adequately with the less invasive, gentler ring, donut, Gehrung, or Marland pessary (Bioteque America, Fremont, CA). More severe or exteriorized lesions, however, may require the Gellhorn (Milex Products, Chicago, IL) or cube device. An intact pelvic outlet consists of a cylindrical, nonfunneled vagina with a well-supported introitus, admitting only two to three fingerbreadths and a thick, long, intact muscular perineum. Many older women with stages III and IV pelvic organ prolapse, however, have a funneled vagina with loss of levator integrity, plus a gaping relaxed vaginal outlet and a markedly deficient perineum. Although all pessaries sit obliquely in the vagina behind the pubic symphysis, the ring, donut, Marland (Bioteque America, Fremont, CA), and Gehrung types rely on a well-supported intact introitus/perineum to stay in the vagina. They will fall out of a funneled vagina with a gaping introitus and deficient perineum with any significant increase in intra-abdominal pressure, such as defecation. The Gellhorn and cube types, conversely, will usually hold up even massive exteriorized lesions with a gaping introitus because they stay in by a different mechanism. The single large dish of the Gellhorn and the multiple cups of the cube pessaries become attached to the vaginal walls by a partial suction effect. This keeps both prolapse and pessary in situ through full activities of daily living.

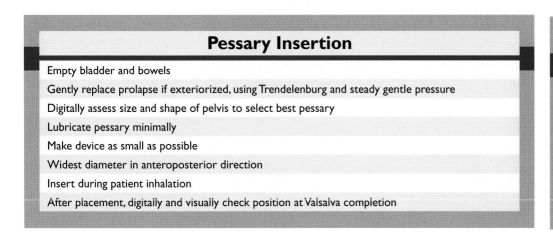

Pessary Insertion

Empty bladder and bowels
Gently replace prolapse if exteriorized, using Trendelenburg and steady gentle pressure
Digitally assess size and shape of pelvis to select best pessary
Lubricate pessary minimally
Make device as small as possible
Widest diameter in anteroposterior direction
Insert during patient inhalation
After placement, digitally and visually check position at Valsalva completion

Figure 10-7. General pessary insertion.

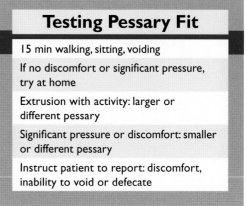

Testing Pessary Fit

15 min walking, sitting, voiding
If no discomfort or significant pressure, try at home
Extrusion with activity: larger or different pessary
Significant pressure or discomfort: smaller or different pessary
Instruct patient to report: discomfort, inability to void or defecate

Figure 10-8. Testing the fit and comfort.

Nonsurgical Management of Pelvic Organ Prolapse 191

Pessary Care
Topical creams
Estrogen cream, metronidazole gel
Self-insertion and removal
Follow-up
Time varies with pessary type
Remove and wash device, inspect vagina
Mild vaginitis: irrigate, betadine painting
Severe vaginitis, erosion, or ulceration: discontinue temporarily

Figure 10-9. Pessary care.

Pessary Complications
Vaginal odor and/or discharge (dilute vinegar or betadine douche)
Severe anaerobic vaginitis
Urinary or fectal retention, pressure
Urinary tract infections
Ulceration, erosion, laceration
Entrapped, embedded pessary
Recto- or vesicovaginal fistulas [17]
Cytologic atypias, vaginal or cervical cancers [18]

Figure 10-10. Complications of pessary use.

SELECTION OF PESSARIES

RING PESSARY

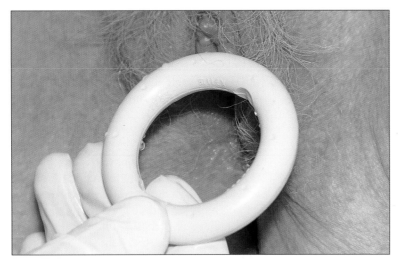

Figure 10-11. Ring pessary. The ring pessary is available with or without a supportive membrane for mild to moderate (stages II and III) prolapse. It is the least invasive and rarely causes heavy discharge. It requires infrequent visits (up to annually), allows easy self-insertion and removal, and without the supportive membrane permits coitus. This ring is used in a very healthy, independent, 80-year-old, multiparous woman with symptomatic stage II utero-vaginal prolapse. She had a strong desire to avoid pelvic surgery if possible and also a well-supported perineum and intact introitus. This was achieved with a folding ring pessary, which is cleaned and reinserted every 6 months.

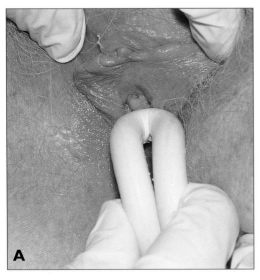
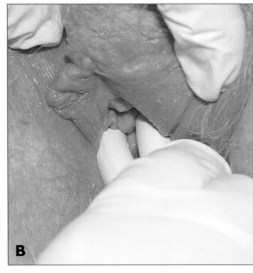
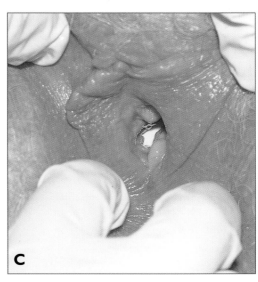

Figure 10-12. Insertion. **A**, Index finger and thumb grasp the ring opposite the notches. Pressure causes the ring to fold in half. **B**, This semicircle is inserted over the perineum, through the introitus with the convexity upward while the nondominant hand holds the labia apart. **C**, Once the lubricated pessary has slipped into the vagina, it is released. It will open up into its semirigid circular form and assume an oblique axis. Its distal rim sits anteriorly just cephalad to the pubic symphysis. Its proximal rim sits posteriorly behind the cervix. Rotate the notch 90° so that it will not flex on its own and spontaneously extrude. This demonstrates a well-positioned pessary.

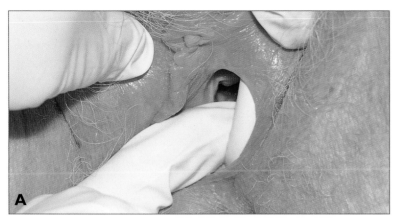

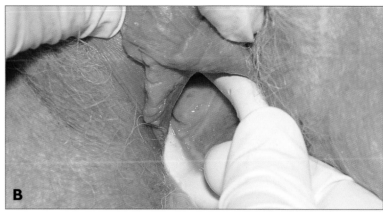

Figure 10-13. Removal. **A**, To remove, insert an index finger inside the ring and find the notch located along the inner surface. **B**, Gently pulling down and out while turning will fold the ring, decreasing its diameter and easing removal.

DONUT PESSARY

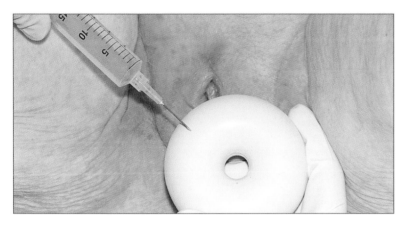

Figure 10-14. Donut pessary. If the ring fails, the donut pessary can be the next choice. It requires outlet integrity and occludes the upper vagina to support prolapse. After approximating the most appropriate size, the air is removed via a 21-gauge needle and a syringe. With the plunger out, the pessary is compressed, and after maximally deflating, the needle is removed.

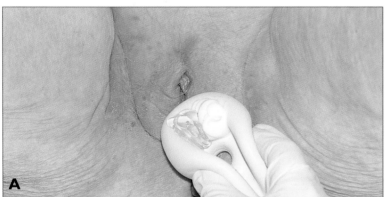

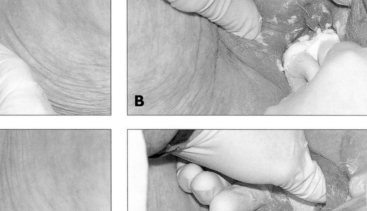

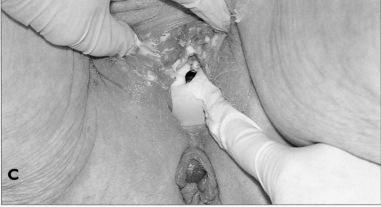

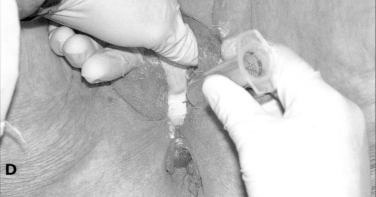

Figure 10-15. Insertion. **A**, The deflated donut occupies less space. **B**, When lubricated, the donut is very easily inserted through the separated labia. **C**, Once the widest part of the donut enters the vagina through the introitus, it tends to slip away from the physician's grasp. **D**, It is held near the introitus with an index finger in the donut's hole so that the needle and syringe without plunger can again be inserted through the silicone wall. The pessary reinflates by equilibrating with room atmosphere. The needle is removed and the pessary slides apically.

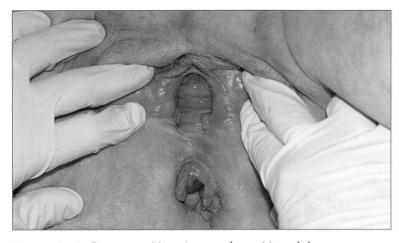

Figure 10-16. Correct position. A properly positioned donut pessary in a 91-year-old woman with massive stage IV uterovaginal prolapse. This patient has been completely asymptomatic through 9 years of treatment with a donut pessary. Generally, patients are seen every 3 months or as needed.

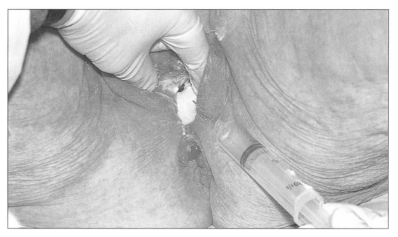

Figure 10-17. Removal. Atraumatic removal is facilitated by first removing the air. The intravaginal donut is grasped with an index finger in the donut hole and brought down near the introitus. The needle and syringe, now with plunger in, are used to draw out the 30 to 60 mL of air. This now deflated donut can be gently and easily removed with simple traction.

GEHRUNG PESSARY

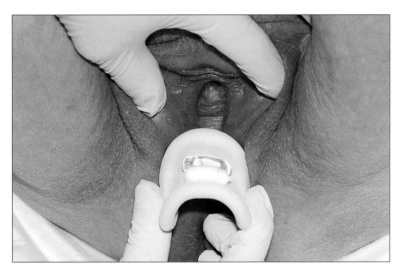

Figure 10-18. Gehrung pessary. This type of pessary is specifically designed for cystocele but may also be used for rectocele. It sits as a double arch under the anterior wall with its legs directed posteriorly. The patient is seen every 3 months for the first year, then bianually. The Gehrung pessary with lubricant is positioned outside the introitus as it will sit intravaginally to treat cystocele. Its two arches will act as a bridge to support the anterior wall. This 68-year-old morbidly obese woman with a symptomatic stage III isolated cystocele and severe anxiety regarding surgery was successfully treated using a Gehrung pessary.

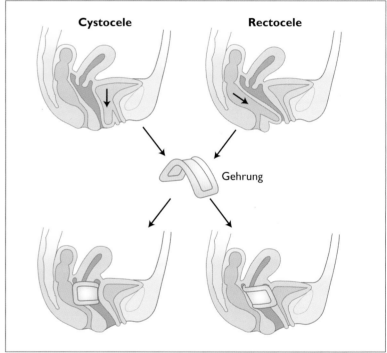

Figure 10-19. Position schematic. The Gehrung pessary with its semirigid double arches sits perpendicular to the long axis of the vagina and is designed specifically as a bridge to support isolated anterior (cystocele) or posterior (rectocele) defects.

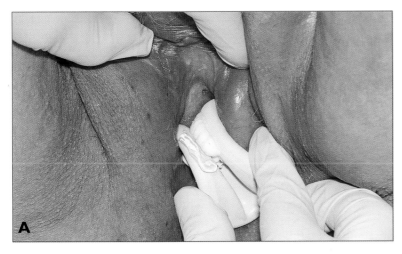

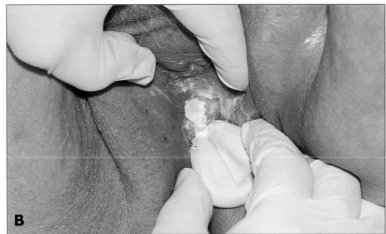

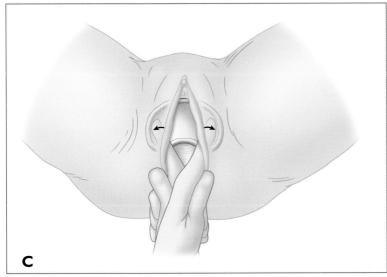

Figure 10-20. Insertion and position. **A**, The two arches are pushed together to decrease its overall size. As such, its insertion is similar to that of a folded ring pessary. **B**, It is slipped into the vagina, convexity upward over the posterior fourchette. It is then rotated 90° so that the more distal arch sits transversely behind the symphysis and the more proximal arch sits transversely under the anterior vaginal apex. **C**, Final adjustment of the Gehrung. Widening the arch: wrists crossed, index fingers inside arch supports push laterally until supports approximate ischiopubic rami. This tends to keep pessary intravaginal and in proper position.

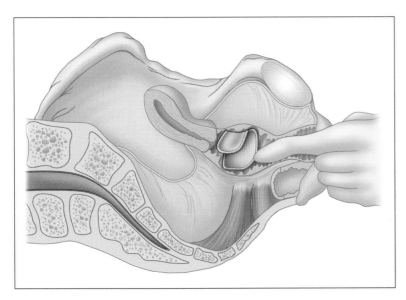

Figure 10-21. Removal. To remove the pessary, insert the index finger and gently turn the pessary as you pull its presenting part down toward, through, and out of the introitus. It will compress as it is twisted.

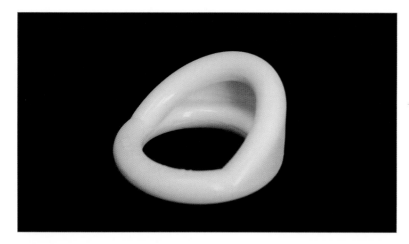

Figure 10-22. The Marland (Bioteque America, Fremont, CA) is a ring pessary with a perpendicular flange coming off one half of the ring. This right angularity will keep the pessary behind the symphysis, preventing slippage. When a ring with or without support membrane slips out of the patient, the Marland pessary (Bioteque America, Fremont, CA) is an excellent choice.

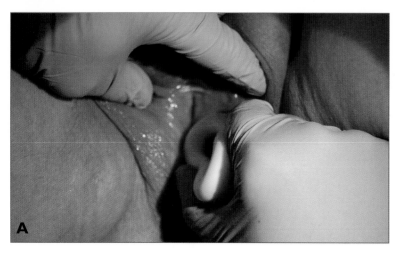

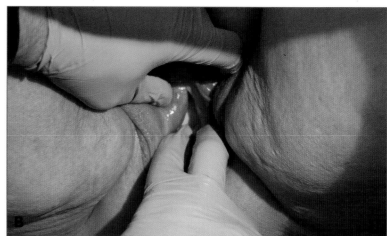

Figure 10-23. Insertion. **A,** Just as the ring is folded, so is the Marland (Bioteque America, Fremont, CA). As shown, the compressed ring part of the Marland is eased through the introitus via the edge opposite the flange. It is then corkscrewed fully into the vagina. **B,** Once in, two fingers inside the ring can adjust the pessary so that the flange sits parallel and just behind the symphysis. The ring part will automatically be in the same oblique position it would be without the flange; *ie,* anterior lip of ring behind symphysis, midring arching obliquely posterior and apical, and posterior rim posterior to cervix.

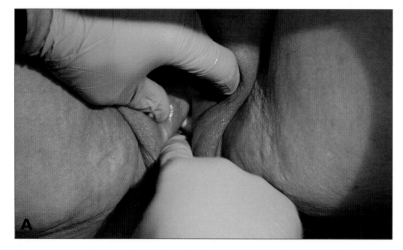

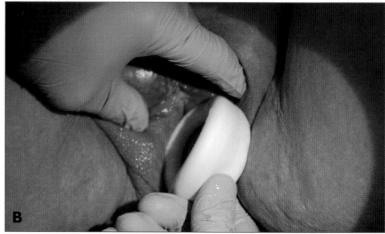

Figure 10-24. Removal. **A,** The Marland pessary (Bioteque America, Fremont, CA) is removed in a manner similar to removing a ring pessary. The dominant index finger is inserted into the ring part. Gentle traction will bring the pessary toward the introitus as the ring compresses. **B,** As traction is slowly continued the pessary is turned to ease its outward motion.

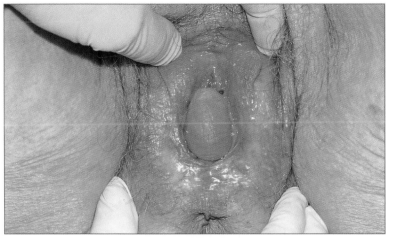

Figure 10-25. Gellhorn pessary. A Gellhorn pessary (Milex Products, Chicago, IL) is an effective device, especially for stages III and IV prolapse. It is strong and supportive because of its size, structure, and partial suction effect. It is successful in those with less outlet support, but its insertion and removal can be difficult. Careful attention to details will minimize patient discomfort. Cleanings are necessary every 2 weeks initially, and then every 1 to 2 months. This 92-year-old patient has stage III vaginal vault prolapse and has been unable to hold a ring or donut pessary. The bulge is very bothersome to her and definitive reconstructive surgery is not an option. In the PESSRI study, Cundiff et al. [19] showed that the ring with support and Gellhorn pessaries are effective and equivalent in relieving symptoms of protrusion and voiding dysfunction.

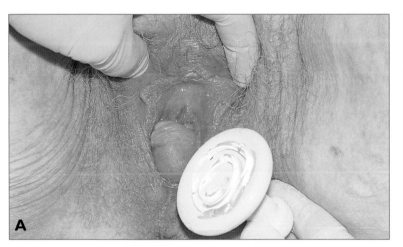

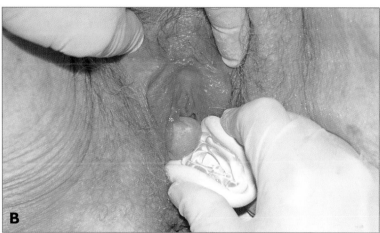

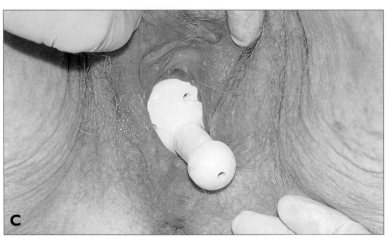

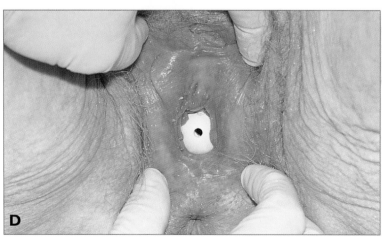

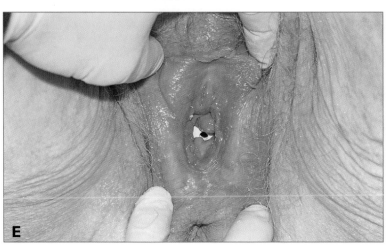

Figure 10-26. Insertion and position. A, Lubricant is applied to the Gellhorn pessary (Milex Products, Chicago, IL). Small Gellhorns like the one pictured (2 ¼ in) can be inserted directly with the dish parallel to the anteroposterior diameter of the introitus, inserting the side of the dish first. B, Alternatively, and particularly with larger Gellhorns, the dish can be pinched or folded to compress its size and inserted obliquely through the vulva held open with the nondominant hand. C, Once the dish is in the vagina, it will spontaneously and easily turn into the proper axis. It should sit obliquely with the dish positioned under the vaginal apex and the horn pointing toward the perineum. D, After the patient is given a chance to relax, the pessary is pushed up into the vaginal apex. E, A properly positioned Gellhorn pessary has its horn pointing down toward the perineum and just barely visible with the vulva held apart and the patient performing a Valsalva maneuver. Gellhorns are also available with a short horn for use in patients with short vaginas.

Nonsurgical Management of Pelvic Organ Prolapse 197

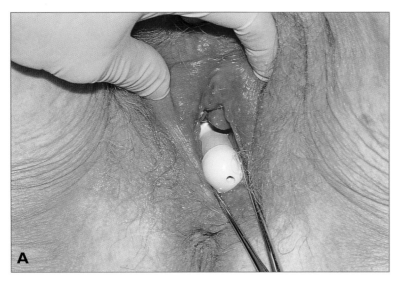 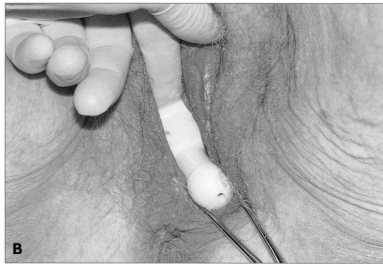

Figure 10-27. Removal. **A**, Removal is facilitated by finding the distal horn with the fingers and grasping it with a single-toothed tenaculum. **B**, Gentle traction on the tenaculum posteriorly will allow an intravaginal index finger of the other hand to slip above the dish and break the suction. Once the suction is broken, the two hands working together will gently guide the Gellhorn pessary (Milex Products, Chicago, IL) down through the vagina and out with the dish in the anteroposterior diameter of the introitus. Significant foreign body–related lesions warrant a temporary moratorium from pessary use until topical estrogen-mediated healing occurs. Vaginal discharge can occur with any pessary and is sometimes quite copious and purulent with the cube and Gellhorn types. After pessary removal and inspection, the vagina can be painted with povidone-iodine–soaked scopettes. With a Gellhorn or cube pessary, epithelial damage is more common. A thorough observation of the entire vaginal epithelium is indicated every time a Gellhorn or cube pessary is changed prior to reinsertion.

━━ CUBE PESSARY ━━━━━━━━━━━━━━━━━━━━━━━━━━━━━━━━━━

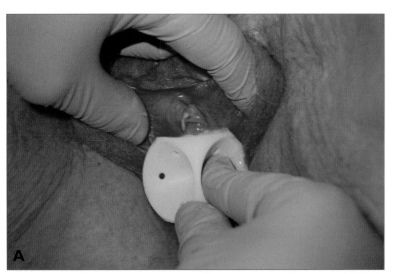 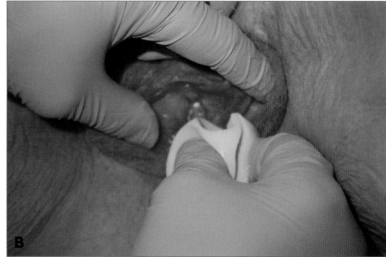

Figure 10-28. Cube pessary. **A**, The cube pessary is a highly effective, space-occupying, soft silicone device that is easily inserted and will support even very large stage III and IV lesions. It does not require introital integrity (well-supported perineum and outlet) and will therefore remain in situ when others fail. It is extremely compressible and with its six suction cups, it is self-positioning. It does create a hypoxic intravaginal environment so that frequent changes are required. If it is removed and cleaned regularly by the patient, she will have no discharge. If not, patients return initially at 1 month and then every 2 months. Although these procedures are seemingly difficult, many elderly women care for their cube pessaries quite successfully. The 84-year-old patient pictured with a stage IV apical prolapse sees her physician for her annual examination. She cares for her cube by removing it nightly, soaking it in soapy water and replacing it in the morning.

B, Insertion is eased by the compressibility of the cube. The lubricated, appropriately sized cube can be eased past the introitus without significant patient discomfort, particularly if she is relaxed and exhaling. Women without marked vaginal outlet relaxation and a vagina of normal size and shape usually accommodate a size 2 to 4 cube. Conversely, women with a capacious introitus and vaginal size may require sizes 5 to 7 and rarely 8 or 9.

Continued on the next page

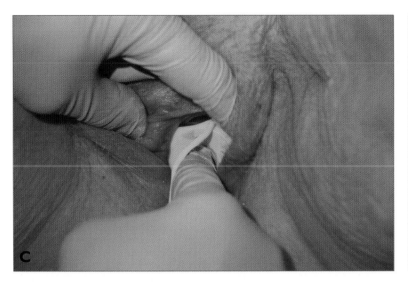

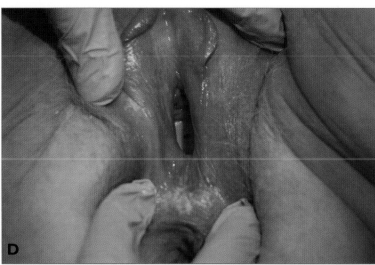

Figure 10-28. *(Continued)* **C**, With the cube in the lower vagina, the patient is asked to relax. Then, again during exhalation, one or two fingers push the cube cephalad into the apex. **D**, The suction cups of the cube in the vaginal apex will attach themselves to the vaginal walls. Shown here, Valsalva effort with labial/perineal separation demonstrates the cube to be stabilized in the vaginal apex with no descent.

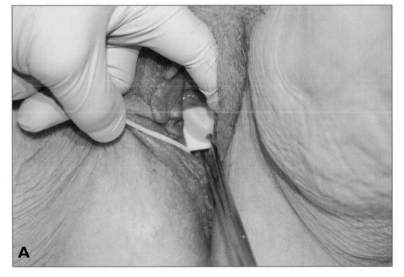

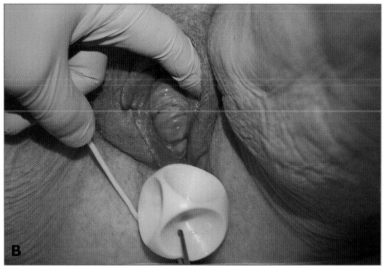

Figure 10-29. A, Clinical cube removal is easily accomplished using the index finger of one hand and a tenaculum in the other. The labia are parted and a single-toothed tenaculum grasps the most accessible cube lip. The opposite index finger placed above the cube in the vaginal apex breaks the cube's seal as gentle traction on the tenaculum in the direction of the vaginal axis eases the cube's downward motion. **B**, Downward and outward motion is continued until the cube is eased out between the labia. Careful inspection of the vaginal epithelium is indicated to rule out ulcerations, abrasions, and lacerations. It is generally wise to irrigate the vaginal walls with betadine.

Patient self-care. Patients who are willing and able to care for their cube pessaries at home will be instructed to remove the cube at any frequency from nightly to twice monthly in order to wash the cube and rest the vagina. To remove the pessary the most accessible position for the individual patient should be used—standing with one foot on a step, sitting on the toilet, or squatting or lying on a bed in the frog position. The tail is retrieved and grasped and traction is applied until the patient is able to insert the opposite finger to break the cube suction and ease out the pessary. Reinsertion by the patient is just the same as by the health care provider as described here.

Guide to Commonly Used Pessaries

Pessary	Mechanics	Requires Vaginal Outlet Integrity	Coitus Possible with Pessary In Situ	Self-Removal and Insertion	Vaginitis	Follow-Up*	Tips/Comments
Ring with or without membrane	Fits obliquely behind pubic symphysis	X	X	Easiest	None to mild	Initially 3 mo, then q 6 mo	Least invasive. Use ring with support membrane for procidentia, which may prolapse through open ring
Donut	Occludes upper vagina by filling the space to support prolapse	X		No	Moderate	q 3 mo	Removing the air from the donut with a syringe will markedly facilitate insertion and removal
Inflato	Occludes upper vagina by filling space to support prolapse	X		Yes (specifically designed for self-care)	None to mild	prn	Patient pumps air in or lets it out with beaded stem and grenade. Inserted for activity, removed at rest
Gehrung	Sits as a double arch under the anterior wall, legs directed posteriorly	X	X	Yes	Mild	q 3 mo	Designed especially for cystoceles (turn over for rectoceles)
Marland	See "Ring"	X		No	Mild	Initially I mo, then q 3–6 mo	
Gellhorn	Shallow cup is directed anteriorly and obliquely holding up the prolapse while the horn is directed toward the posterior fourchette			No	Moderate to severe	Initially I mo then q 2 mo	Removal is not always easy and may be aided with single-tooth tenaculum traction on the horn while opposite index finger breaks suction cup with apex to gently ease it out
Cube	Size fills vagina and suction cups adhere to vaginal walls			Yes	Severe except with self-care	Initially I mo, then q 2 mo Self-care: annually or prn	It will remain intravaginal, relieving significant external protrusions, despite a gaping introitus and deficient perineum when all others are extruded. Encourage self-care

*If patient is not self-removing.

Figure 10-30. Guide to commonly used pessaries: Inflato, Gehrung, and Gellhorn (Milex Products, Chicago, IL); Marland (Bioteque America, Fremont, CA). Pessaries are extremely useful devices to prepare for, postpone, or prevent pelvic reconstructive surgery. With minimal experience any obstetrician-gynecologist can become comfortable in the use of pessaries. Many patients with prolapse, hesitant to undergo surgery, will become more receptive after an initial trial of conservative pessary treatment. There are almost no contraindications to pessary use other than a noncompliant patient. A neglected pessary may be trapped behind a rigid vaginal cicatrix. A severely neglected pessary, especially of the Gellhorn variety, may cause deep ulceration and can even, on rare occasion, cause a fistula into the bladder or rectum [17]. However, with proper care an extremely valuable clinical function can be served by the lowly vaginal pessary. prn—as needed.

References

1. Kegel AH: Progressive resistance exercise in the functional restoration of the perineal muscles. *Am J Obstet Gynecol* 1948, 56:238–249.

2. Bo K: Pelvic floor muscle training is effective in treatment of female stress urinary incontinence, but how does it work? *Int Urogynecol J* 2004, 15:76–84.

3. Jarvis SK, Hallam TK, Lujic S, *et al.*: Peri-operative physiotherapy improves outcomes for women undergoing incontinence and or prolapse surgery: results of a randomized controlled trial. *Aust N Z J Obstet Gynaecol* 2005, 45:300–303.

4. Bo K, Kvarstein B, Nygaard I: Lower urinary tract symptoms and pelvic floor muscle exercise adherence after 15 years. *Obstet Gynecol* 2005, 105:999–1005.

5. Bo K: Vaginal weight cones: theoretical framework, effect on pelvic floor muscle strength and female stress urinary incontinence. *Acta Obstet Gynecol Scand* 1995, 74:87–92.

6. Herbison P, Dean N: Weighted vaginal cones for urinary incontinence. Cochrane Incontinence Group. *Cochrane Database Syst Rev* 2008, 2.

7. Trowbridge ER, Fenner DE: Conservative management of pelvic organ prolapse. *Clin Obstet Gynecol* 2005, 48:668–681.

8. Bo K, Larsen S, Oseid S, *et al.*: Knowledge about and ability to correct pelvic floor muscle exercises in women with urinary incontinence. *Neurourol Urodyn* 1988, 7:261–262.

9. Bo K: Can pelvic floor muscle training prevent and treat pelvic organ prolapse? *Acta Obstet Gynecol Scand* 2006, 85:263–268.

10. Lang JH, Zhu L, Sun ZJ, Chen J: Estrogen levels and estrogen receptors in patients with stress urinary incontinence and pelvic organ prolapse. *Int J Gynaecol Obstet* 2003, 80:35–39.

11. American College of Obstetricians and Gynecologists: Pelvic organ prolapse. ACOG practice bulletin No. 79. *Obstet Gynecol* 2007, 109:461–473.

12. Albertazzi P, Sharma S: Urogenital effects of selective estrogen receptor modulators: a systematic review. *Climacteric* 2005, 8:214–220.

13. Ballagh SA: Vaginal hormone therapy for urogenital and menopausal symptoms. *Semin Reprod Med* 2005, 23:126–140.

14. Estrogen and progestogen use in peri- and postmenopausal women: March 2007 position statement of The North American Menopausal Society. *Menopause* 2007, 14:168–182.

15. Handa VL, Garrett E, Hendrix S, *et al.*: Progression and remission of pelvic organ prolapse: a longitudinal study of menopausal women. *Am J Obstet Gynecol* 2004, 190:27–32.

16. Miller DS: Contemporary use of the pessary. In *Gynecology and Obstetrics*, vol 1. Edited by Sciarra JJ. Philadelphia: JB Lippincott; 1995:1–12.

17. Goldstein I, Wise GJ, Tancer ML: A vesicovaginal fistula and intravesical foreign body. *Am J Obstet Gynecol* 1990, 163:589–591.

18. Jain A, Majoko F, Freites O: How innocent is the vaginal pessary? Two cases of vaginal cancer associated with pessary use. *J Obstet Gynecol* 2006, 26:829–830.

19. Cundiff GW, Amundsen CL, Bent AE, *et al.*: The PESSRI study: symptom relief outcomes of a randomized crossover trial of the ring and Gellhorn pessaries. *Am J Obstet Gynecol* 2007, 196:405.e1–8.

11

Surgical Management of Pelvic Organ Prolapse

Douglass S. Hale

S urgery for pelvic organ prolapse (POP) is one of the most common gynecologic procedures in the United States, accounting for nearly 300,000 cases each year at a cost of over $1 billion [1]. It is estimated that a woman living in the United States has an 11.1% lifetime chance of undergoing a single surgery for POP or urinary incontinence during her lifetime [2]. Studies estimate that over the next 30 years, there will be a 45% increase in women seeking care for these disorders as a result of the population aging [3]. When treating these problems, the philosophy to address the pelvic floor as a whole and not fragment it into separate, unrelated compartments has been realized [4]. Rarely do defects in one area of the pelvic floor exist alone. More often, multiple defects are present. In a study of 100 consecutive patients referred for radiographic evaluation of POP, 95% were found to have defects in all three vaginal vault compartments [5].

Failure to identify all defects may stem from practitioner oversight or ineffective evaluative techniques. In either case, incomplete repair of the pelvic floor at the time of prolapse surgery risks an unsatisfactory result and potential need for secondary repair. The goal of the pelvic surgeon should be relief of patient symptoms balanced with compensation of anatomy and function.

Realization of the symbiotic relationship between the neuromuscular system and the connective tissue support system is leading to a change in prolapse procedures. Oversimplification of the etiology and pathology of prolapse has led surgeons to believe that treatments are also simple. Like most medical problems, prolapse requires the identification and addressing of risk factors. Surgery attempts to compensate for the end stage of the problem; it does not cure the problem, which generally is neuromuscular in origin. Incomplete understanding of normal versus abnormal, parous versus nulliparous, and symptomatic versus asymptomatic contributes to the confusing state of prolapse evaluation and management. Sorely lacking are scientific studies that are standardized in regard to evaluation, management, and follow-up. Our knowledge is largely drawn from case series and expert opinions, among the weakest types of scientific evidence. It is rare to find such a study that does not claim excellent results. Recent reviews help to merge the data from these studies but are still limited by the nature of the studies with which they have to work [6]. In one of the few prospective randomized studies that has been conducted comparing surgical techniques for POP, abdominal reconstructive procedures had twice the success rate when compared with vaginal procedures for pelvic prolapse [7]. Despite the arguments, this study was less about approach and more about native tissue versus synthetic graft. This is not a discussion germane only to POP. Hernia data have shown over twice the success rate when a synthetic material is used as compared with relying on native tissue alone [8]. However, the vaginal vault is not the abdominal wall, and adopting widespread use of synthetic mesh for prolapse repair is not warranted given the present state of knowledge. Likewise, the high failure rates of traditional anterior and posterior colporrhaphies should spur new ideas and approaches for more successful treatments. These repairs were described more than 100 years ago and have changed little. Attention to the complete support of the vaginal vault and perineal body combined with an understanding of the patient's neuromuscular pelvic floor function and the demands that are placed on this system are emerging at the forefront of prolapse surgery.

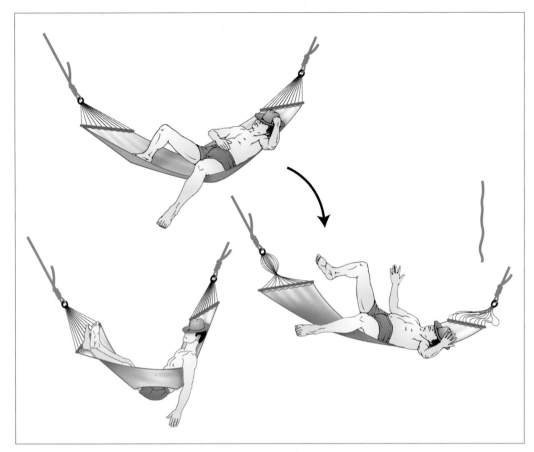

the anterior vaginal wall laterally while the arcus tendineus fascia rectovaginalis supports the posterior wall laterally. The perineal membrane and crura of the levator ani muscles offer level III support (*see* Chapter 1) [10]. In addition, the vaginal muscularis and rectovaginal septum must be in continuity with this endopelvic connective tissue for proper pelvic organ support.

When organs are prolapsed, the defect lies not in the organ but in the support network of muscle and connective tissue. Damage can result from injury to the nerve, muscle, connective tissue, or all three of these components that compromise the support system's ability to resist intra-abdominal pressure increases. As one or all of the components fail, the organs that rely on them for their support prolapse. An analogy between a hammock and this network can be made. The rope support of the hammock can be cut and the person in the hammock falls. This "defect" may be at the ends of the hammock, analogous to any of the three levels of endopelvic support, or the defect may be in the body of the hammock itself, analogous to defects in the surrounding musculofascial shell. Lastly, a slow stretching of the whole system may lead to loss of hammock support, analogous to loss of levator ani support. The problem is not with the person, but with the supporting hammock structures. Likewise, with a cystocele, enterocele, rectocele, or uterovaginal prolapse, the pathology results in a "defect" in the enveloping or supporting musculofascial connective tissue. These defects lead to displacement of the overlying organ.

Figure 11-1. The vaginal vault should be thought of as an epithelial-lined tube surrounded by a musculofascial connective tissue shell. In the past, a layer separate from the vaginal muscularis has been described. However, the pubovesicocervical fascia, which is often described grossly, has not been a layer that can be demonstrated histologically [9]. The vaginal muscularis envelops the epithelial tube and blends with a vast endopelvic connective tissue network, the fascia endopelvina. This blending of tissue creates a "shell" around the vagina, which is supported at the different levels. True ligamentous support of the vaginal vault and uterus does not exist. These connective tissue structures, along with the levator ani, provide an active platform of support and are interdependent. At level I, the cardinal and uterosacral ligaments support the upper vaginal vault and uterus. This area represents the "keystone" of the vaginal arch. At level II, the arcus tendineus fascia pelvis supports

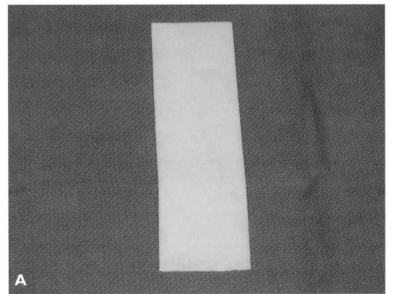

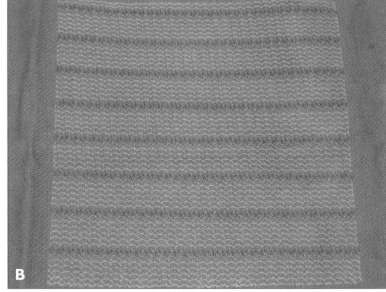

Figure 11-2. Examples of graft material. **A,** Cross-linked porcine dermis. **B,** Polypropylene macroporous mesh.

Continued on the next page

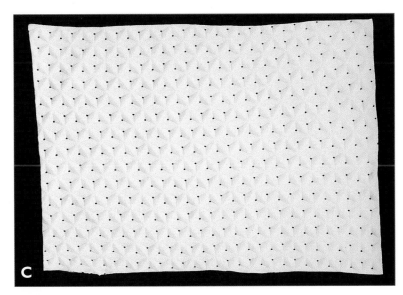

Figure 11-2. *(Continued)* **C,** Gore-tex mesh.

Many times, defects in the supporting tissues can be recognized and repaired. However, at other times this tissue is of such poor quality that its use in a repair is unacceptable. In these instances, substitution of this tissue with an autograft, allograft, or synthetic material may be necessary. The ideal support material that eliminates erosion, infection, and foreign body reaction is still awaiting development. Autografts of rectus fascia or fascia lata have been reported. Often, the sizes needed for pelvic reconstructive procedures make the use of autografts impractical. Allografts of fascia lata, rectus fascia, dura mater, patellar tendon, and Achilles tendon are available. Xenografts, mostly from porcine donors, are used. In general, studies of biologic grafts have not shown good long-term results in prolapse repair [11]. Tissue preparation techniques (radiation, dehydration, lyophilization, cross-linking) differ, which may impact graft performance. Examples of synthetic grafts include, but are not limited to, polyethylene terephthalate (Mersilene), polypropylene (Marlex, Prolene, Gynemesh, Pelvitex, Atrium), polytetrafluoroethylene (Teflon), and expanded polytetrafluoroethylene (Gore-tex). Erosions or exposures are the major problem, occurring in 3% to 11% of cases [12]. These numbers have decreased with advances in mesh design. Experts have recommended that macroporous, monofilament, polypropylene meshes be used currently. Until definitive answers are found, the limitations and risks of each material should be discussed with patients before selecting materials for use.

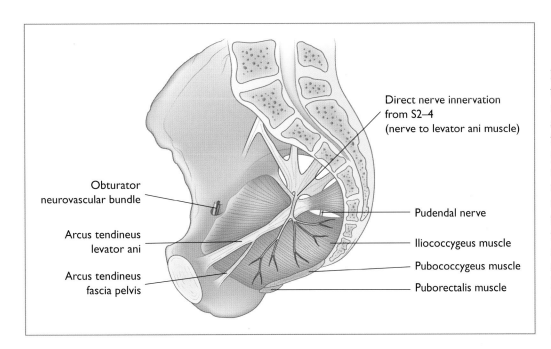

Figure 11-3. Levator ani showing innervation. Musculature of the pelvic diaphragm requires intact innervation to provide an active platform that aids the connective tissue in supporting the pelvic organs. For proper support of pelvic organs, both the muscular floor (pelvic diaphragm) and the musculofascial connective tissue network must be intact. Often, after reconstructive efforts, little or no attention is paid to the rehabilitation of the levator ani, which misses an opportunity to address a major contributing factor to pelvic organ prolapse. Persistent weakness in the levator ani places a greater stress on the surgical repair, whereas a strong levator ani can augment the surgical repair.

ANTERIOR WALL PROLAPSE

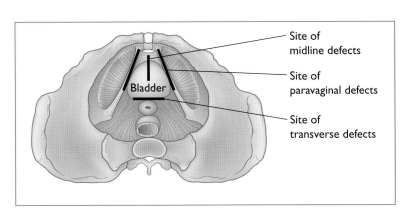

Figure 11-4. Reported sites of defects in the anterior vaginal wall. A loss of anterior vaginal wall support can result in cystocele, urethrocele, or anterior enterocele. The most commonly reported sites for defects in the anterior vaginal wall are shown [13]. Paravaginal cystoceles have been cited as the most common, although no large epidemiologic study exists to confirm this. Recent studies have focused on the high incidence of apical defects as a component of cystoceles, an assessment with which most experts agree [14]. Other sites include the transverse and midline defects. Site-specific analysis examining the lateral sulci, apex, and midline is needed to identify these different areas. The defect theory has come into question due to an inability to demonstrate these defects histologically, and this theory probably does oversimplify prolapse. However, it allows a systematic evaluation of support by the clinician, which is important because not all cystoceles have the same cause and different procedures are needed to correct them.

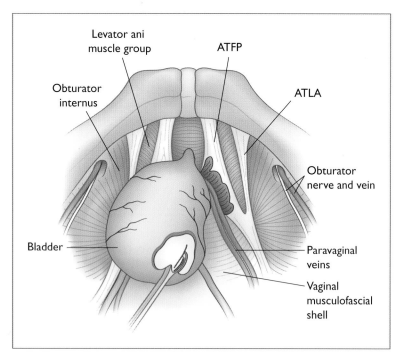

Figure 11-5. Paravaginal defect repair—abdominal approach. Opening the transversalis fascia enters the space of Retzius. The obturator internus muscle is located laterally with the accompanying obturator

canal and obturator neurovascular bundle. The levator ani muscle is identified originating from the arcus tendineus levator ani (ATLA), a fascial thickening of the obturator internus muscle. The ATLA is fused posteriorly with the arcus tendineus fascia pelvis (ATFP). The ATFP begins approximately 1 cm superior and 1 cm lateral to the inferior margin of the pubic symphysis, extending posteriorly to the ischial spine. The ATFP is the lateral support for vaginal level II. The paravaginal veins serve as a border for the lateral margin of the bladder. These vessels run in an anteroposterior direction and are differentiated from the vessels of the bladder, which usually run in a more transverse direction. Paravaginal cystoceles would be expected to begin at the apex and progress distally, which has been shown in an observational study [15]. Intra-abdominal pressures leading to prolapse would be transmitted to the apex of the vagina and proceed distally. In a paravaginal defect, the vaginal musculofascial shell has torn away from the ATFP at level II. On physical examination, the lateral vaginal sulcus is absent and central vaginal rugation is maintained.

Several variations of a paravaginal defect may exist. The ATFP may remain attached to the pelvic sidewall with the vagina torn away medially, as shown in this figure. Alternatively, the ATFP may be found on the vaginal wall, having torn away from the pelvic sidewall. Lastly, the ATFP may be split in two. In any of these cases, repair of the paravaginal defect is accomplished by reapproximating the vagina and the ATFP in their correct anatomic location. Surgeons must remember to address the apical component as well.

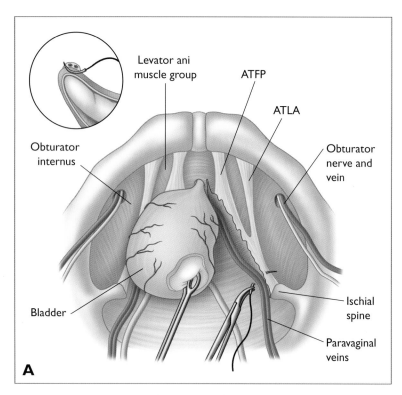

A

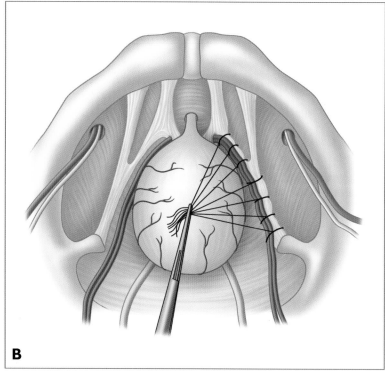

B

Figure 11-6. Correction of paravaginal cystocele. **A,** With the surgeon's nondominant hand intravaginally, the extent of the defect is palpated. The bladder is gently retracted medially over the vaginal hand, exposing the glistening white musculofascial tissue of the vagina. Before suture placement, pressure should be removed temporarily from the vaginal hand to ensure that a vein is not being entered. **B,** Sutures are then placed close to the bladder medially, either encircling the paravaginal veins or placed just lateral to them. A full-thickness vaginal suture is used. The suture is completed by

placement in the arcus tendineus fascia pelvis (ATFP) on the sidewall or in the anatomic location of the ATFP if it has torn away. Successive sutures are placed extending from the ischial spine to the urethrovesical junction. When repairing a bilateral defect, the first side should be tied down before proceeding with the second side to prevent overcorrecting of the anterior vaginal wall. As the sutures are tied, the surgeon should feel the lateral vaginal sulci returning and a correction of the cystocele occurring. ATLA—arcus tendineus levator ani.

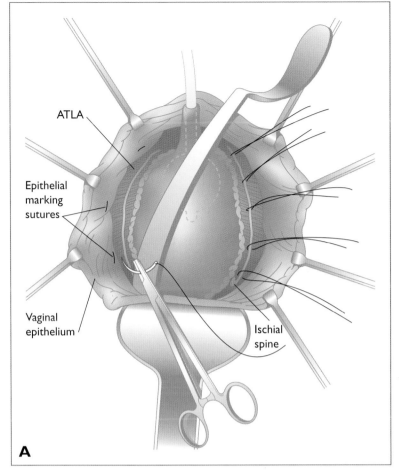

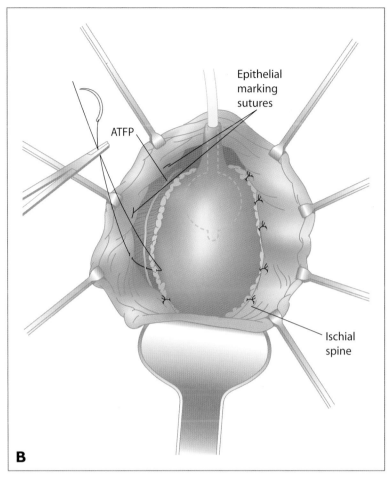

Figure 11-7. Vaginal–paravaginal cystocele repair—marking sutures and vaginal suture placement into arcus tendineus fascia pelvis (ATFP). Although technically more difficult and somewhat controversial in the literature, a vaginal approach to paravaginal cystoceles has been described. Several vaginal incisions including a midline, parasagittal, or an inverted U incision may be used to gain access to the space of Retzius. A midline incision is known to cause damage to the perineal nerve, which may affect urethral sphincter function. The other incisions have not been studied with respect to perineal nerve damage. Before any incision is made, marking sutures are placed in the vaginal epithelium to approximate the final location of the vaginal wall. This will aid in suture placement once the vaginal epithelium is opened. Typically, three marking sutures are used: anterior to the level of the ischial spine, midway between the spine and the symphysis, and close to the symphysis.

A, The space of Retzius is entered and the bladder is retracted medially and superiorly. Breisky–Navratil retractors along with a lighted suction irrigation device aid in visualization. The vaginal musculofascial tissue may be dissected into a separate layer or left intact on the vaginal epithelium. The ATFP is located and sutures are placed along it extending from just anterior to the ischial spine to the insertion of the ATFP on the pubis.

B, Sutures are then placed through the musculofascial connective tissue shell and the vaginal epithelium at the level of the marking sutures. Sequential tying begins with the deepest suture working toward the symphysis. The repair is completed with epithelial closure. ATLA—arcus tendineus levator ani.

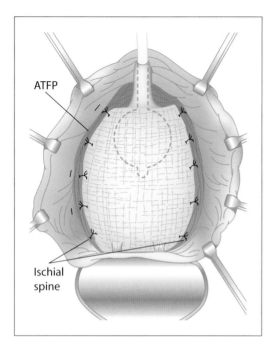

Figure 11-8. Anterior vaginal wall graft for multiple defects—graft in the anterior vaginal wall. If paravaginal defects exist with a central defect, an alternative to correcting each site individually is to use a graft. The repair is exactly the same as that used for a vaginal–paravaginal repair, with the exception of the intervening graft. The superior edge of the graft should be sutured to the supported vaginal apex and include the uterosacral–cardinal complex. A double-layer vaginal wall closure over the graft may help prevent graft erosion. Alternatively, transobturator tension-free graft repairs are being developed (*see* Figure 11-19**B**). ATFP—arcus tendineus fascia pelvis.

ANTERIOR COLPORRHAPHY FOR CENTRAL DEFECTS

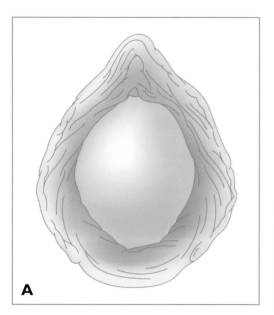

A

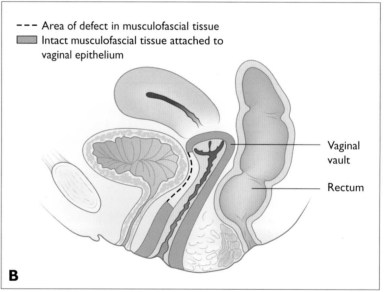

--- Area of defect in musculofascial tissue
▨ Intact musculofascial tissue attached to vaginal epithelium

Vaginal vault

Rectum

B

Figure 11-9. Anterior colporrhaphy for central defects—bladder "herniation" in a central defect. The anterior colporrhaphy is used to correct a central vaginal wall defect. The extent of the defect can often be appreciated by looking for the presence or absence of vaginal rugae, because rugae indicate vaginal epithelial attachment to the underlying musculofascial tissue. With a central vaginal wall defect, the lateral sulci (paravaginal attachment) will be intact as will support to the vaginal cuff. **A,** The bladder can be visualized herniating through the central defect in the vaginal muscularis, which leads to bladder muscularis in direct contact with vaginal epithelium. **B,** Area of defect in musculofascial tissue and intact musculofascial tissue attached to vaginal epithelium.

In an anterior colporrhaphy, repair begins with a midline or an inverted U anterior vaginal epithelial incision. A subepithelial injection of saline or a dilute vasoconstricting solution may aid in this dissection. The extent of the defect is identified and the separated musculofascial connective tissue is reapproximated while reducing the herniating bladder. Vaginal epithelial trimming should be limited as this adds little to the support and may lead to vaginal shortening.

Procedures for support of the vaginal apex involve restoring the continuity of level I vaginal support. Choices for apical support include the use of the native uterosacral–cardinal complex, a graft material substitute for native connective tissue, or an alternative support site such as the sacrospinous ligament or levator plate. A Cochrane review concluded that abdominal sacral colpopexy had a lower recurrence rate than vaginal sacrospinous colpopexy, but that finding must be considered in light of the fact that the vaginal procedure has a lower morbidity [6].

ABDOMINAL SACRAL COLPOPERINEOPEXY

This procedure allows for simultaneous correction of multiple vaginal wall defects and has evolved from the abdominal sacral colpopexy [16–18]. The basic premise is rebuilding the vaginal musculofascial "shell" using a graft to envelop the vagina epithelium and then recreate the vaginal levels of support. Two leaves are involved in graft placement. A posterior graft restores the continuity of the rectovaginal septum, correcting the descending perineum, rectocele, and entero-

cele. This graft extends support from the perineal body to the sacrum, recreating the natural support of the rectovaginal septum, musculofascial shell, and the uterosacral ligaments. An anterior graft is placed into the vesicovaginal space from just above the level of the trigone and vaginal apex to the sacrum. This corrects the cystocele component of the prolapse. Additional support may need to be added to level II with a paravaginal repair.

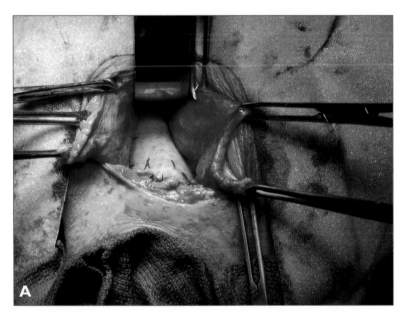

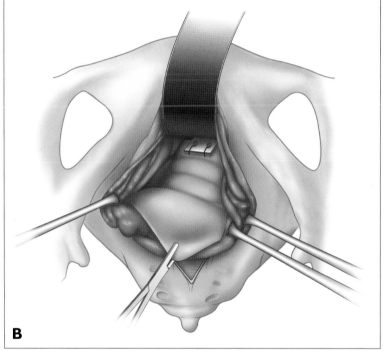

Figure 11-10. A, Perineal body graft attachment. Graft attachment to the perineal body is achieved through a vaginal approach, a laparoscopic approach, or an abdominal route. This decision is based on the degree of perineal body descent and the need for a perineorrhaphy. If there is significant perineal descent and a perineorrhaphy is required, a vaginal route is useful, which allows secure graft fixation to the perineal body and also perineorrhaphy simultaneously. If there is good perineal body support and no need to narrow the introitus, an abdominal or laparoscopic approach is used. If a perineorrhaphy is required, a diamond-shaped area of vaginal and perineal epithelium is removed from the vaginal introitus allowing a two to three finger-breadth introital opening. If no perineorrhaphy is required, a midline introital incision is used. A posterior midline vaginal incision is made to the top of the rectovaginal septum, allowing entrance through the enterocele or the cul-de-sac peritoneum without a full-length posterior vaginal wall incision. The vaginal epithelium is mobilized laterally along the levator ani to the level of the ischial spine.

The lateral graft margins are sutured to the fascia overlying the levator muscles. The most proximal sutures are placed 1 cm below the ischial spine into this fascia. The maximum graft width is 6 to 8 cm at this level, which is then tapered superiorly and inferiorly to fit the patient's anatomy. Progressing distally, the graft is next attached to a point on the levator fascia midway between the perineal body and original proximal suture. Lastly, the graft is attached to the perineal body. The apical portion of the graft is then passed through the enterocele sac opening to be retrieved during the abdominal or laparoscopic portion of the case.

B, Adhesions or other pathology may prevent safe entry into the cul de sac. In these cases, the graft can still be placed vaginally and left in the rectovaginal space for later abdominal retrieval. After a vaginal approach to place the graft, the orthopedic fracture plate is attached to the graft apex and placed just beneath the cul-de-sac peritoneum. The plate will help locate the graft abdominally, especially in obese patients. The vaginal epithelium is closed and perineorrhaphy is performed as necessary. The abdominal portion is begun and appropriate exposure is gained.

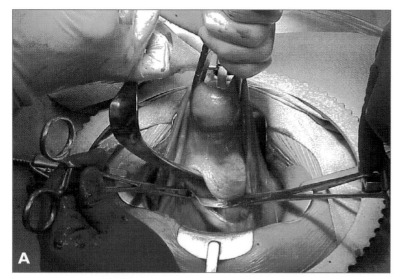

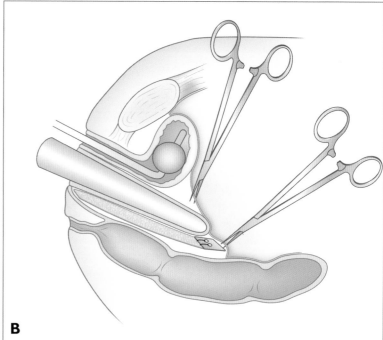

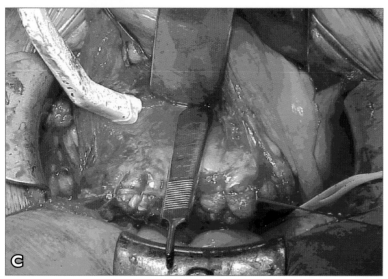

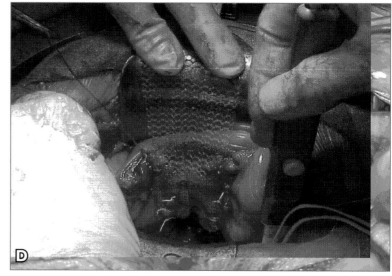

Figure 11-11. Graft placement. **A,** If cul-de-sac entry and distal graft placement were begun vaginally, the graft will be lying in the cul de sac upon entering the abdomen. **B,** If the cul de sac could not be entered vaginally, the peritoneum overlying the orthopedic plate and graft is incised and they are recovered. Appropriate anatomy is identified including the common iliac vessels and their bifurcation, the sacral promontory, and ureters. A peritoneal incision extending from the promontory to the cul de sac is made, which will allow for complete graft retroperitonealization. A lucite stent placed vaginally helps dissect the vesicovaginal space and, if needed, the rectovaginal space. Dissection into the vesicovaginal space will separate the bladder from the underlying white musculofascial tissue of the vagina and can extend to just above the level of the trigone.

C, The dissection should be bloodless; significant bleeding indicates wrong tissue planes. Laterally, this dissection extends to the bladder pillars and must respect the course of the ureters. The vagina has now been isolated and is ready for graft placement.

D, If the posterior graft placement had begun vaginally, it is now continued with the aid of the lucite stent. The graft is spread as widely as possible and fixed laterally and to the vaginal apex. Sutures are placed 2 cm apart vertically and as widely as possible on the posterior wall, which typically results in a total of eight to 10 sutures holding the posterior graft in place.

Continued on the next page

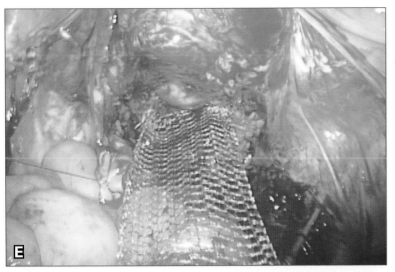

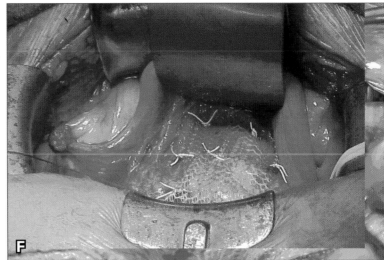

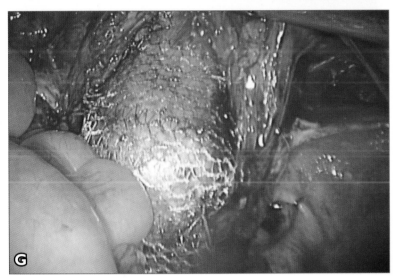

Figure 11-11. *(Continued)* **E,** If a laparoscopic or abdominal approach was used for posterior graft attachment, this view will be seen after attachment to the perineal body. The remaining graft will be attached to the posterior wall, as shown in **D. F** and **G,** The anterior graft is secured by placing gentle retraction on the bladder following dissection of the vesicovaginal space. With the lucite rod serving as a guide, the graft is fixed to the anterior vaginal wall as laterally and as distally as possible. Typically, three or four rows of two sutures each are placed to secure this graft. **F,** laparotomy view and **G,** laparoscopic view.

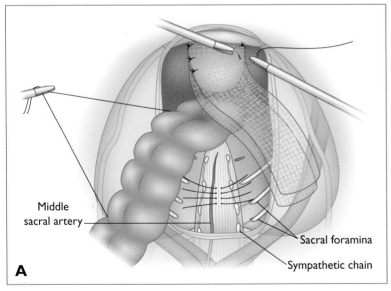

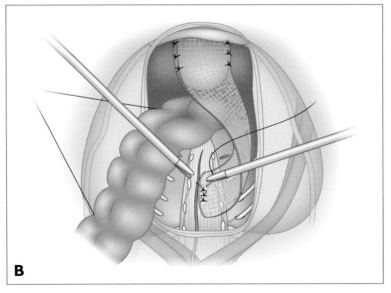

Figure 11-12. A, The open presacral space is now further explored. The sacral promontory is located and the sigmoid colon is retracted to the left. Landmarks to identify include the middle sacral vessels, sacral foramina and nerves, terminal portion of the sympathetic chain, and the possibility of anomalous structures that may be present. At the level of S2–3, successive sutures on a heavy needle are placed through the midline into the anterior longitudinal ligament. At this level, the anterior longitudinal ligament becomes attenuated but is still available for secure suture fixation. This is confirmed by strong

upward traction on the suture after placement. A double-armed suture is helpful, as both suture ends will eventually be placed through both leaves of the graft. A total of three or four sacral sutures are placed.

B, Appropriate tension is then placed on the graft to provide support. Too much tension on the graft is avoided to prevent suture pullout and potential pain postoperatively. Both leaves of the graft are cut to the appropriate length and secured to the sacrum with the previously placed sacral sutures.

Continued on the next page

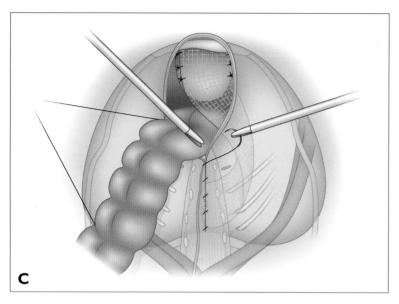

Figure 11-12. *(Continued)* **C,** The grafts are wrapped around the rectosigmoid retroperitoneally, eliminating the posterior cul de sac and treating any posterior enterocele or sigmoidocele. Graft attachment to the rectosigmoid may also help in cases of rectal prolapse. Copious irrigation helps dilute any bacteria introduced to the graft during its vaginal fixation. The peritoneum is closed to complete graft retroperitonealization.

UTEROSACRAL SUPPORT TO THE APEX

The native vaginal level I support is to the uterosacral–cardinal ligament complex. If identified, they can be used to reconstruct apical support abdominally, vaginally, or laparoscopically. In any of these cases, identifying ureters and surrounding vasculature is critical. A hysterectomy is performed for indicated reasons. The uterosacral ligaments are appropriately shortened and reattached to the vagina, most often in several areas.

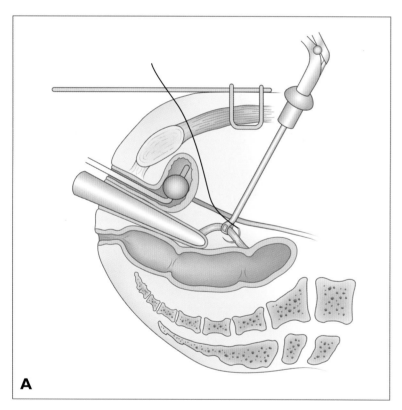

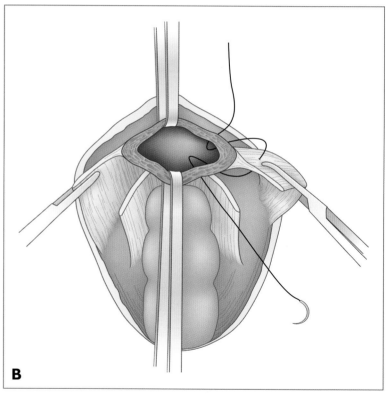

Figure 11-13. A, Abdominal approach to uterosacral support. If a concomitant hysterectomy is being performed, strong upward traction on the uterus will delineate the uterosacral ligaments. If a hysterectomy has already been performed, the vaginal vault can be placed on traction with a stent helping to delineate the ligaments. Following the ligaments back to the sacrum with a Babcock clamp is often helpful.

With traction now applied to the uterus toward the sacrum, the proper segment of uterosacral ligament that is needed for support will become evident. The longer the vagina, the more proximal is the area on the ligament that is used. A tagged suture is placed around this area of the ligament for later use. The hysterectomy is performed and the cuff closed. **B,** Strong cardinal support should be provided to the angles.

Continued on the next page

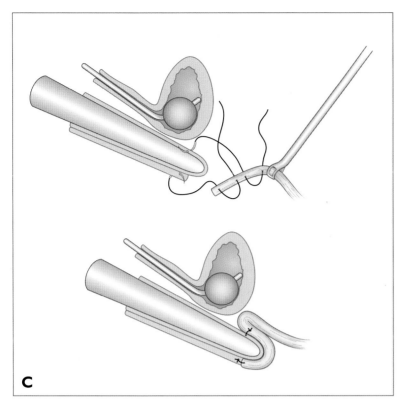

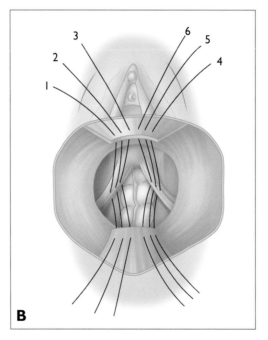

Figure 11-13. *(Continued)* **C,** A lucite rod placed intravaginally allows dissection of the vesicovaginal space anteriorly and the rectovaginal septum posteriorly. The uterosacral ligaments are freed distally to the previous tagged area. The most distal uterosacral segment is attached to the rectovaginal septum and the most proximal portion of the ligament is placed to the anterior vaginal wall just inferior to the cuff. Remaining sutures are placed along the posterior vaginal wall as needed. This technique will provide support to both the anterior and posterior apexes.

Laparoscopic approach: this technique is performed exactly as above with the exception of a laparoscopic-assisted vaginal hysterectomy if indicated. As others have stated, the laparoscope is a means of access. It should not mean changing the way the basic procedure is done. There are no long-term data on this procedure but it should be used to provide some support to the cuff when hysterectomy is performed.

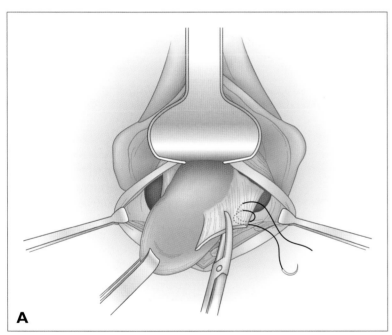

Figure 11-14. Vaginal approach to uterosacral support. **A,** The vaginal approach involves the same identification of the uterosacral ligaments. It is made easier if the uterus is still intact to provide traction and help trace the course of the uterosacral ligaments. If the uterus has been removed, outward and upward traction applied to the vaginal apex will help delineate the ligaments. As in all support procedures, ureteral location is critical. Location of the ureters may be through palpation or direct visualization, or a laparoscope can be passed through the cul de sac vaginally to help with their localization. Typically, the ligaments run 1 cm below the ischial spine and posteriorly and inferiorly to the sacrum.

B, The ligament is tagged at the level needed to support the apex and restore normal anatomic location over the levator plate. Three double-armed sutures are placed on each side. The most distal uterosacral suture is placed most laterally into the vaginal muscularis and the most proximal (highest) is placed near the midline of the cuff.

Continued on the next page

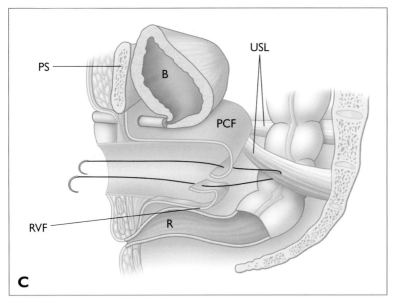

C

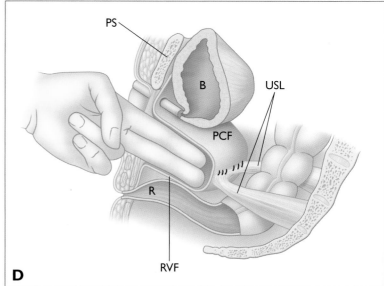

D

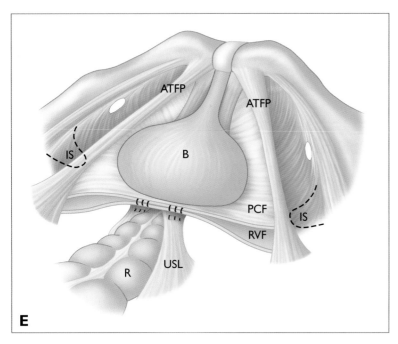

E

Figure 11-14. *(Continued)* **C–E,** The anterior portion of the suture is placed through the anterior vaginal muscularis and held. The posterior suture is passed through the posterior peritoneum and posterior vaginal wall muscularis.

If absorbable sutures are being used, full-thickness vaginal wall sutures are placed. Sutures are placed from distally on the uterosacral ligament and laterally on the vaginal apex to proximally on the ligament and more medially on the vaginal apex. Ureteral integrity is ensured after tying the sutures. Good medium-term success has been reported with this technique [20]. ATFP— arcus tendineus fascia pelvis; B—bladder; IS—ischial spine; PCF—pubocervical fascia; PS—pubic symphysis; R—rectum; RVF—rectovaginal fascia; USL—uterosacral ligament. (**B** *adapted from* Shull et al. [19].)

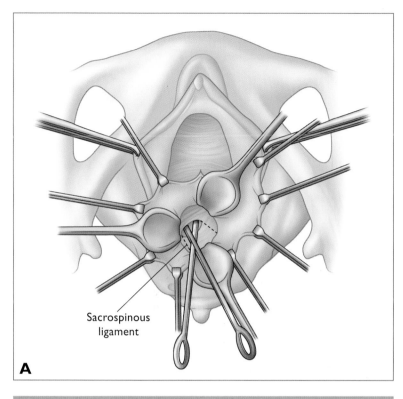

Sacrospinous
ligament

A

B	**Instruments for Sacrospinous Vault Suspension**	
Instrument	**Manufacturer**	
Shutt punch [24]	ConMed Linvatec, Largo, FL	
Endo stitch [25]	Autosuture Co., US Surgical Corp., Norwalk, CT	
Miya hook [26]	Boston Scientific, Natick, MA	
Capio suture device	Boston Scientific, Natick, MA	

Figure 11-15. Sacrospinous ligament fixation. This has been the most popular vaginal approach to correction of apical prolapse since its introduction to the United States in 1971 [21]. Various modifications using surrounding fascial points of attachment have also been described. Difficulties with supporting the anterior apical wall are seen with this technique.

The sacrospinous ligament can be approached through a midline vertical incision or a midline apical incision [22,23]. Some authors propose bilateral sacrospinous vault suspension, although the utility of this has not been proven. In addition, the bilateral technique depends on adequate vaginal length and depth.

Marking sutures placed on the epithelium at the anticipated site of attachment are recommended. The vaginal epithelium is separated from the underlying musculofascial tissue and the dissection taken to the level of the ischial spine. The rectal pillars, which separate the vagina from the sacrospinous ligament, are perforated with an atraumatic clamp gaining access to the sacrospinous–coccygeus ligament complex.

A, The ligament complex is visualized using Breisky retractors to retract the bladder superiorly and the rectum medially. Under direct visualization, a permanent suture is placed approximately 3 to 4 cm medial to the ischial spine. Generally, at least two sutures are placed. Alternatively, the Michigan four wall technique may be used [23]. **B,** Numerous devices are now available for this suture placement. The surgeon must be aware of surrounding anatomic structures, including the superiorly located inferior gluteal vessels and nerve. The lumbosacral plexus lies on the piriformis muscle just above the ligament complex. Just deep to the ligament complex are the pudendal vessels and nerves, sciatic nerve, and accompanying nerves of the lumbosacral plexus. Nerves running in the sacrospinous–coccygeus ligament complex may result in postoperative pain [24].

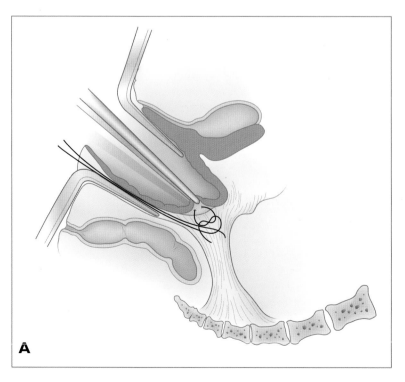

A

Figure 11-16. A, Pulley suture. After the sutures are secured to the ligament complex, a pulley suture is placed at the site of the vaginal marking suture.

Continued on the next page

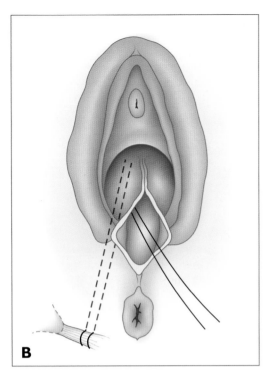

Figure 11-16. *(Continued)* **B,** Before these are tied down securely, the vaginal apex is partially closed in order to prevent difficulty reaching the apex once the pulley stitches are tied down. Suture bridging is avoided as the pulley sutures are secured, bringing the vagina in direct apposition to the sacrospinous–coccygeus ligament complex.

Pulley sutures are also used in the iliococcygeus vault suspension, which uses the iliococcygeus fascia or the levator plate as points of vaginal fixation [28,29]. The approach is similar to that of the sacrospinous vault suspension with a midline posterior vaginal wall incision. The epithelium is separated from the rectovaginal septum and the dissection is extended laterally and superiorly to the levator muscles. The iliococcygeus fascia is located lateral to the rectum and anterior to the ischial spine. Sutures are anchored in this fascia as the rectum is retracted medially. Pulley sutures are used for fixation and secured after partial closure of the midline incision.

UTERINE PRESERVATION AND OBLITERATIVE PROCEDURES

In general, childbearing should be completed before the patient undergoes major reconstructive pelvic surgery for POP. However, uterine preservation may be indicated in women desiring fertility or in patients whose body self-image does not permit them to undergo a hysterectomy. Study numbers for uterine preservation with POP are small but several techniques have been used and may be discussed with patients. Abdominal and vaginal approaches can be used and are similar to the procedures described for apical support. These include use of the uterosacral ligaments [30], sacrospinous ligament [31], sacral hysteropexy [32], or grafts to the anterior abdominal wall [33].

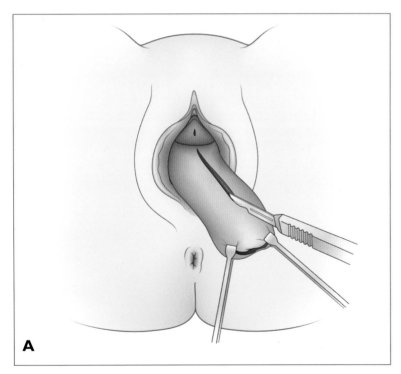

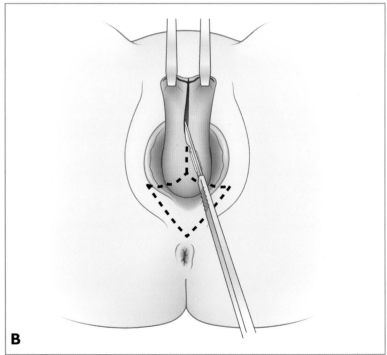

Figure 11-17. Obliterative surgery. This surgery is reserved for patients who no longer desire sexual intercourse or in whom body self-image is not an issue. A LeFort colpocleisis may be used if the uterus is still present. This technique is simpler and results in less blood loss [34]. An alternative approach uses a vaginal hysterectomy, if the uterus is still present, combined with a complete colpocleisis [35] and levator plication.

A, After a vaginal hysterectomy is performed, the vaginal epithelium is undermined with a subepithelial solution of saline. Kocher clamps placed at the vaginal angles help to maintain orientation as the dissection proceeds. Either a circumferential epithelial incision just inside the hymen can be made or a standard midline anterior and posterior incision is used. **B,** A wide perineorrhaphy is made by removing a large diamond-shaped area of perineum and distal vaginal epithelium.

Continued on the next page

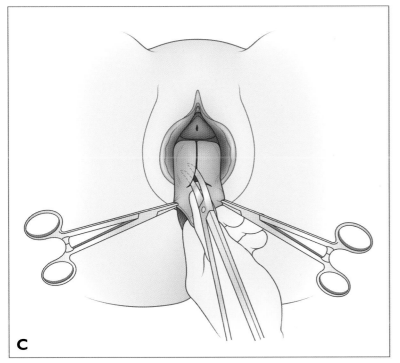

C

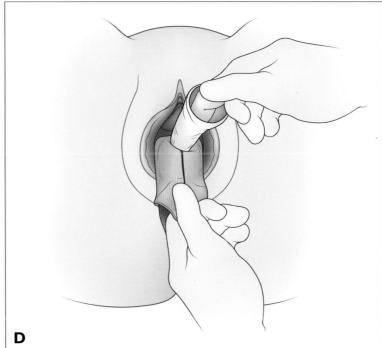

D

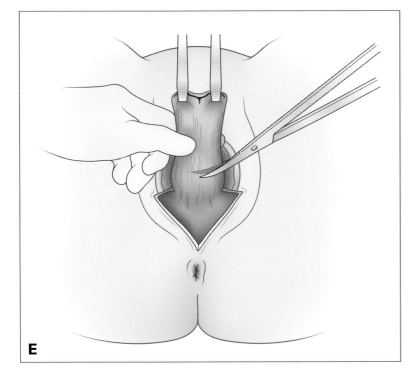

E

Figure 11-17. *(Continued)* **C–E**, Using sharp and blunt dissection, the vaginal epithelium is dissected away from the underlying musculofascial tissue. The bladder, enterocele, and rectocele are all freed from the vaginal epithelium.

The surgeon's nondominant hand is placed immediately on the vaginal epithelium and an assistant places countertraction on the prolapsing organs and musculofascial tissue. Metzenbaum scissors are used to sharply divide the vaginal epithelium. The epithelium is removed, leaving behind the prolapsing structures.

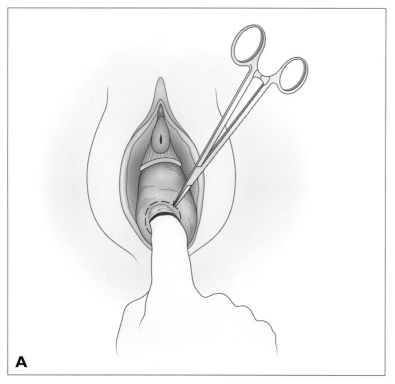

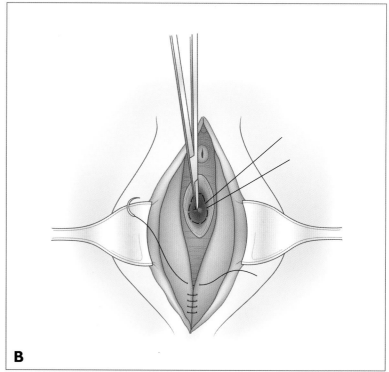

Figure 11-18. A, Suturing. The leading edge of the prolapse is identified and a pursestring suture is placed around it. As the suture is tied down and the tissue reduced, a hemostat is placed on the knot and the suture is cut. The next pursestring suture is then placed with the tagged suture serving as the center. The hemostat helps to reduce the tissue as the next suture is tied. This process is repeated until the prolapsing tissue is above the level of the levator plate.

B, The levator muscles are palpated and approximated using a #0 or #1 permanent or delayed absorbable suture. The muscle should be closed from above the rectum to the level of the urethrovesical junction (UVJ). The ureters must be clear of the levator muscles and the surgeon should place a finger rectally to help with suture placement. A Kelly-type plication at the UVJ helps prevent downward traction on the UVJ from the levator plication. A tight perineorrhaphy is performed so that at most one fingerbreadth can be placed below the urethra. At completion the typical vaginal vault will be reduced to 3 cm in length and only one finger should fit below the urethra to the posterior fourchette.

POSTERIOR VAGINAL WALL

Defects in the posterior vaginal wall may be enterocele, rectocele, or sigmoidocele. Ancillary imaging such as dynamic cystoproctography may be helpful in differentiating these entities. Patient symptoms vary widely with posterior wall defects, a fact that underscores the importance of discussing patient and physician expectations of surgery. Successful correction of the bulging does not always equate with relief of patient symptoms.

Several methods have been described for rectocele correction, including a defect repair, graft replacement, traditional posterior colporrhaphy, rectal wall imbrication, and trans-anal repair. No single method has proven to be superior. The Cochrane review on prolapse [6] concluded that the vaginal approach was associated with a lower rate of recurrent rectocele or enterocele than the transanal approach. However, other data were too few to draw conclusions. A recent randomized trial of three rectocele repair techniques found the worst outcomes with a defect repair reinforced with a specific biograft (46% anatomic failure; FortaGen, Organogenesis, Canton, MA) whereas traditional posterior colporrhaphy (14% failure rate) and site-specific defect repair (22%) were statistically similar for anatomic failure.

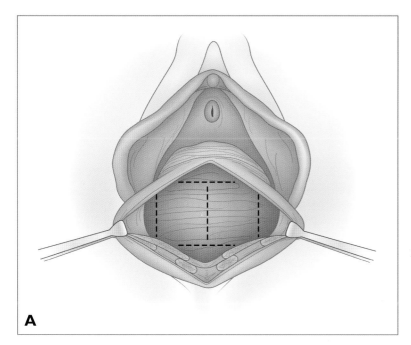

A

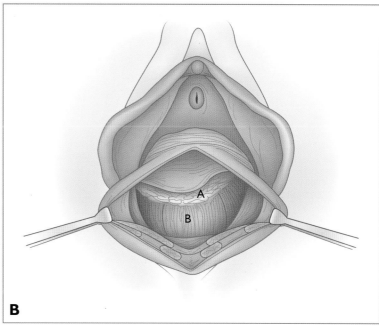

B

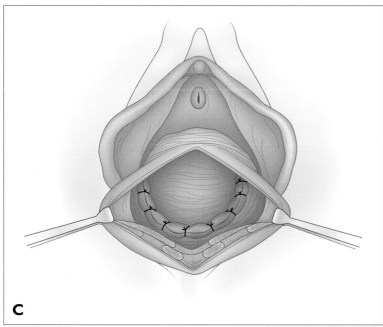

C

Figure 11-19. Defect repair [36]. **A,** Sites of rectovaginal septal defects. The defect approach to rectocele repair involves identifying the defect in the musculofascial tissue or the rectovaginal septum and correcting it, avoiding the mass closure technique of the posterior colporrhaphy. The support tissue may be torn at the perineal body, lateral sidewall, or apex. The concept is the same as that for defects involved in the anterior wall. **B,** The dissection is begun in the posterior midline and carried out laterally. The dissection should be kept as thin as possible below the vaginal epithelium. A finger placed rectally will aid in this dissection and help delineate the margins of the defect. *Point A* shows the torn rectovaginal septum and *point B* the rectal muscularis. **C,** Once identified, the defect is repaired with interrupted suture and the epithelium closed.

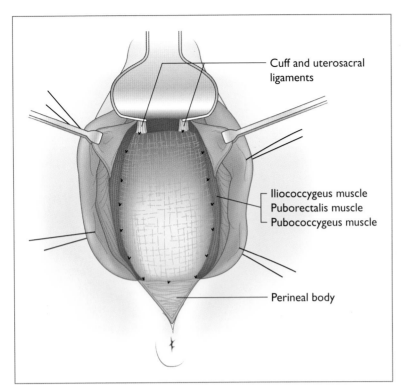

Figure 11-20. Graft replacement of rectovaginal septum. When the rectovaginal septum is inadequate for repair, a graft can be substituted. Studies indicate that the rectovaginal septum does not reach the vaginal apex and may in fact be only 2 to 3 cm in length [37]. This makes the native septum too short to reach the vaginal apex; its use will result in a markedly foreshortened vagina. In these cases a graft can be used. The dissection is begun in the posterior midline and widened laterally to the level of the levator muscles. Vaginal apical support is also identified. The graft is measured and sutured to the perineal body and vaginal apex and laterally to the levator muscles, recreating a full-length rectovaginal septum. Long-term studies are lacking. At times, a voluminous rectum may require some imbrication before the graft can be laid. Kit graft repairs are described later (*see* Figure 11-28).

POSTERIOR COLPORRHAPHY

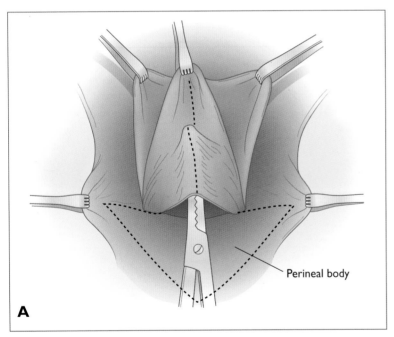

A

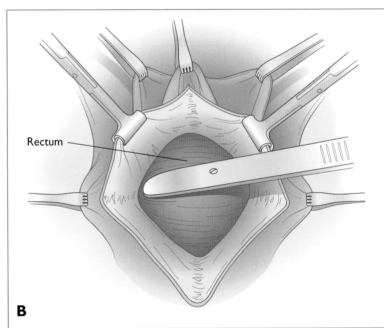

B

Figure 11-21. Posterior colporrhaphy [38]. **A,** The extent of the rectocele is ascertained and a posterior midline incision is made through the vaginal epithelium only. Loss of rugation may indicate separation of the epithelium from the underlying musculofascial tissue and rectovaginal septum. **B,** The dissection is taken laterally to the crura of the levator muscles and superiorly as far as needed. A rectal finger delineates the deficient support tissue.

Continued on the next page

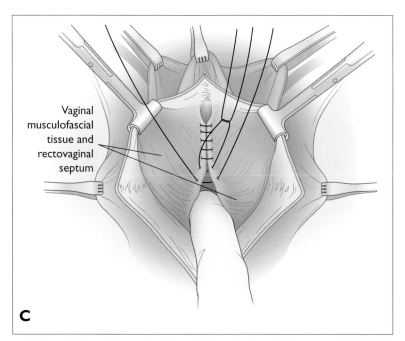

Vaginal
musculofascial
tissue and
rectovaginal
septum

C

Figure 11-21. *(Continued)* **C,** The lateral musculofascial tissue and rectal vaginal septum are plicated in the midline, rebuilding this tissue. Epithelial trimming is done to remove redundant tissue only. The epithelium is closed and a perineorrhaphy completed as needed. Some surgeons recommend incorporating the levator muscles into this midline plication. This levator plication does not represent normal anatomy and should be avoided in the sexually active patient, as a 30% rate of dyspareunia or apareunia following this repair has been reported [39].

RECTAL WALL IMBRICATION

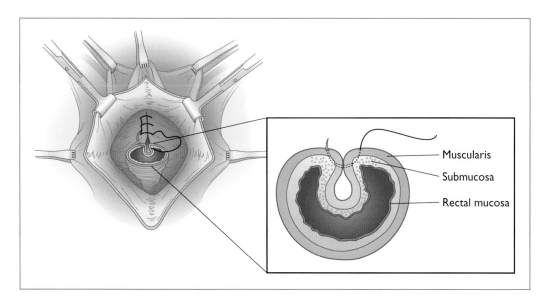

Muscularis

Submucosa

Rectal mucosa

Figure 11-22. Rectal wall imbrication has been reported in few series [40,41]. A transvaginal or transanal approach may be used: the transvaginal repair is shown here. A posterior midline incision into the rectovaginal space is made and the rectal muscularis and submucosa are plicated for the length of the rectocele with a running interlocking suture. The width of suture placement depends on the size of the rectocele, resulting in a ridge of rectal mucosa and muscularis inverted into the rectal lumen, which purportedly undergoes necrosis that narrows the rectum. In the transanal approach, a running interlocking suture is placed through the rectal mucosa, submucosa, and superficial muscularis. The incorporated tissues slough and scarring results, narrowing the rectal lumen.

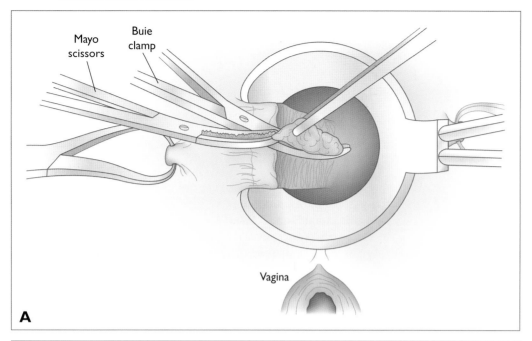

A, Mayo scissors, Buie clamp, Vagina

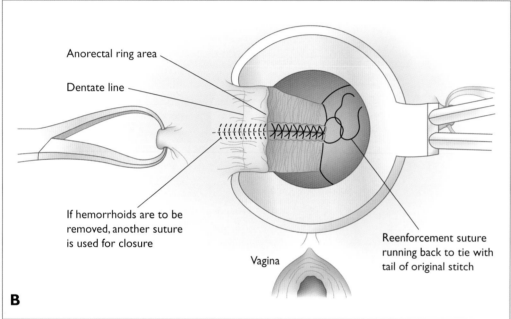

B, Anorectal ring area, Dentate line, If hemorrhoids are to be removed, another suture is used for closure, Vagina, Reenforcement suture running back to tie with tail of original stitch

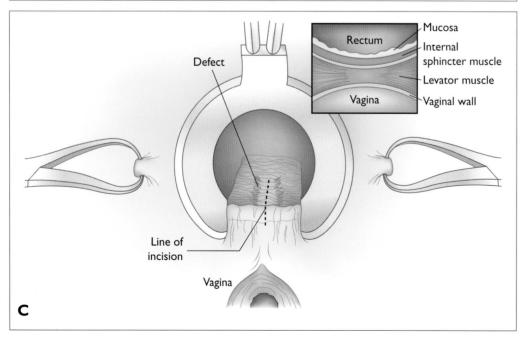

C, Defect, Line of incision, Vagina, Rectum, Mucosa, Internal sphincter muscle, Levator muscle, Vaginal wall, Vagina

Figure 11-23. Transanal repair [42,43]. The transanal rectocele repair is unfamiliar to many gynecologic surgeons; however, it is well known to colorectal surgeons. The patient is placed in the jack-knife position. **A,** Lubricated rectal dilators are used to allow the passage of a Fansler speculum or Hill–Ferguson rectal retractors. Using a long, slightly curved clamp, redundant rectal mucosa is pulled into the clamp. **B,** The excess mucosa is trimmed and a running suture is placed around the clamp from proximal to distal. A suture tail is left at the proximal end. The clamp is removed and the suture is run back from distal to proximal for reinforcement and is tied. Excision is performed in from one to three quadrants, depending on the amount of mucosal redundancy. **C,** Lastly, the anterior rectal wall is addressed. A mucosal incision is made superiorly from the dentate line (7–8 cm).

Continued on the next page

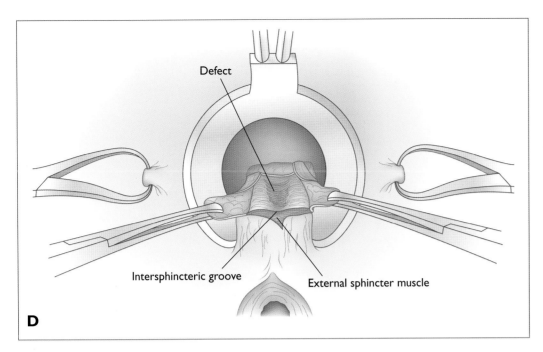

Defect

Intersphincteric groove   External sphincter muscle

D

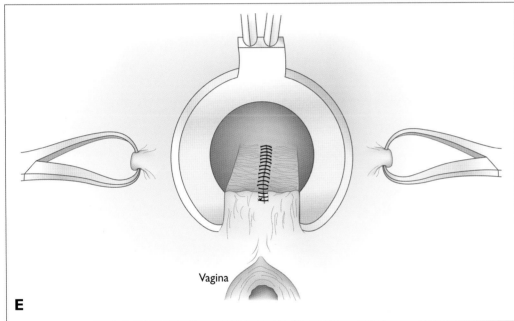

Vagina

E

Figure 11-23. *(Continued)* **D,** The rectal mucosa is mobilized for 1 to 2 cm on each side of the midline incision. **E,** The rectal muscularis and rectovaginal septum are plicated with horizontal mattress sutures and the rectal mucosa is closed with a running suture. Newer techniques using staplers to remove the excess tissue lack data and are not shown.

ENTEROCELE

Cul-de-sac depth may have little to do with the finding of an enterocele. An enterocele is formed when the cul de sac and contents herniate through the levator hiatus impinging on the posterior wall. In any repair of enterocele, the vaginal axis must be restored over the levator plate. Three techniques are often used for enterocele repair, although data supporting them are lacking.

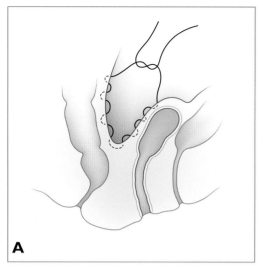
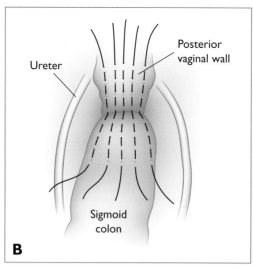
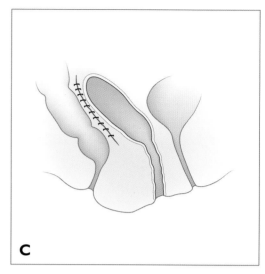

A **B** **C**

Figure 11-24. Halban repair [44]. **A,** In this abdominal approach, successive vertical sutures are used to obliterate the cul de sac. The repair is begun at the S2–3 level of the serosa overlying the sigmoid colon, continuing on across the cul de sac, and finally up the posterior vaginal wall. The first suture serves as the midline, with the remaining being placed to the right and left. **B,** Sutures should be placed approximately 1 cm apart and end 1 cm medial to the ureters. The sutures should also taper in, as the posterior vaginal wall is approached to avoid crossing the ureter as it dives below the cardinal ligament. **C,** Appropriate apical support should be restored as needed and the Halban sutures tied down.

MOSCHCOWITZ REPAIR

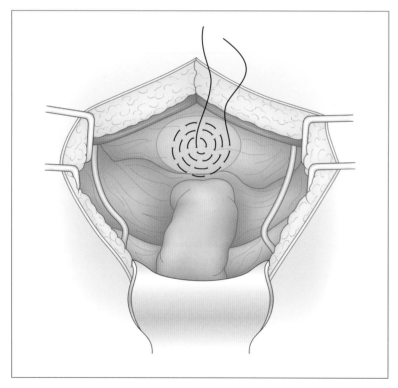

Figure 11-25. The Moschcowitz repair [45] involves successive purse-string sutures placed around the cul de sac through the peritoneal and serosal surfaces only. The most superior suture should be 1 cm below the ureter to prevent kinking. Moschcowitz sutures can be placed on either side of the sigmoid as shown or across the sigmoid as a single suture. The Halban and Moschcowitz procedures possess little intrinsic strength themselves and vaginal axis restoration over the levator plate is needed in order for these to be successful.

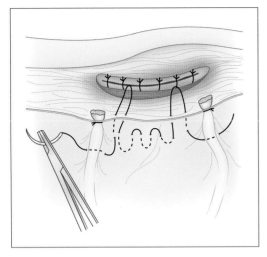

Figure 11-26. McCall culdoplasty [46]. Originally described for vaginal approach cul-de-sac closure, this technique may also be modified for an abdominal approach. The uterosacral ligament is appropriately shortened, brought through the ipsilateral posterior vaginal wall, reefed across the cul de sac and through the contralateral posterior vaginal wall, and lastly brought through the contralateral uterosacral ligament. Excessive bunching of tissue in the midline should be avoided as it can lead to dyspareunia.

PERINEORRHAPHY

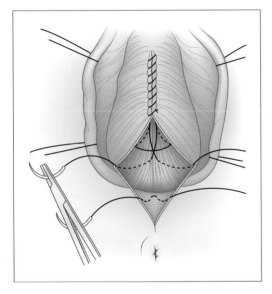

Figure 11-27. Perineorrhaphy. An enlarged introitus and perineal body disruption often accompany pelvic organ prolapse. Allis clamps are placed laterally on the introital opening so that, when brought together, they approximate the new opening, typically two to three fingerbreadths in size. A diamond-shaped incision is made, incorporating the perineal body and posterior vaginal wall, and the epithelium is removed. After other vaginal repairs are completed, the perineorrhaphy is begun. At approximately the level of the hymen, the transverse vaginae muscle is approximated along with the inferior parietal fascia of the pubococcygeus. A modified crown suture is used to join the bulbocavernosus muscle and introital epithelium. The rectovaginal septum and anterior capsule of the anal sphincter are placed together followed by the transversus perinei muscle. A subcuticular stitch is used to close the epithelium.

PROLAPSE REPAIR KITS

Currently Available Prolapse Repair Kits

Kit Name	Manufacturer
Apogee/Perigee	American Medical Systems, Minnetonka, MN
Avaulta/Avaulta Plus	Bard Urologic Division, Covington, GA
Prolift	Women's Health and Urology, Somerville, NJ

Figure 11-28. Prolapse repair "kits." In an attempt to duplicate the success of midurethral slings, prolapse "kits" with precut grafts and vaginal delivery systems have been marketed. These kits make use of a transobturator approach for correction of anterior prolapse and a perianal approach for posterior and apical support. These kits include anterior grafts, posterior grafts, and combined or total grafts. Unfortunately, materials are changing too quickly for sound scientific studies to keep pace: before the first generation can be studied, the next generation has already been released. To date, little clinical evidence exists to support using these products. Registries are being developed to help address these issues.

Limited and cautious use of these kits is recommended until further data are available. Some experts are adamantly opposed to use of these kits until data are presented. These procedures are too new to have recommendations concerning coincident hysterectomy or uterine preservation if the uterus is still present. An increased graft-exposure incidence with hysterectomy incision has been shown in the European literature [47]. Surgeons should discuss the lack of data with their patients and make appropriate decisions on an individual basis if these kits are used.

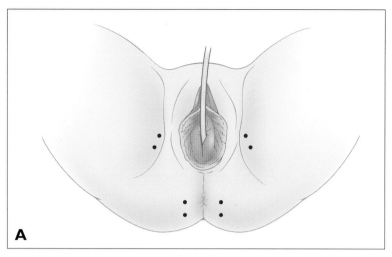

A

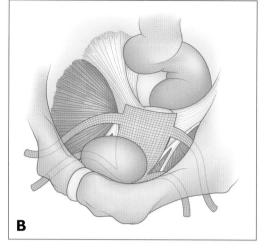

B

Figure 11-29. The anterior approach typically involves a midline vaginal incision starting just above the urethral vesical junction and extending proximally for 4 cm. Keeping this incision small will help reduce future graft exposure. Prior to making the incision, a dissecting solution is injected into the true vesicovaginal space. The bladder is separated from the vaginal wall and access to the space of Retzius is gained. This space may be more easily entered closer to the ischial spine and then gentle traction should be used, advancing more distally toward the pubic symphysis. If possible, the arcus tendineus fascia pelvis (ATFP) is left intact on the pelvic sidewall musculature. The obturator anatomy is identified, including the obturator foramina, obturator canal, and levator muscles. Alternatively, passes may be made below the arcus without entering the retropubic space. Two transobturator passes are made.

A, The first incision is made at or slightly below the level of the urethra in the superomedial aspect of the obturator foramen adjacent to the pubic ramus. It is guided through the foramen with the surgeon's finger protecting the bladder and urethra within the space of Retzius. **B,** The second incision is made 1 cm lateral and 2 cm inferior to the first. The trocar is passed laterally to the levator ani in the ischiorectal fossa and guided to the ischial spine. The tip of the trocar is palpated and the distance between the first distal trocar

pass (distal) and the current proximal pass is estimated, which will help to adjust the second pass so that adequate space is created between the two trocars. This overlooked step can result in rolling of the mesh due to inadequate distance between the passes. After the location of the second trocar along the proximal ATFP is settled, the tip is penetrated medially with the surgeon's finger in the space of Retzius to protect the bladder. Care is taken not to tear the levator muscle or arcus with overrotation of the trocar. The same sequence is repeated on the contralateral side. The graft can be attached at the vaginal apex and distally just above the urethrovesical junction. The graft arms are attached to their respective trocars and pulled through. The graft should lay tension free, without folds or wrinkles. Copious irrigation is followed by closure of the vagina with little to no vaginal trimming. Final positioning is completed and the graft arm is cut at the skin level. A vaginal packing may be placed for up to 24 hours.

Posteriorly, no agreement on the best incision has been reached. Some surgeons prefer a 4- to 5-cm posterior wall incision made above the rectovaginal septum (3 cm proximal to the posterior fourchette) whereas others use a standard incision as described for a perineorrhaphy and posterior repair. In either case, the shortest incision that allows safe trocar passage is used.

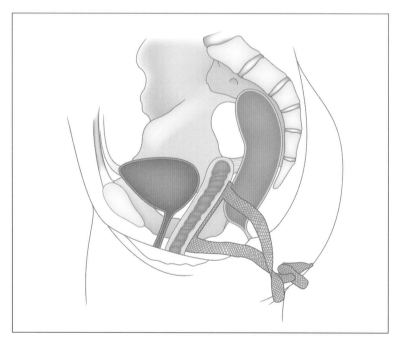

Figure 11-30. Incisions are made 3 cm lateral and 3 cm inferior to the mid anus (*see* Figure 11-29A). Trocars enter the ischiorectal fossa below the inferior hemorrhoidal neurovascular bundle and lateral to the levator ani. The trocars are guided to either the proximal end of the arcus rectovaginalis just distal to the ischial spine or through the inferior half of the sacrospinous ligament complex, two fingerbreadths medial to the ischial spine. A rectal examination confirms integrity of the rectum. The graft is attached to the vaginal apex and then the arms are pulled through. The graft is cut to the appropriate length and attached to the rectovaginal septum or perineal body. Some kits have separate distal posterior arms that are pulled through the perineal body. Appropriate graft tensioning and vaginal closure follow copious irrigation. Other than to freshen the edges, trimming vaginal epithelium is avoided. Final positioning is completed and confirmed with a rectal examination. A vaginal packing may be placed for up to 24 hours. If a posterior graft is to be placed, the posterior dissection should be performed first to avoid potentially obscuring bleeding from the anterior dissection.

CONCLUSION

The future of prolapse surgery depends on the development of well-designed studies controlled for evaluation, management, and treatment. Biases must be eliminated and honest follow-up provided so that the level of care for these patients will continue to rise. It cannot be overemphasized that prolapse is not the problem; it is the result of the problem, just as in a cardiac bypass patient, surgery is part of the treatment, but far from the whole treatment. The patient is never "cured" and most therapies must be combined to effect long-term success. In patients with prolapse, addressing risk factors is critical to successful surgery; we must identify these factors using a scientific approach instead of arbitrary limitations. Lastly, embracing new techniques and technology before data are available to support them is a risk about which the patient and physician must be well informed.

REFERENCES

1. Subak LL, Waetjen LE, van den Eeden S, *et al.*: Cost of pelvic organ prolapse surgery in the United States. *Obstet Gynecol* 2001, 98:646–651.

2. Olsen A, Smith VJ, Bergstrom JO, *et al.*: Epidemiology of surgically managed POP and urinary incontinence. *Obstet Gynecol* 1997, 89:501–506.

3. Luber K, Boero S, Choe JY: The demographics of pelvic floor disorders: current observations and future projections. *Am J Obstet Gynecol* 2001, 184:1496–1501.

4. Wall LL, DeLancey JOL: The politics of prolapse: a revisionist approach to disorders of the pelvic floor. *Perspect Biol Med* 1991, 34:486–496.

5. Maglinte DDT, Kelvin FM, Fitzgerald K, *et al.*: Association of compartment defects in pelvic floor dysfunction. *AJR Am J Roentgenol* 1999, 172:439–444.

6. Maher C, Baessler K, Glazener CMA, *et al.*: Surgical management of pelvic organ prolapse in women. *Cochrane Database Syst Rev* 2007, 3:CD004014.

7. Benson JT, Lucente V, McClellan E: Vaginal versus abdominal reconstructive surgery for the treatment of pelvic support defects: a prospective randomized study with long-term outcome evaluation. *Am J Obstet Gynecol* 1996, 175:1418–1422.

8. Scott N, Go PM, Graham P, *et al.*: Open mesh versus non-mesh for groin hernia repair. *Cochrane Database Syst Rev* 2001, 4:CD002197.

9. Webber AM, Walters MD: Anterior vaginal prolapse: review of anatomy and techniques of surgical repair. *Obstet Gynecol* 1997, 89:311–318.

10. Delancey JOL: Anatomic aspects of vaginal eversion after hysterectomy. *Am J Obstet Gynecol* 1992, 166:1717–1728.

11. Culligan PJ, Blackwell L, Goldsmith LJ, *et al.*: A randomized controlled trial comparing fascia lata and synthetic mesh for sacral colpopexy. *Obstet Gynecol* 2005, 106:29–37.

12. Iglesia CB, Fenner D, Brubaker L: The use of mesh in gynecologic surgery. *Int Urogynecol J* 1997, 8:105–115.

13. Richardson AC: Pelvic support defects in women (urethrocele, cystocele, uterine prolapse, enterocele, and rectocele). In *Hernia: Surgical Anatomy and Technique*. Edited by Skandalakis J, Gray S, Mansberger A Jr., *et al*. New York: McGraw-Hill; 1989:238–263.

14. Rooney K, Kenton K, Mueller ER, *et al.*: Advanced anterior vaginal wall prolapse is highly correlated with apical prolapse. *Am J Obstet Gynecol* 2006, 195:1837–1840.

15. DeLancey JO: Fascial and muscular abnormalities in women with urethral hypermobility and anterior vaginal wall prolapse. *Am J Obstet Gynecol* 2002, 187:93–98.

16. Cundiff GW, Harris RL, Coates K, *et al.*: Abdominal sacral colpoperineopexy: a new approach for correction of posterior compartment defects and perineal descent associated with vaginal prolapse. *Am J Obstet Gynecol* 1997, 177:1345–1355.

17. Fischer JR, Hale DS, Benson JT, *et al.*: Combined rectocele repair and abdominal sacralcolpopexy: a new method for repair of Denonvillier's fascia. Paper pesented at the American Urogynecologic Society 18th Annual Scientific Meeting. Tucson, AZ, September 25–28, 1997.

18. Timmons MC, Addison WA, Addison SB, *et al.*: Abdominal sacral colpopexy in 163 women with posthysterectomy vaginal vault prolapse and enterocele: evolution of operative techniques. *J Reprod Med* 1992, 37:323–327.

19. Shull BL, Capen CV, Riggs MW, *et al.*: Bilateral attachment of the vaginal cuff to iliococcygeus fascia: an effective method of cuff suspension. *Am J Obstet Gynecol* 1993, 168:1669–1677.

20. Silva W, Pauls R, Segal, J, *et al.*: Uterosacral ligament vault suspension: five-year outcomes. *Obstet Gynecol* 2006, 108:255–263.

21. Randall CL, Nichols DH: Surgical treatment of vaginal inversion. *J Obstet Gynecol* 1971, 38:327–332.

22. Nichols DH: Sacrospinous fixation for massive eversion of the vagina. *Am J Obstet Gynecol* 1982, 142:901–904.

23. Morley GW, DeLancey JOL: Sacrospinous ligament fixation for eversion of the vagina. *Am J Obstet Gynecol* 1988, 158:872–881.

24. Barksdale PA, Gasser RF, Gauthier CM, *et al.*: Intraligamentous nerves as a potential source of pain after sacrospinous ligament fixation of the vaginal apex. *Int Urogynecol J* 1997, 8:121–125.

25. Sharp TR: Sacrospinous suspension made easy. *Obstet Gynecol* 1993, 82:873–875.

26. Watson JD: Sacrospinous ligament colpopexy: new instrumentation applied to a standard gynecologic procedure. *Obstet Gynecol* 1996, 88:883–885.

27. Miyazaki FS: Miya hook ligature carrier for sacrospinous ligament suspension. *Obstet Gynecol* 1987, 70:286–288.

28. Shull BL, Capen CV, Riggs MW, *et al.*: Bilateral attachment of the vaginal cuff to iliococcygeus fascia: an effective method of cuff suspension. *Am J Obstet Gynecol* 1993, 168:1669–1677.

29. Zaccharin RF: Abdomino-perineal repair of large pulsion enterocele. In *Pelvic Floor Anatomy and the Surgery of Pulsion Enterocele*. Edited by Zaccharin RF. New York: Springer-Verlag Wien; 1985:135–155.

30. Williams BFP: Surgical treatment for uterine prolapse in young women. *Am J Obst Gynecol* 1966, 95:967–971.

31. Kovac SR, Cruikshank SH: Successful pregnancies and vaginal deliveries after sacrospinous uterosacral fixation in five of nineteen patients. *Am J Obstet Gynecol* 1993, 168:1778–1786.

32. Arthure HE, Savage D: Uterine prolapse and prolapse of the vaginal vault treated by sacral hysteropexy. *J Obstet Gynaecol Br Emp* 1957, 64:355–360.

33. Durfee RB: Suspension operations for treatment of pelvic organ prolapse. *Clin Obstet Gynecol* 1966, 9:1047–1061.

34. Fitzgerald MP, Richter HE, Siddique S, *et al.*: Colpocleisis: a review. *Int Urogynecol J Pelvic Floor Dysfunct* 2006, 17:261–271.

35. DeLancey JOL, Morley GW: Total colpocleisis for vaginal eversion. *Am J Obstet Gynecol* 1997, 176:1228–1235.

36. Richardson AC: The rectovaginal septum revisited: its relationship to rectocele and its importance in rectocele repair. In *Clinical Obstetrics and Gynecology*. Edited by Pitkin RM, Scott JR, DeLancey JOL. Philadelphia: JB Lippincott; 1993:977.

37. Kuhn RJP, Hollyock VE: Observations on the anatomy of the rectovaginal pouch and septum. *Obstet Gynecol* 1982, 59:445–447.

38. Jeffcoate TNA: Posterior colpoperineorrhaphy. *Am J Obstet Gynecol* 1959, 77:490–502.

39. Kahn MA, Stanton Sl: Posterior colporrhaphy: its effects on bowel and sexual function. *Br J Obstet Gynecol* 1997, 104:82–86.

40. Benson JT: Rectocele, descending perineal syndrome, enterocele. In *Female Pelvic Floor Disorders: Investigation and Management*. Edited by Benson JT. New York: WW Norton; 1992:384.

41. Block IR: Transrectal repair of rectocele using obliterative suture. *Dis Colon Rectum* 1986, 11:707–711.

42. Sullivan ES, Leaverton GH, Hardwick CE: Transrectal perineal repair: an adjunct to improved function after anorectal surgery. *Dis Colon Rectum* 1968, 11:106–114.

43. Sehapayak S: Transrectal repair of rectocele: an extended armamentarium of colorectal surgeons, a report of 355 cases. *Dis Colon Rectum* 1985, 28:422–433.

44. Halban J: *Gynakologische Operationslehre*. Berlin: Urban and Schwarzenberg; 1932.

45. Moschcowitz AV: The pathogenesis, anatomy, and cure of prolapse of the rectum. *Surg Gynecol Obset* 1912, 15:7.

46. McCall ML: Posterior culdoplasty: surgical correction of enterocele during vaginal hysterectomy: a preliminary report. *Obstet Gynecol* 1957, 10:595.

12

Urethral Diverticula and Genitourinary Fistulas

Patrick J. Woodman

Urethral diverticula and genitourinary fistulas are uncommon and difficult conditions to treat. The uncontrollable leakage of urine, recurrent vaginitis or cystitis, and negative effects that accompany these conditions make them devastating for patients. Because of the infrequent incidence of these conditions, research studies of high quality are also rare, and much of what we know is drawn from retrospective case series and anecdotal reports. The epidemiology of these conditions reveals a variety of causative diseases, treatments, and surgeries, which further complicate consolidating the data into a meaningful analysis [1].

URETHRAL DIVERTICULA

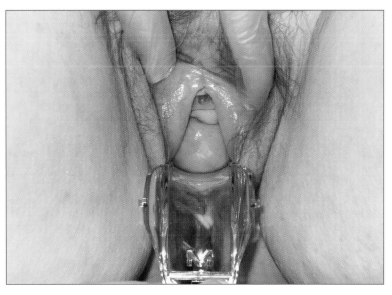

Figure 12-1. Urethral diverticulum in a 57-year-old white woman. Urethral diverticula are cystic, suburethral swellings of the paraurethral or Skene's glands. Their incidence depends on clinical suspicion and the subsequent work-up to establish the diagnosis, typically listed as 3% (ranging from 0.6% in general necropsy specimens to 6% in certain gynecologic patient populations) [2–7]. There are notable associations with female sex and African American race. In patients with a history of recurrent urinary tract infections, the incidence is as high as 16% to 40%. Approximately 500 to 3400 surgeries are performed in the United States annually for the treatment of urethral diverticula [8].

Frequency of Common Presenting Symptoms in Patients Presenting with a Urethral Diverticulum		
Symptom	**Range, %**	**Mean, %**
Frequency	63–70	66
Burning	35–79	53
Rucurrent urinary tract infections	9–61	38
Urinary incontinence	25–49	37
Dysuria	9–55	30
Urgency	21–38	28
Urethral pain	6–40	28
Vaginal mass	6–27	18
Dyspareunia	6–24	15
Hematuria	9–20	15
Voiding dysfunction (difficult urination/dribble)	4–32	20
Urinary retention	2–19	8

Figure 12-2. Frequency of urethral diverticula symptoms. This condition is commonly associated with inflammation and patients subsequently complain of pelvic discomfort, urinary frequency, and other irritative voiding symptoms. "Dysuria," "dyspareunia," and the "dribbling" of urine that can represent muscle-induced or gravity-associated drainage of the diverticulum represent the three classic "D" symptoms that should make the practitioner think immediately of urethral diverticulum. The frequency of common presenting symptoms in patients presenting with a urethral diverticulum is listed. (*Data from* Wharton and Kearns [2], Sogor [3], MacKinnon *et al.* [4], Davis and Robinson [5], Hoffman and Adams [6], and Aspera *et al.* [7].)

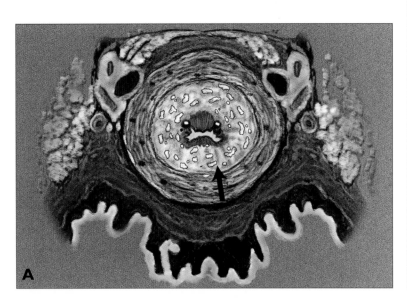

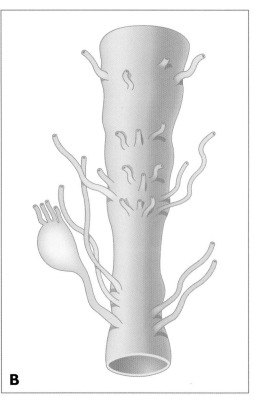

Figure 12-3. Anatomy of the urethra. **A,** A histologic cross-section of the urethra shows the area where diverticula tend to form (*arrow*). **B,** Small branches of the paraurethral ducts course somewhat parallel to the urethra, traverse the lamina propria, and empty into the urethra proper.

The anatomy of the urethra has been described by Huffman [9] and others [10,11]. Using wax necropsy specimens and serial histologic sections, Huffman showed that most paraurethral glands originate in the middle one third of the urethra, track caudally,

and then communicate with urethral lumen. Histologic sampling of these glands ranges from squamous epithelium close to the meatus to cuboidal to transitional near the bladder [9]. The Skene's glands are not found universally but when present they dump into the distal one third of the urethra, near the meatus. One or more urethral diverticula may be present, since the inflammation that causes occlusion of one paraurethral duct may certainly cause occlusion of others [3]. Urethroscopic investigation should focus on locating all diverticula ostia.

Proposed Etiologic Causes of Urethral Diverticula

Congenital	Acquired
Gartner's duct cyst	Infection
Wolffian duct cyst	Birth or other trauma
Failure of urethral primal fold union	Instrumentation
Sequestration of periurethral cell rests	Obstruction
	Urethral stone impaction
	Urethral stricture
	Urethral or vaginal surgery
	Malignancy

Figure 12-4. Etiology of urethral diverticula. Both congenital and acquired theories have been proposed to explain the etiology of urethral diverticula [12].

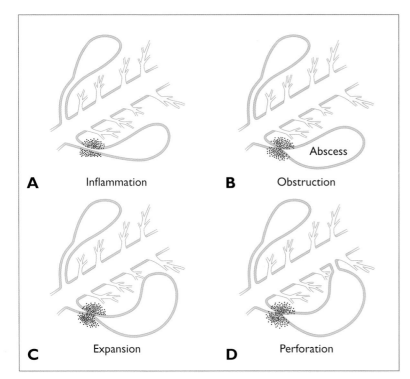

Figure 12-5. Hypothetical mechanism of acquired suburethral diverticulum. **A,** An initial inflammatory response occurs in Skene's duct or one of the paraurethral ducts. **B,** An abscess forms within the gland or duct, leading to obstruction of the gland neck. **C,** Expansion

of the abscess. **D,** Perforation of the abscess into the urethral, leading to diverticulum formation.

The predominant theory of causes of urethral diverticula is infection: either by sexually transmitted disease, such as *Neisseria gonorrhoeae* or *Chlamydia trachomatis*, or by more traditional genitourinary bacteria. Inflammation from the infection leads to abscess formation, expansion under pressure, then release of that pressure as the abscess drains into the urethra. Chronic inflammation in the abscess cavity can lead to epithelialization and the formation of a mature diverticulum. Birth trauma, or trauma from gynecologic surgery that disrupts normal blood flow and anatomy of the urethra, can lead to necrosis or can redirect the normal arrangement of paraurethral glands. For similar reasons, pelvic trauma and the vasculitis associated with radiation can also disrupt normal anatomy. Congenital theories suggest either a disordered fusion of the urethral primal folds or persistence of cell rests around the urethra.

Patients with urethral syndrome have similar subjective complaints without suburethral swelling [13]. This may represent an early manifestation on a continuum that includes periurethritis through urethral diverticulum, in which the diverticular sac arises from repeated infection and abscess formation [7]. The obstructed glands rupture into the urethral lumen and the resultant outpouching epithelializes. These conditions have been likened to a female prostatitis [13] and histologic work confirms the presence of glands and even anti–prostate-specific antigen, suggesting that the paraurethral glands collectively may represent a homologue to the prostate gland [9,13]. (*Adapted from* Sogor [3].)

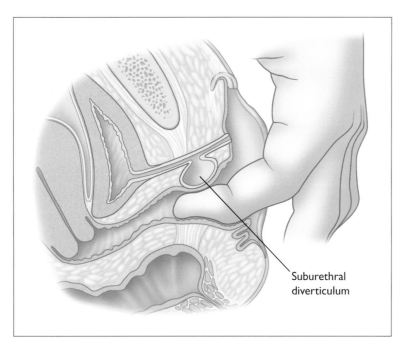

Suburethral
diverticulum

Figure 12-6. Palpation of the urethra. This should be done with the clinician's finger along and bilateral to the urethra against the pubic bone in order to elicit localized tenderness or swelling. Digital palpation of the urethra against the flat of the pubic bone is important and is the step most missed by gynecologists. This assessment of swelling, tenderness, and the expression of pus or urine may be facilitated with the presence of a sound or a cystoscope in the urethra. (*Adapted from* Wheeless [14].)

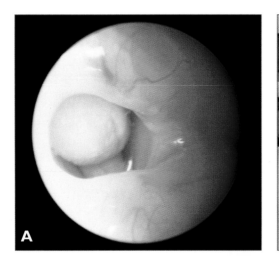

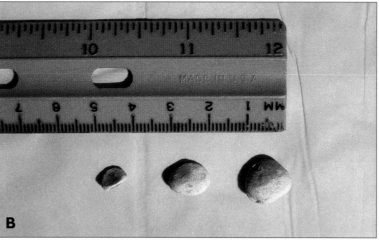

Figure 12-7. Urethral calculi. The diagnosis of urethral diverticula can be suggested by a thorough history and physical. The presence of irritative voiding symptoms (urgency, frequency, dysuria, and voiding dysfunction) with a suburethral mass and a history of "recurrent urinary tract infections" should suggest diverticula. The key feature with such a history is that the condition is refractory to adequate medical treatment [3]. Using these signs, Davis and TeLinde [15] were able to correctly diagnose diverticula in 63% of cases in their series. Local supersaturation of urine within the diverticulum can lead to stone formation. **A,** Diverticular calculi occur after many years of incomplete emptying and recurrent infection. **B,** Stone size can vary, depending on the size and shape of the diverticulum and the length of time the patient has had the diverticulum.

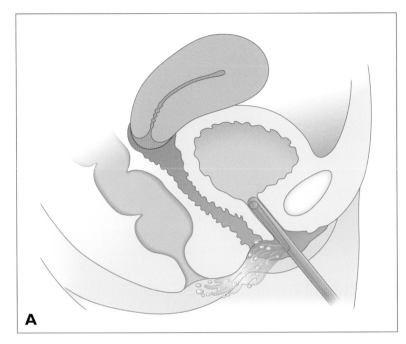

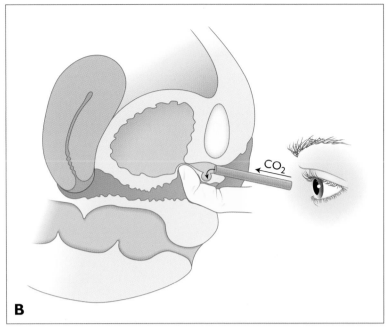

Figure 12-8. Cystourethroscopic examination. **A,** Up to 50% of diverticula have been previously examined either once or many times without the diagnosis being made. **B,** Urethroscopy is essential for diagnosis. Carbon dioxide, normal saline, or sterile water may be used for a distention medium. The examiner's fingers in the vagina push the vesical neck against the symphysis to expand the urethra.

Direct visualization of the diverticular ostia under cysto-urethroscopic guidance is the classic method for diagnosing a urethral diverticulum. By pinching the bladder neck against the scope or cystoscopic sheath, fluid is allowed to temporarily fill an empty diverticular cavity.

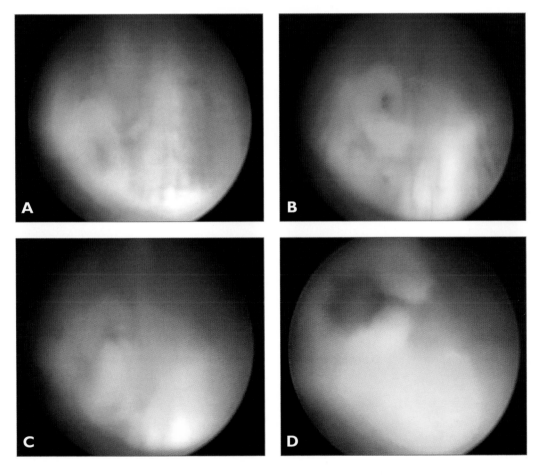

Figure 12-9. Urethroscopic examination of the urethra. **A,** At first glance, there appears to be one ostium in the left lower quadrant of the mid-urethra. Notice the epithelialization of the diverticular tract. **B,** On further examination, the clinician can see two distinct ostia. **C,** With palpation, a small amount of pus can be seen extruding from the diverticular ostia. **D,** More vigorous manipulation results in much more pus drainage.

Compressing the anterior vaginal wall may reveal the location of the diverticular ostia and express pus or urine into view. If pus is not evident, the practitioner can inject indigo carmine or methylene blue into the diverticulum proper, to assist in endoscopically locating the ostia. Unfortunately, cysto-urethroscopy can miss up to 30% to 40% of diverticula [7].

Urethral Diverticula and Genitourinary Fistula 233

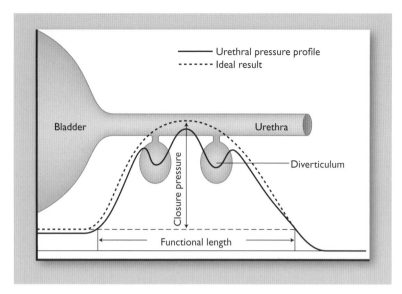

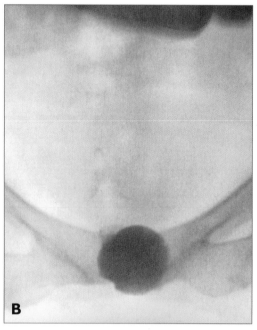

Figure 12-10. Urethral closure pressure profile, with superimposed diverticular ostia proximal and distal to maximal urethral closure pressure (MUCP). Suburethral diverticula can result in a dip in pressure on urethral pressure profilometry (UPP), which can sometimes be used to localize the diverticulum in relation to the area of MUCP. If the diverticulum is located within the high-pressure zone, then an attendant decrease in urethral pressure will be seen on the UPP. It has been suggested that UPP has an accuracy of 72% in diagnosing urethral diverticula [3]. (*Adapted from* Bent [16].)

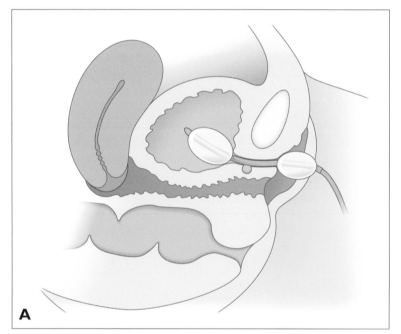

Figure 12-11. Double-balloon catheterization (positive-pressure) urethrogram. **A,** Davis and Tratner catheters occlude the urethrovesical junction and urethral meatus to allow positive-pressure urethrography (PPUG). **B,** A urethral diverticulum fills with contrast agent during this PPUG study.

Various radiographic studies have been used to delineate the cystic structure of the diverticulum. Since the introduction of retrograde injection of iodized oil into the urethra (retrograde urethrography) in the 1930s, improved techniques have improved the ability to make a diagnosis. Voiding cystourethrography (VCUG), performed under cinefluoroscopy, has improved the diagnostic yield by 40% [3]. Davis and Cian [17] described positive-pressure urethrography (PPU), with a double-balloon catheter to force contrast medium into even smaller urethra ostia. They noted that several diverticula can coexist, as well as have more than one ostial opening. However, PPU can be quite uncomfortable and difficult to perform, despite accuracy as high as 90% [16].

Ultrasonography of the urethral diverticulum has been described via transvaginal, transperineal, and endourethral approaches. When compared with VCUG, ultrasound has comparable diagnostic ability and provides more information about the extent and location of the diverticular neck [7]. However, ultrasonography is limited, mainly by being dependent on surgeons and technicians. More recently, MRI has been used to diagnose diverticula, performing better than urethrography and urethroscopy in one trial [18]. VCUG is also limited by concomitant procedures, revealing a positive predictive value of 60% when performed following PPU [19]. Yet PPU was able to detect all 22 diverticula missed on VCUG at a comparable cost.

When compared with all other modalities, PPU was found to have the highest accuracy and sensitivity [20]. However, one other small series suggested that MRI outperforms PPU [21]. MRI certainly provides several ways to image the urethra in women: endoluminal, endorectal, and endovaginal and external coils can enhance the difference between the viscous organs and fluid-filled structures, but it is expensive. The reader must also keep in mind that all diagnostic tests have both a false-positive and false-negative rate, and a combination of modalities may be necessary to diagnose urethral diverticula.

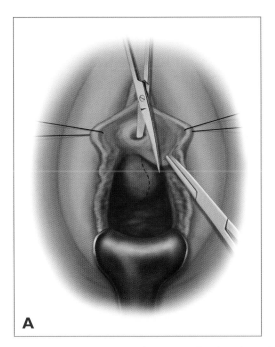

A

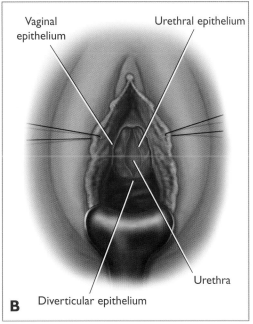

Vaginal epithelium

Urethral epithelium

Diverticular epithelium

Urethra

B

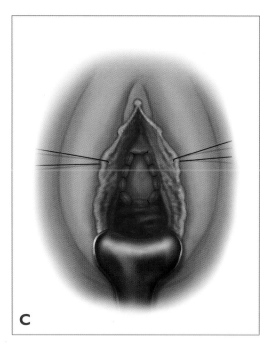

C

Figure 12-12. Marsupialization of a distal urethral diverticulum (Spence procedure). **A,** The dotted line indicates an incision along the posterior urethral and anterior vagina from the external urethral meatus to proximal diverticulum. **B,** Exteriorized diverticulum showing continuous urethral and diverticular epithelia surrounded by vaginal epithelium. **C,** Marsupialization completed with a continuous running locked suture.

Spence procedure for treatment of a urethral diverticulum: Treatment includes preoperative antibiotics (particularly when treating an acutely infected diverticular abscess), local heat, and incision and drainage of the diverticular cavity. When deciding which antibiotic to use, consider the most likely causative agent, risks for sexually transmitted disease, previous therapy, and the length of symptoms. In a reproductive-age female patient with more than one partner, priority should be given to a broad-spectrum cephalosporin or fluoroquinolone, then 7 days of doxycycline, 100 mg twice daily. However, 30-day use of a fluoroquinolone has also been advocated, which is similar to the treatment of chronic prostatitis [13]. Some consideration should be given to prophylactic treatment with an antifungal agent.

The type of surgery recommended depends on the location of the diverticulum. A distal urethral location makes marsupialization via meatotomy quite an attractive choice [22]. Spence's procedure is 90% to 100% effective at treating the diverticulum, with rare complication [23]. The procedure is performed distally to the high-pressure zone that is associated with continence, so very few patients later present with de novo incontinence. Straight Mayo or tenotomy scissors are placed within the urethral meatus and worked down into the base of the diverticulum. The other blade of the scissors is kept outside the vaginal epithelium. Carefully, the intervening tissue is cut along the long axis of the urethra. The resulting defect allows the surgeon to gain access to the diverticular sac and to marsupialize it to the vaginal epithelium, in a running, locked fashion. (*Adapted from* Lichtman and Robertson [23].)

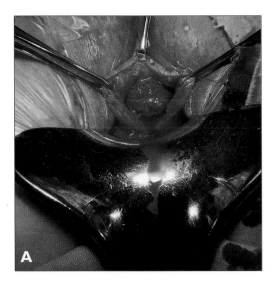

A

Figure 12-13. Direct urethrovaginal fistula repair; excision of a mid-urethral diverticulum. **A,** Gross appearance of a dissected urethral diverticulum.

Continued on the next page

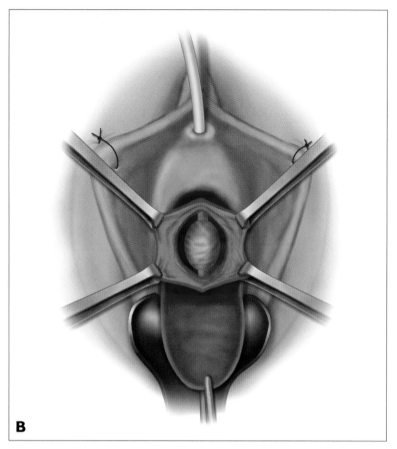

B

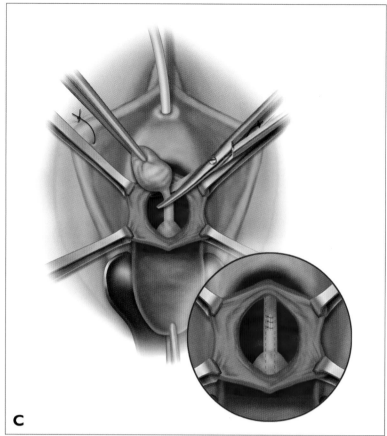

C

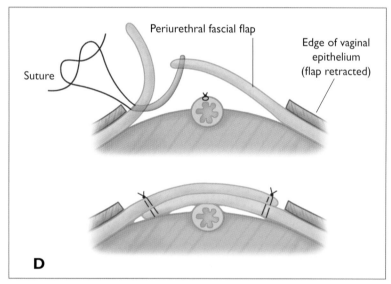

Periurethral fascial flap

Edge of vaginal epithelium (flap retracted)

Suture

D

Figure 12-13. *(Continued)* **B,** Diverticulum exposed. **C,** Diverticulum excised at its base and the urethra repaired perpendicular to the tube to avoid constriction. **D,** Periurethral fascia closed in a "double-breasted" fashion.

Midurethral diverticula should be treated with a direct fistulectomy; the predominant procedure is the manner described by Hoffman and Adams [6]. These authors stressed the importance of complete removal of the diverticular sac to prevent recurrent accumulation and diverticula formation, and the identification of all ostia. An inverted U-shaped incision or midline incision is made through the epithelium at the level of the diverticulum and is dissected away from the underlying fascial layer. A linear incision is made parallel to the urethra, exposing the diverticular sac. This is completely circumcised from the urethra and the defect in the urethra is closed in a transverse fashion. The fascia has likely been stretched by the sac and the surgeon's manipulations, so this can be closed in a "double-breasted vest" fashion to interrupt overlapping

of the suture lines. Finally, the skin is closed. This procedure has been reported as 92% effective, with a 5% complication rate [6].

Proximal diverticula are more problematic. Not only do these diverticula lie in the urethral high-pressure zone (threatening continence), but because the operative field is so far away from the operator and so close to the bladder, cystotomy and fistulization are much more likely. To modify the surgical technique for this, Tancer *et al.* [24] recommended a partial ablation technique. The diverticular sac is dissected out vaginally, incised longitudinally, and entered. The main portion of the diverticulum is excised, but no effort is made to completely excise the neck of the diverticular sac. The urethral defect is closed in two layers, imbricating the urethral incision. The periurethral fascia is then closed in a double-breasted fashion. The authors found no cases of urinary incontinence or fistula formation in 34 cases over 10 years when utilizing this technique [24].

Considering the various types of surgical repair, the overall complication rate runs at approximately 17% for diverticulectomy, including issues such as inadvertent cystotomy, subsequent urethrovaginal fistulas, recurrent diverticula, de novo stress incontinence, urethral strictures, dyspareunia, and persistent irritative voiding symptoms [23]. For instance, close to 4% of diverticula repairs result in urethrovaginal fistulization, subsequent to infection or poor healing [3]. Risk factors for diverticula recurrence include active urethral infection, difficult dissection, and excessive suture-line tension [7].

Postoperative management includes double drainage (urethral and suprapubic catheters) for 10 to 14 days to decompress the bladder and act as a urethral stent for healing. Patients remain on antibiotics for 2 weeks and an anticholinergic for bladder spasms, after which time a voiding cystourethrography (VCUG) is done to rule out extravasation of radio-opaque dye. Voiding trials can begin after it is confirmed that there is no extravasation and the Foley catheter is removed. If extravasation is seen, another week of bladder rest is prescribed and another VCUG should be done to confirm closure. Physical restrictions include vaginal rest from tampons, douches, and intercourse for 4 to 6 weeks. (**B–D** *adapted from* Sogor [3].)

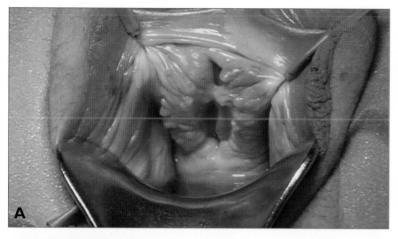

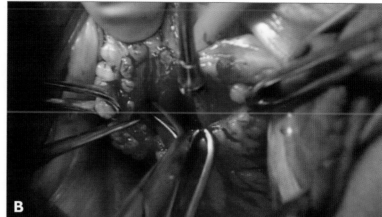

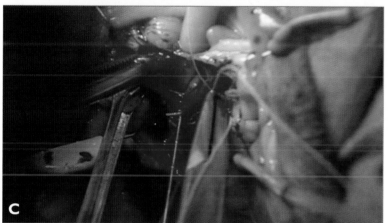

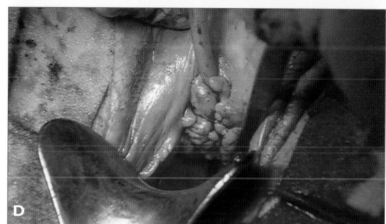

Figure 12-14. Direct urethrovaginal fistula repair. **A,** Gross appearance of a linear urethrovaginal fistula, which was caused by posterior urethral disruption. **B,** Urethral muscle is mobilized. **C,** Muscle is reapproximated over a Foley catheter stent. **D,** Vaginal epithelium is closed over urethral repair. A Martius fat-pad flap can be interposed between the urethral repair and vaginal epithelium to avoid overlapping suture lines.

Urethrovaginal fistula (UVF) can be a complication of urethral diverticulectomy, a result of either birth or surgical trauma, or a result of either local inflammation or invasion. UVF most commonly are caused by direct trauma or pressure necrosis to the anterior wall of the vagina and can leave the patient with a condition from intermittent leakage of small amounts to near-total incontinence with constant leakage into the vagina as soon as urine is produced.

Only several hundred UVFs have been reported in the medical literature since the early 20th century [25–37]. In one large tertiary referral center, the rate of UVF occurrence as a complication of gynecology cases was 0.012% over nearly 25,000 cases and 15 years [25]. Traditionally, the classic risk factor for fistula formation has been obstructed labor, but this has been replaced by complications from urologic or gynecologic surgery (urethral diverticula, anterior repair, and bladder neck suspension) as the most common causes of UVF. In cases of vaginal hysterectomy combined with an anterior colporrhaphy, the incidence is as high as 1.05% [30]. Other causes include trauma, irradiation, and cancer [27,33,34,36,37].

Because the incidence of UVS is rare, many case series include only two to five repairs per year. However, it seems clear that certain conditions predispose patients to failure: pelvic irradiation, complicated fistulas, and posterior urethral disruption. In the face of posterior urethral destruction, success rates hover around 71%, compared with 87% for a more limited defect [36]. Surprisingly, patients with previous failed repairs have as much success as those with primary repairs, depending on the center.

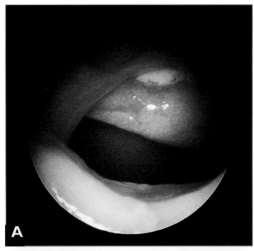

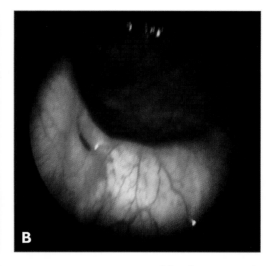

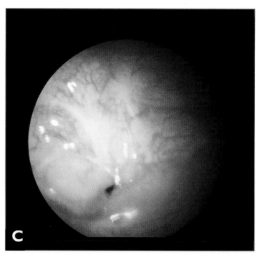

Figure 12-15. Vesicovaginal fistulas. **A,** Fistula seen from the vaginal side. **B,** Vesicovaginal fistula (VVF) seen from the vesical side. **C,** Intravesical view of a small VVF that was secondary to hysterectomy. The patients in panels **B** and **C** reside in developing countries and are devastated; families shun them and very few hospitals can treat them. In Africa, many young women commit suicide as a result of this diagnosis. **D,** Intravesical view of a large VVF. In Africa, India, and China, unattended births are common. If the infant cannot be delivered, the uterus ruptures and the woman is left with a huge hole in her bladder.

The etiology of VVF is varied but usually involves pelvic trauma. In developing countries, this trauma usually takes the form of obstructed labor or ritualistic cuts of the vagina. In industrialized countries, the most common cause is gynecologic surgery for benign conditions. Although fistulas can be congenital, other causes include malignancy, radiation, infections, stones and foreign bodies (such as neglected pessaries), urethral or uterine instrumentation, bowel surgery, and surgical delivery. The most common surgical procedure associated with VVF is hysterectomy, with 65% of reported injuries resulting in VVF [38]. The reported bladder injury rate of 1.3 per 1000 procedures results in a VVF rate of 0.8 per 1000 procedures.

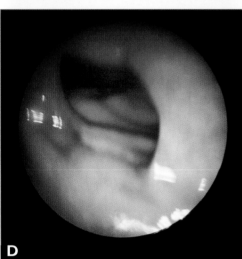

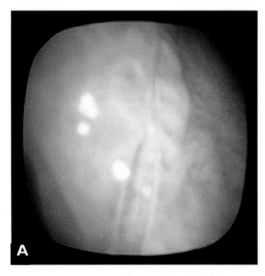

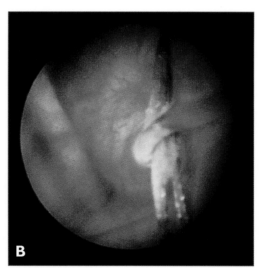

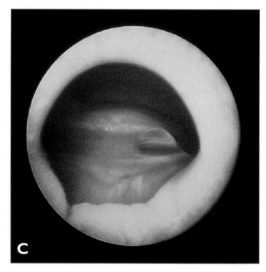

Figure 12-16. Suture through the bladder. **A,** Cystoscopy at the end of surgery is important to ensure that postoperative problems will not develop. **B,** This postoperative problem would not have occurred if cystoscopy had been accomplished before the patient left the operating room. **C,** An important reason for cystoscopy at the end of surgery is to know that the ureters are intact and functioning. If ureteral damage is discovered in the operating department, these patients do well. This is true even if the ureter has to be transplanted.

Continued on the next page

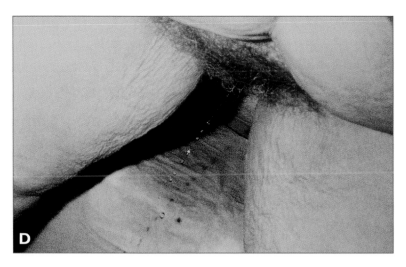

Figure 12-16. *(Continued)* **D,** A common problem is that the diverticulum has been closed, but the patient is incontinent because she had undiagnosed stress incontinence. The author starts these patients on Kegel exercises preoperatively and continues postoperatively.

Although it is attractive to blame the majority of these injuries on stray sutures that breech a bladder due to a poorly retracted bladder flap, there is evidence that this is not the only culprit. Meeks *et al.* [39] used a rabbit vagina and bladder model and purposefully placed a stitch in the bladder during the cuff closure after hysterectomy and found that no animal developed fistulization by 4 weeks after surgery. Clearly, there is something else going on, possibly unrecognized laceration of the bladder, crush, or electrocautery injuries at the time of hysterectomy with subsequent necrosis, or erosion due to cuff cellulitis or abscess.

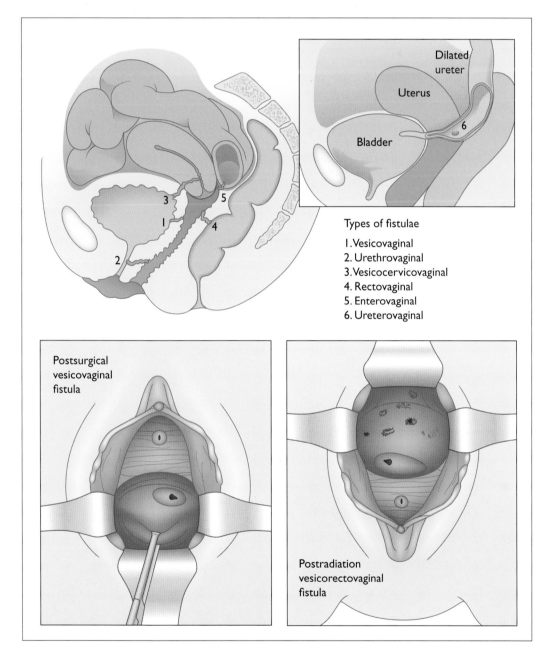

Types of fistulae

1. Vesicovaginal
2. Urethrovaginal
3. Vesicocervicovaginal
4. Rectovaginal
5. Enterovaginal
6. Ureterovaginal

Postsurgical vesicovaginal fistula

Postradiation vesicorectovaginal fistula

Figure 12-17. Classification of fistulas. On the vaginal side, the fistula tends to be just above the scar and on the vesical side, it is just above the interureteric ridge.

Urinary tract or gastrointestinal fistulas are named by their location. Although diagrams such as this are useful in counseling patients, it is helpful to provide the patient with a picture or diagram of her specific defect. Diagnosis can be made through a variety of in- and outpatient manipulations that are designed to highlight the tract. In cases of large fistula, the defect may be obvious. For smaller fistulas, this may not be so clear. Oral phenazopyridine, intravenous indigo carmine, and intravesical methylene blue or sterile milk can help the clinician delineate between the various types of fistula. Placement with subsequent examination under direct visualization can sometimes reveal a stained fistula tract or visualization of stained urine directly into the vagina. These medications can also be used if a fistula tract is not macroscopically visible.

For instance, simultaneous administration of oral phenazopyridine and intravesical indigo carmine or methylene blue, followed by a tampon placed in the vagina, can help distinguish between ureterovaginal and vesicovaginal fistulas. Provocative maneuvers, followed by careful removal of the tampon, may show a high and orange staining of the tampon, suggesting ureteral involvement. A high blue stain may suggest vesicovaginal fistula, whereas a distal blue stain may suggest urethral involvement. Care must be taken to rule out urinary incontinence through the urethral meatus, and complex multichannel urodynamics may be useful in documenting coexistent urodynamic stress incontinence. Endoscopy with cystoscopy or proctoscopy can be helpful in recording the number and placement of the position of the fistulous tract(s).

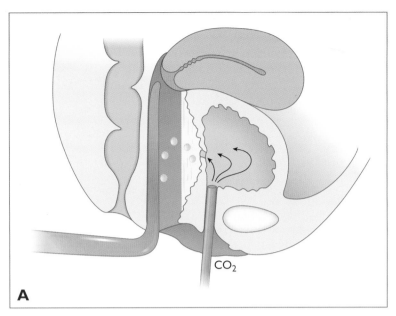

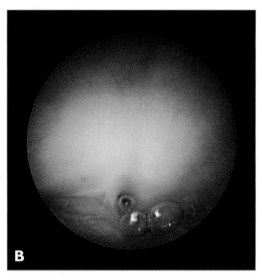

Figure 12-18. Diagnostic tips: the "flat-tire" technique. **A,** For those who use CO_2 as a distention medium for cystourethroscopy, this technique can assist in the location of small urinary tract fistulas. When CO_2 is instilled in the bladder, a patient in the knee-chest position should start to leak CO_2 bubbles through the fistula once it is under pressure. **B,** A small amount of sterile water or saline in the vagina can show the practitioner these bubbles, in stark contrast to the fluid, and a location of the fistulous opening vaginally [40].

Along with a proper history and physical, an intravenous urogram is required for a comprehensive examination of the urogenital fistula.

In up to 10% of fistulas, ureteral involvement is discovered [41]. Extravasation, hydronephrosis, or a persistent column of contrast may suggest the presence of ureteral involvement. Cystoscopy can help determine the size, number, and location of the fistulous openings on the bladder side. In many cases, a postoperative vesicovaginal fistula (VVF) is located along the anterior vaginal wall and interureturic ridge of the trigone. Other testing modalities that help in outlining VVFs are oblique and lateral cystograms, vaginograms, and contrast CT scans that can show extravasation into the vagina. Ultrasound and MRI have limited utility in the diagnosis of VVF.

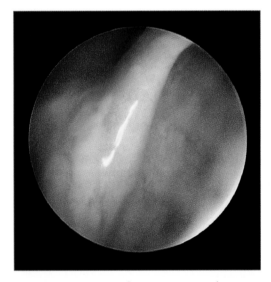

Figure 12-19. Steroid pretreatment of a postoperative urogenital fistula. An endoscopic view of the fistula after cortisone treatment shows its clean edge. If the edges are not clean, then it is necessary to wait until they are. This is preferable to having a set time for repair, such as 3 months.

Pretreatment for urethrovaginal and vesicovaginal fistulas includes optimizing the condition of vaginal tissues with vaginal estrogen administration for 4 to 6 weeks. Some surgeons recommend pretreatment with steroids such as cortisone to help speed the resolution of inflammation [42]. Recommendations for timing the repair suggest at least 8 to 12 weeks after injury in nonradiated patients and 6 months to 1 year in those with radiation. Bypass drainage via a transurethral or suprapubic catheter can divert the

constant flow of urine sometimes seen with fistulas, allowing the vagina to heal further and relieving clinical symptoms. Of course, antibiotic coverage for concurrent lower urinary tract or vaginal infections may be necessary. Preoperative antibiotics should cover both urinary tract and gastrointestinal bacteria. Ureteral stents should be considered if ureteral involvement is suspected, or if the location of the fistula falls within 1 to 2 cm of the ureteral orifices.

Small fistulas (less than a few millimeters) can sometimes respond to prolonged bypass drainage, with the catheter acting as a stent. Other minimally invasive techniques include the use of fibrin glue in fistulas smaller than 3 mm or the use of electrocautery application to the tract, but results have been disappointing. Distal fistulas can sometimes be treated with a urethral meatotomy, if the contractile portion of the urethra is not affected (*see* Figure 12-11). Although urethral defects can usually be closed longitudinally without fear of stricture, larger defects may be so extensive that this may not be possible. If minimal tissue destruction is present, the muscular layer may need to be closed side-to-side. If significant tissue destruction has occurred (the muscular layer is poor, weakened, or sloughed), an autograft or xenograft patch over the urethral musculature may be necessary to prevent stenosis of the urethra. In either closure, it is important to mobilize the urethral musculature enough to ensure a tension-free closure, usually a 2:1 ratio. Interrupted 2-O or 3-O absorbable sutures are typically used. Although a second layer is usually used to imbricate and reinforce the first, this can significantly decrease the caliber of the urethra. In a situation in which the proximal, high-pressure zone of the urethra is damaged and stress incontinence is expected, a staged procedure should be considered to allow the urothelium to heal adequately.

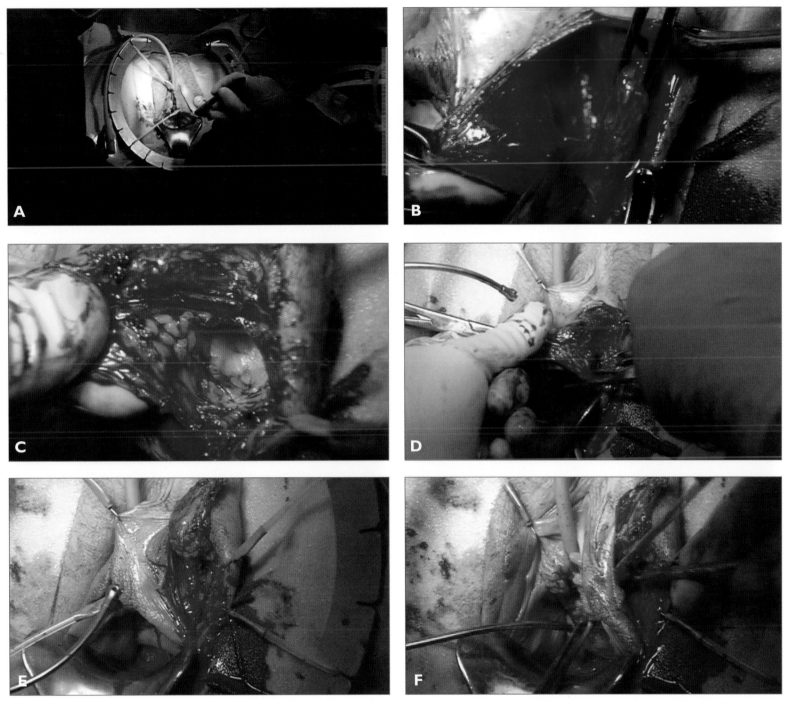

Figure 12-20. Development of a Martius fat-pad flap. **A,** Fat-pad harvest incision site outlined between the labia minora and labia majora. **B,** The fat pad is dissected down to the bulbospongiosus muscle. **C,** The base of the flap is exposed. **D,** The blood supply is sacrificed either cephalad or caudally. **E,** Hemostasis is achieved. **F,** A subepithelial tunnel is made to pierce the plane between the repair and the vaginal epithelium at the apex of the repair.

Continued on the next page

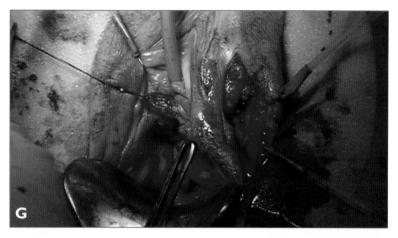

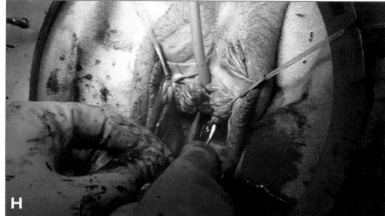

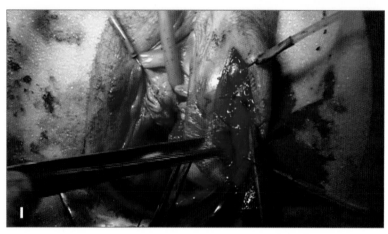

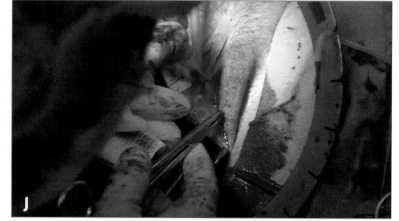

Figure 12-20. *(Continued)* **G,** The fat pad is passed through the subepithelial tunnel. **H,** The fat-pad flap is tacked over the repair site. **I,** The subcutaneous space is closed and a subcutaneous drain can be placed if hemostasis is not meticulous. **J,** The harvest-site incision is closed with a subcuticular closure.

In instances of complex urethrovaginal fistula repair, an interposition graft should also be considered. Blood supply to the labial fat pad is supplied from the external pudendal above, internal pudendal below, and perforating obturator vessels laterally. Sacrifice of the anterior or posterior blood supply allows a well-vascularized pedicle to be mobilized and fixed underneath the length of the urethral repair through a subepithelial tunnel. The Martius flap provides a well-vascularized pedicle to interrupt the integrity of the genitourinary fistulous tract. Reports of urethrovaginal fistula repair with Martius flap interposition success rates vary from 74% to 92% [29].

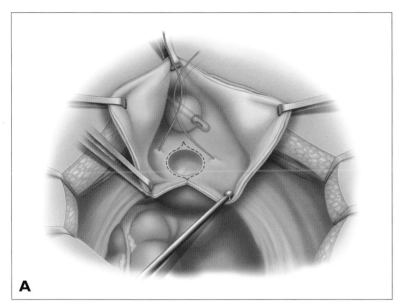

A

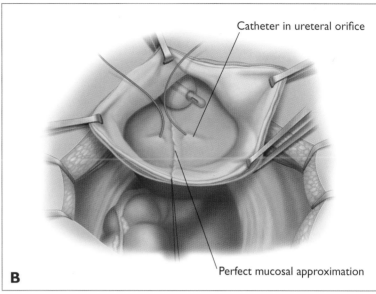

Catheter in ureteral orifice

Perfect mucosal approximation

B

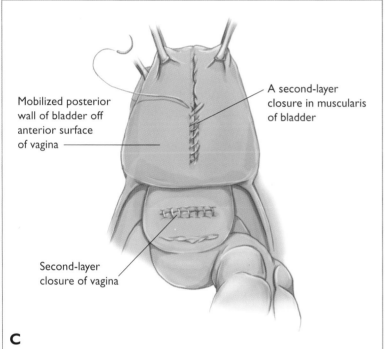

Mobilized posterior wall of bladder off anterior surface of vagina

A second-layer closure in muscularis of bladder

Second-layer closure of vagina

C

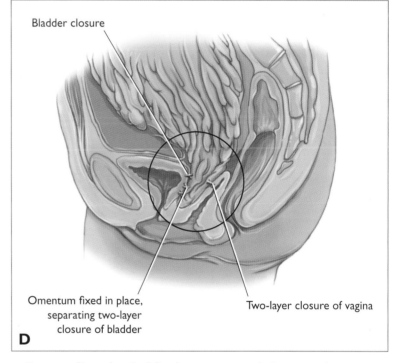

Bladder closure

Omentum fixed in place, separating two-layer closure of bladder

Two-layer closure of vagina

D

Figure 12-21. Abdominal repair of a vesicovaginal fistula (VVF). **A,** The bladder is bivalved in the plane to include the fistulous tract during repair, after freshening the edges. **B,** The mucosal edges are reapproximated. **C,** The muscularis is closed in two more layers to imbricate the bladder repair. Adequate mobilization between the vesicovaginal plane is necessary in order to make room for an interposition graft. **D,** A posterior or lateral segment of intact peritoneum, or the omentum, can be mobilized and tacked into place between the vaginal and bladder sides of the repair.

Although not the first surgeon to successfully close a VVF in the United States, J. Marion Sims's treatise on VVF repair became a foundation for the reconstructive pelvic surgery to follow. Sims [43] emphasized proper exposure and positioning, as well as wound edge opposition, both not yet well understood in the late 1840s. As layered closures and interposition grafts were introduced, VVF repair became more and more successful [41].

For complicated, apical fistulas, an open technique may be necessary. Particularly with large fistulas, fistulas with ureteral or trigonal involvement, those with previous failed repairs, or those caused by radiation, the abdominal approach is the one of choice. O'Conor *et al.* [44] recommended ureteral stenting and praised the surgical exposure. This group and others have found a success rate of 85% even though these patients have some of the most serious and difficult fistulas to repair. A suprapubic incision is made and a laparotomy is performed. The vagina wall is mobilized from the bladder as much as possible, and the bladder is then bivalved at the dome. Ureteral catheters can be placed, if necessary. The incision is continued until continuity with the fistula is achieved. The fistulous tract is excised and the bladder and vagina are closed in separate layers. The bladder repair (high-pressure side) is then imbricated in one or two more layers. Suprapubic tube placement can be accomplished through a separate, lateral bladder incision, before closure of the abdomen. (*Adapted from* Hurt [38].)

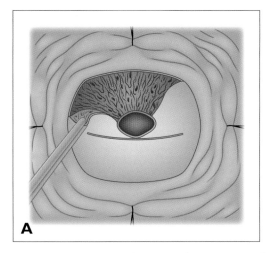 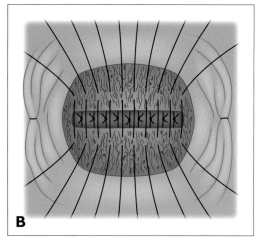

A

B

Figure 12-22. A, Latzko procedure (proximal colpocleisis) is recommended for small, apical vesicovaginal fistulas (VVFs) located above the trigone. **B,** Essentially a partial,

proximal colpocleisis, it closes the bladder defect in at least three layers, sequentially imbricating the repair [45]. With clamps or stay-sutures placed approximately 2 cm from the fistula in four quadrants, a curvilinear incision is made around the fistula and then the epithelium is removed. An appropriate-sized Foley catheter can assist in dissection if placed through the fistulous tract, so it can be placed on tension. The first layer is closed with absorbable suture, with two layers of interrupted delayed-absorbable suture. The simplicity of the repair allows most simple VVFs through a vaginal approach. Authors have reported surgical success rates of 93% to 100% for simple VVFs [40,45,46].

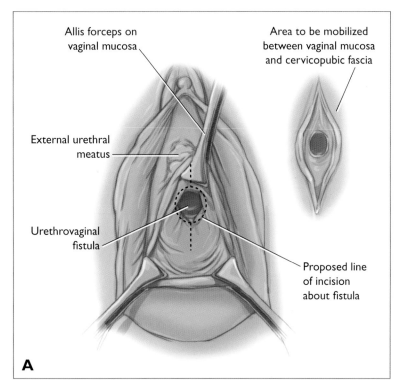

Allis forceps on vaginal mucosa

Area to be mobilized between vaginal mucosa and cervicopubic fascia

External urethral meatus

Urethrovaginal fistula

Proposed line of incision about fistula

A

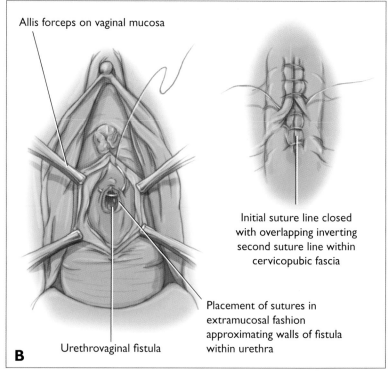

Allis forceps on vaginal mucosa

Initial suture line closed with overlapping inverting second suture line within cervicopubic fascia

Placement of sutures in extramucosal fashion approximating walls of fistula within urethra

Urethrovaginal fistula

B

Figure 12-23. Vaginal repair is the mainstay of vesicovaginal fistula (VVF) repairs, allowing the appropriate closure of even large fistulas. **A,** An elliptical incision is made around the fistula and can be extended laterally or along the midline to assist in dissection and exposure. **B,** Once the vaginal epithelium is mobilized widely, the fistulous tract can then be either closed without excision or removed

with subsequent urothelial closure at this time. A muscular layer imbrication is then performed, followed by a fascial closure. Any excess vaginal epithelium is trimmed at this time, allowing more excision on one side than the other, so the closure does not override the bladder repair.

Continued on the next page

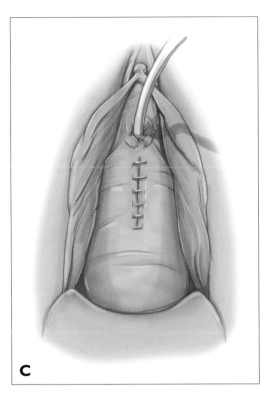

C

Figure 12-23. *(Continued)* **C,** The vaginal epithelium is closed. The reported success rates range from 90% to 100% [47–49]. More complicated, distal fistulas can be closed and reinforced with a Martius interposition graft placement, as described above or, with a variety of skin or muscular flaps, the scope of which is beyond this chapter [50].

Overall, success rates for VVF repair range from 67% to 100%. Urinary tract fistula repairs can be complicated by ureteral injury, ileus, urethral shortening, stress incontinence, and fistula persistence or recurrence, in addition to infectious conditions and diverticula formation [28].

Postoperative care includes dependent drainage for 10 to 14 days and anticholinergic medication to prevent bladder spasms. After ureterovesical junction (UVJ) repairs, transurethral catheterization is imperative to act as a stent and prevent unwanted urethral stricture due to scarification. The author uses a single prophylactic daily dose of urinary tract–specific antibiotics while any urinary catheter or ureteral stent is in situ. On removal of the catheter, voiding cystography is mandatory to exclude extravasation and persistent fistulization. Physical restrictions are meant to prevent pain, bladder spasms, and unintended removal of the catheters, such as with brisk physical activity or careless removal of clothing. *(Adapted from* Hurt [38].]

REFERENCES

1. Committee on Female Pelvic Medicine and Reconstructive Surgery: *Guide to Learning in Female Pelvic Medicine and Reconstructive Surgery*, edn 2. Dallas, TX: American Board of Obstetrics & Gynecology and American Board of Urology; 2003:18–19.

2. Wharton LR, Kearns W: Diverticula of the female urethra. *J Urol* 1950, 63:1063–1076.

3. Sogor L: Suburethral diverticula. In *Urogynecology and Reconstructive Pelvic Surgery*, edn 2. Edited by Walters MD, Karram MM. St. Louis: Mosby; 1999:367–375.

4. MacKinnon N, Pratt JH, Pool TL: Diverticulum of the female urethra. *Surg Clin North Am* 1959, 39:953–962.

5. Davis BC, Robinson DG: Diverticula of the female urethra: assay of 120 cases. *J Urol* 1970, 204:850–853.

6. Hoffman MJ, Adams WE: Recognition and repair of urethral diverticula. *Am J Obstet Gynecol* 1965, 92:106–111.

7. Aspera AM, Rackley RR, Vasavada SP: Contemporary evaluation and management of the female urethral diverticulum. *Urol Clin North Am* 2002, 29:617–624.

8. Burrows LJ, Howden NL, Meyn L, Weber AM: Surgical procedures for urethral diverticula in women in the United States, 1979–1997. *Int Urogynecol J Pelvic Floor Dysfunct* 2005, 16:158–161.

9. Huffman J: The detailed anatomy of the paraurethral ducts in the adult human female. *Am J Obstet Gynecol* 1948, 55:86–100.

10. Strohbehn K, Quint LE, Prince MR, *et al.*: Magnetic resonance imaging anatomy of the female urethra: a direct histological comparison. *Obstet Gynecol* 1996, 88:750–756.

11. Skene AJC: The anatomy and pathology of 2 important glands of the female urethra. *Am J Obstet* 1880, 13:265–270.

12. Johnson C: Diverticula and cyst of the female urethra. *J Urol* 1938, 39:506–516.

13. Gittes RF: Female prostatitis. *Urol Clin North Am* 2002, 29:613–616.

14. Wheeless C: Suburethral diverticulectomy via the double-breasted closure technique. In *Atlas of Pelvic Surgery*, edn 3. Edited by Wheeless CR. Baltimore: Williams & Wilkins; 1997:108–109.

15. Davis HJ, TeLinde RW: Urethral diverticula: an assay of 121 cases. *J Urol* 1958, 80:34–39.

16. Bent AE: Disorders affecting the urethra. In *Ostergard's Urogynecology and Pelvic Floor Dysfunction*, edn 5. Edited by Bent AE, Ostergard DR, Cundiff GW, Swift SE. Philadelphia: Lippincott Williams & Wilkins; 2003:245–260.

17. Davis J, Cian L: Positive pressure urethrography: a new diagnostic method. *J Urol* 1956, 75:753–757.

18. Kim B, Hricak H, Tanagho EA: Diagnosis of urethral diverticula in women: value of MR imaging. *AJR Am J Roentgenol* 1993, 161:809–815.

19. Wang AC, Wang CR: Radiologic diagnosis and surgical treatment of urethral diverticulum in women: a reappraisal of voiding cystourethrography and positive pressure urethrography. *J Reprod Med* 2000, 45:377–382.

20. Fortunato P, Schettini M, Gallucci M: Diagnosis and therapy of the female urethral diverticula. *Int Urogynecol J Pelvic Floor Dysfunct* 2001, 12:51–57.

21. Neitlich JD, Foster HE, Glickman MG, Smith RG: Detection of urethral diverticula in women: comparison of a high-resolution fast spin echo technique with double balloon urethrography. *J Urol* 1998, 159:408–410.

22. Spence H, Duckett J: Diverticulum of the female urethra: clinical aspects and presentation of a single operative technique for cure. *J Urol* 1970, 104:432–437.

23. Lichtman A, Robertson J: Suburethral diverticula treated by marsupialization. *Obstet Gynecol* 1976, 47:203–206.

24. Tancer ML, Mooppan MU, Pierre-Louis C, *et al.*: Suburethral diverticulum treatment by partial ablation. *Obstet Gynecol* 1983, 62:511–513.3

25. Lee RA, Symmonds RE, Williams TJ: Current status of genitourinary fistula. *Obstet Gynecol* 1988, 72:313–319.

26. Hedlund H, Lindstedt E: Urovaginal fistulas: 20 years of experience with 45 cases. *J Urol* 1987, 137:926–930.

27. Kliment J, Berats T: Urovaginal fistulas:experience with the management of 41 cases. *Int Urol Nephrol* 1992, 24:119–124.

28. Tehan TJ, Nardi JA, Baker R: Complications associated with surgical repair of urethrovaginal fistula. *Urology* 1980, 15:31–35.

29. Leach GE: Urethrovaginal fistula repair with Martius labial fat pad graft. *Urol Clin* 1991, 18:409–413.

30. Gray L: Urethrovaginal fistulas. *Am J Obstet Gynecol* 1968, 101:28–36.

31. Creatsas G, Deligeoroglou E, Sakellariou P, *et al.*: Reconstruction of urethro-vaginal fistula and vaginal atresia in an adolescent girl after an abdomino-perineal-vaginal pull-through procedure. *Fert Steril* 1997, 68:556–559.

32. Fall M: Vaginal wall bipedicled flap and other techniques in complicated urethral diverticulum and urethrovaginal fistula. *J Am Coll Surg* 1995, 180:150–156.

33. Tancer ML: A report of thirty-four instances of urethrovaginal and bladder neck fistulas. *Surg Gynecol Obstet* 1993, 177:77–80.

34. Keettel WC, Sehring FG, de Prosse CA, Scott JR: Surgical management of urethrovaginal and vesicovaginal fistulas. *Am J Obstet Gynecol* 1978, 131:425–431.

35. Krogh J, Kay L, Hjortrup A: Treatment of urethrovaginal fistula. *Br J Urol* 1989, 63:555.

36. Symmonds RE, Hill LM: Loss of urethra: a report on 50 patients. *Am J Obstet Gynecol* 1978, 130:130–138.

37. Marshall VE: Vesicovaginal fistulas on one urological service. *J Urol* 1979, 121:25–29.

38. Hurt WG: Vesicovaginal and ureterovaginal fistulae. In *Ostergard's Urogy-necology and Pelvic Floor Dysfunction*, edn 5. Edited by Bent AE, Ostergard DR, Cundiff GW, Swift SE. Philadelphia: Lippincott Williams & Wilkins; 2003:433–446.

39. Meeks GR, Sams JO, Field KW, *et al.*: Formation of vesicovaginal fistula: the role of suture placement into the bladder during closure of the vaginal cuff after transabdominal hysterectomy. *Am J Obstet Gynecol* 1997, 177:1298–1304.

40. Robertson JR: Vesicovaginal fistula, urethrovaginal fistula, and urethral diverticulum. In *Atlas of Clinical Gynecology: Urogynecology and Recon-structive Pelvic Surgery*. Edited by Stenchever MA, Benson JT. Philadelphia: Current Medicine; 2000:10.1–10.12.

41. Huang WC, Zinman LN, Bihrle, III W: Surgical repair of vesicovaginal fistulas. *Urol Clin North Am* 2002, 29:709–724.

42. Collins C, Pent D, Jones F: Results of early repair of vesicovaginal fistula with preliminary cortisone treatment. *Am J Obstet Gynecol* 1960, 80:1005–1012.

43. Sims J: On the treatment of vesico-vaginal fistula. *Am J Med Sci* 1852, 23:59–82.

44. O'Conor VJ Jr, Sokol JK, Bulkley GJ: Suprapubic closure of vesicovaginal fistula. *J Urol* 1973, 109:51–54.

45. Latsko W: Postoperative vesicovaginal fistulas: genesis and therapy. *Am J Surg* 1942, 58:211–228.

46. Elkins T, Thompson J: Lower urinary tract fistulas. In *Urogynecology and Reconstructive Pelvic Surgery*. Edited by Walters M, Karram M. St. Louis: Mosby; 1999:355–366.

47. Elkins TE, Drescher C, Martey JO: Vesicovaginal fistula revisited. *Obstet Gynecol* 1988, 72:307–312.

48. Margolis T, Mercer LJ: Vesicovaginal fistula. *Obstet Gynecol Surg* 1994, 49:840–847.

49. Raz S: *Female Urology*. Philadelphia: WB Saunders; 1993:373–377.

50. Zinman L: Muscular, myocutaneous, and fasciocutaneous flaps in complex urethral reconstruction. *Urol Clin North Am* 2002, 29:443–466.

13 Rectovaginal Fistulas

Patrick J. Woodman

Rectovaginal fistulas (RVFs) can be even more distressing than their genitourinary counterparts. The passage of small amounts of air, stool, and mucus into the vagina, and subsequent vaginal discharge, cause a distress that easily outweighs the severity of the problem. These and other symptoms, such as recurrent vaginal and urinary tract infections, vulvitis, and perineal skin excoriation, may cause the patient to consult her physician. Concurrent anal incontinence due to anal sphincter separation is common and can confuse the picture of RVF. Patients may also complain of dyspareunia and pelvic pain, dyscopria, and pain when sitting. Often the fear of odor and embarrassment will cause the patient to alienate herself from others, which adversely affects self-esteem and sexual relationships.

Classification of Rectovaginal Fistulas

	Location	Diameter	Environment	Surgery
Simple	Low- or mid-vaginal	< 2.5 cm	Trauma or infection	None previous
Complex	High-vaginal	> 2.5 cm	IBD, radiation, or neoplasm	Multiple failed repairs

Figure 13-1. Classification of rectovaginal fistula (RVF). RVFs can occur anywhere along the rectovaginal septum, from the posterior vaginal fornix to the dentate line. If the internal opening occurs distally to the dentate line, it should be classified as an anorectal fistula. Classification of RVF is most commonly defined according to location, as low (rectal opening at or just above the dentate line, with the vaginal opening close to the introitus), mid (vaginal opening between the introitus and the cervix), or high (vaginal opening behind or close to the cervix) [1]. Fistulas are further dichotomized into simple and complex categories, as shown. IBD— inflammatory bowel disease.

Etiology of Rectovaginal Fistula

Category	Condition	Mechanism
Traumatic		
Obstetric	Prolonged 2nd stage of labor	Pressure necrosis of rectovaginal septum
	Midline episiotomy	Extension directed into rectum
	Perineal lacerations	
Foreign body	Vaginal pessaries	Pressure necrosis
	Violent coitus	Mechanical perforation
	Sexual abuse	Mechanical perforation
Iatrogenic	Hysterectomy	Injury to anterior rectal wall
	Stapled colorectal anastomosis	Staple line includes vagina
	Transanal excision of anterior rectal tumor	Deep margin of resection into vagina
	Enemas	Mechanical perforation
	Anorectal surgery such as incision and drainage of intramural abscesses	Mechanical perforation
Inflammatory	Crohn disease	Transmural inflammation/perforation
	Pelvic radiation	Early tumor necrosis
	Pelvic abscess	Late transmural inflammation
	Perirectal abscess	
Neoplastic	Rectal	Local tumor growth into neighboring structure
	Cervical	
	Uterine	
	Vaginal	
	Primary or recurrent tumors	

Figure 13-2. Etiology of rectovaginal fistula (RVF). Although the predominant cause of genitourinary fistulas has shifted from birth trauma to gynecologic surgery, the most common cause of RVF continues to be damage secondary to vaginal delivery. RVF secondary to obstetric trauma is frequently associated with an anal sphincter injury and fecal incontinence. It has been estimated that the RVF incidence due to obstetric causes is 0.15% in the United States [2]. In large case series of RVFs, 11% to 74% were caused by obstetric complications, 17% to 30% were due to pelvic radiotherapy, 22% were congenital, 16% were due to local malignancy, 11% were due to inflammatory bowel disease, 10% were due to perianal suppurative disease, and 7% were due to operative trauma [3–5]. A full 8% were of unknown cause [2]. The table presents an exhaustive list of RVF etiologies.

Third- and fourth-degree obstetric lacerations and extensions, whether repaired well or not, can result in a localized infection or abscess. Chronic inflammation and the proximity of the vagina to the rectum, especially 3 to 4 cm above the anal verge, make this spot especially vulnerable. Other risk factors for the development of an RVF as a result of vaginal delivery include prolonged labor, high forceps delivery, and shoulder dystocia [6]. Subsets of lower gastrointestinal tract fistulas, such as congenital fistulas and fistulas in situ, are caused by infected anal crypts and are beyond the scope of this chapter.

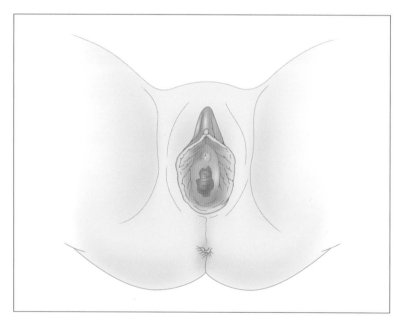

Figure 13-3. Dovetailing of the anal sphincter. Evaluation to diagnose rectovaginal fistula (RVF) should be guided by the patient's history and physical findings. The number of vaginal deliveries should be elicited, as well as a history of birth trauma, forceps usage, proctoepisiotomy, and the temporal relationship of the onset of symptoms. Particular care should be taken to examine the entire length of the rectovaginal septum with an index finger vaginally and rectally. Narrowing of the perineal body, "dovetailing" of the anus, a gaping anus with weak tone and squeeze, or anterior displacement of the anus may also suggest separation of the anal sphincter muscles, which can be complicated by RVF. Palpable masses on rectal examination may suggest malignancy and careful examination should be performed in order to rule out Crohn disease (signs include fleshy skin tags, multiple fissures, or multiple cutaneous fistulous openings) [6]. The surrounding area should be evaluated for condition (ie, induration, inflammation, and radiation). Coexistent abscess detection should be made a priority. Any palpable fistulous opening on examination should be confirmed by direct visualization using anoscopy or endoscopy.

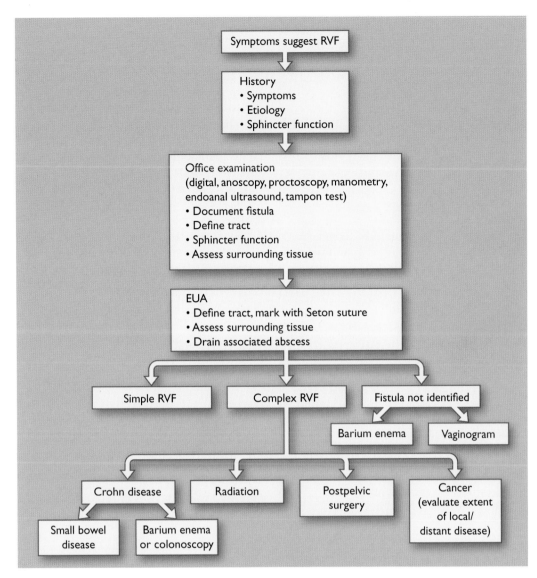

Figure 13-4. Algorithm for the diagnosis of rectovaginal fistula (RVF). Other adjuncts to diagnosis of RVF include efforts to make the fistula tract stand out, such as the placing of a few drops of methylene blue or indigo carmine on the surgeon's examining finger rectally and looking for blue dye vaginally. Soapy water can be used to fill the vagina and the rectum insufflated with air so that bubbles can be seen. Some advocate the use of radiologic tests such as a barium enema, defecography, or ultrasonography. Injecting hydrogen peroxide can increase the diagnostic yield during transanal ultrasonography, revealing the pathway of the fistulous tract [7]. A proposed algorithm for the evaluation of RVF is shown here.

Like genitourinary fistulas, repair is based on a multifactorial list of conditions: the number, size, and location of the fistula openings; whether the anal sphincters are involved or are separated; whether the patient is immunocompromised or has been exposed to radiation; and whether the patient has an inflammatory bowel disease or an associated malignancy. This information is exceedingly important in planning the type and timing of RVF repair, the need for concomitant procedures, and predicting success. For instance, if the surrounding tissue is inflamed, a diverting colostomy may be warranted until the tissue inflammation subsides to optimize success rates. Fecal incontinence due to a lacerated anal sphincter may require concomitant repair in order to cure the patient's symptoms. The fibrosis and vasculitis associated with pelvic radiation may take 6 to 12 months to stabilize before surgical repair. The avenue of approach is chosen based on the level of the fistula, cause, and need for fecal diversion or ancillary procedures.

Patients with inflammatory bowel disease (IBD), such as Crohn disease, require special mention here. Crohn disease is a transmural granulomatous inflammatory disorder that can affect any part of the gastrointestinal (GI) tract from the mouth to the anus [8]. In addition to

the other symptoms of RVF, patients whose disease is caused by IBD can also present with diarrhea, mucus passage, and cramping [9]. Internal fistulas occur in 1% to 40% of patients, and as many as half of those may have multiple fistulas [8,10]. The objective of surgical repair of RVF in the patient with Crohn disease is to restore health and function, while providing respite to allow the withdrawal of steroids. Although there have been numerous advances in the treatment of IBD over the past decade, some of these treatments may hinder the healing of, or have an unknown effect on, an RVF repair [11]. Although the effect of steroids on healing is somewhat predictable, anti–tumor necrosis factor-α agents, cytokine therapies, anti–T-cell activators, growth factors, and adhesion molecule inhibitors have not been well studied in regard to RVF repair. In patients with severe, persistent, or recurrent disease, diverting colostomy is recommended to ensure proper healing.

Radiation-induced RVF can occur as a result of the treatment of urologic, gynecologic, or colorectal cancers. The rectum is the most common GI site of injury due to its proximity to the vagina and its fixed position in the pelvis [12]. Operations on the irradiated rectum have morbidity rates of 12% to 65% and mortality rates of 0% to 13%. Significant risk factors for sequelae include advanced patient age, prior abdominal surgery, and inclusion of the entire pelvis. Characteristic tissue changes include intense hyperemia, mucosal edema and slough, epithelial atypia, intestinal wall fibrosis, serosal thickening, and vascular sclerosis. The prevalence of RVF following radiation treatment approaches 6% and fistulas can recur up to 2 years after treatment [13]. Again, diverting colostomy may be necessary to ensure adequate healing of the RVF repair before reanastomosis is attempted.

Fistulas due to malignant invasion are usually associated with a local rectal mass [14]. En bloc resection of the involved segment, in addition to lymph node dissection and appropriate adjunctive therapy, are typically employed. Subsequent repair of a fistula must ensure that malignant transformation of the tissue surrounding the fistula is not involved, and submission of the excised fistulous tract is recommended as a biopsy of the fistula periphery. EUA—examination under anesthesia.

Management Options for Rectovaginal Fistulas

Symptomatic Relief	Local	Surgical Transposition	Abdominal
Bowel regimen	Fistulotomy	Martius flap	Low anterior resection
Obturator/plug [15]	Vaginal	Bulbocavernosus	Coloanal anastomosis
Fibrin sealant [16]	Transanal	Gracilis muscle	Abdominoperineal resection
Fecal diversion	CARF	Sartorius muscle	Onlay patch anastomosis
	LARF	Gluteus maximus	(Fecal diversion)
	ARS		

Figure 13-5. Management options for the treatment of rectovaginal fistula (RVF). Principles of RVF repair are similar to those of genitourinary fistulas. Wide dissection is recommended to mobilize the tissues at least two times the distance necessary for a closure on no-tension.

The surgeon should avoid two overlapping suture lines to decrease the propensity for persistent fistulization. Any active infection should be drained and treated before attempts at closure are made. Most importantly, the interposition of a well-vascularized tissue pedicle should be made a high priority, especially if a large or complex fistula is encountered. Therapeutic options for RVF are listed in Figure 13-6. ARS—advancement rectal sleeve; CARF—curvilinear advancement rectal flap; LARF—linear advancement rectal flap.

Principles of Rectovaginal Fistula Repair

Excision of fistula tract	Prevent re-epithelialization
Interposition of healthy, well-vascularized tissue	Interrupt fistula tract integrity
No inflammation or infection	Maximize healing potential
Wide dissection, mobilization	Close defect without tension
Do not overlap suture lines	Minimize persistence/recurrence
Anal sphincter defects also repaired	Optimize results/patient satisfaction [17]
Tailor treatments to fistula	Approach, need for diversion [8]

Figure 13-6. Principles of rectovaginal fistula repair.

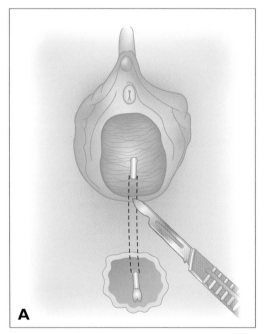

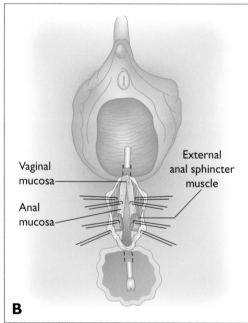

Vaginal mucosa
External anal sphincter muscle
Anal mucosa

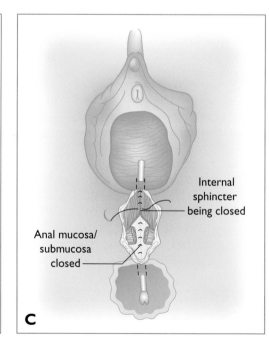

Internal sphincter being closed
Anal mucosa/submucosa closed

A   **B**   **C**

Figure 13-7. Perineoproctotomy. **A,** Surgical correction of low rectovaginal fistula (RVF) can often be performed in one of two ways: distal fistulotomy, with or without a seton (analogous to the Spence procedure), or by laying the tract open and causing an intentional proctoepisiotomy. Often, the former is not chosen because it creates a disruption of the anal sphincter muscles, which is not acceptable to the physician or patient. However, in conjunction with a known disruption, the latter allows excision of the fistulous tract and exposes the sphincter muscles to allow an overlapping repair. Surgical success rates range from 87.5% to 100% [2].

Continued on the next page

Figure 13-7. *(Continued)* As with most anorectal repairs, due to enteric bacteria present in and around the anus despite antibiotic and mechanical bowel preparation, postoperative infection is of concern. Broad-spectrum prophylactic coverage for gram-negative *Enterococcus* and *Bacteroides* organisms should be used. No study has revealed any treatment benefit for continuing antibiotics for more than 24 hours after surgery, unless gross contamination occurs or clinical evidence of infection arises. In the lithotomy position, the patient is prepared, draped, and placed in Trendelenburg position. The fistulous tract is probed to confirm its direction, its number of ostia, and any blind tracts. A lacrimal duct probe or small dilator or probe can be used for this effect. **B,** Utilizing a number 10- or 11-blade scalpel, the intervening skin, perineal musculature, anal sphincter scar, and rectal mucosa are incised and filleted open, creating a proctoepisiotomy. Care is taken to dissect out the epithelial tract and pass this off the field. **C,** The defect is then repaired in multiple layers. Performance of a perineoplasty and an overlapping anal sphincteroplasty *(see* Chapter 8) completes the repair, if necessary. These last steps are particularly important, because persistent anal incontinence after fistula repair affects the risk of the fistula repair breaking down or becoming infected, the patient's perception of the resolution of symptoms, and patient satisfaction [15].

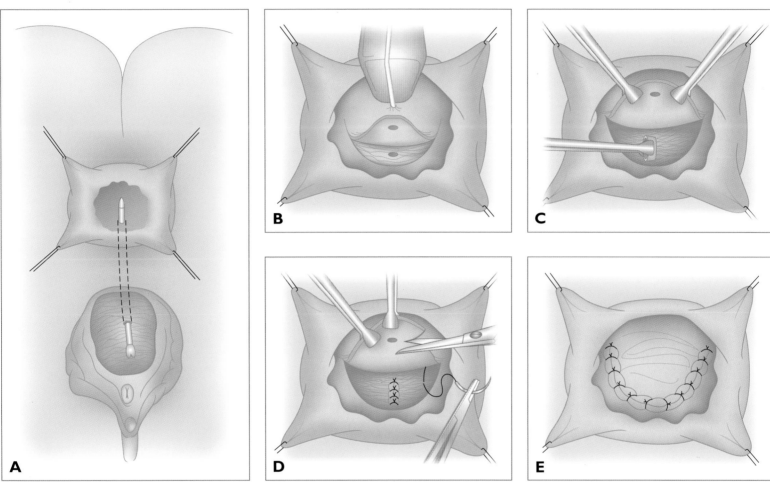

Figure 13-8. Advancement rectal flap repair. Midlevel rectovaginal fistulas (RVFs) are typically repaired by a traditional layered closure or a sliding-wall advancement flap. Closures can be done transvaginally or transanally. **A,** For a transvaginal advancement-flap repair, a longitudinal or transverse/curvilinear elliptical incision is made around the fistulous tract. **B,** The surrounding anal mucosa is elevated off the underlying muscle fascia layer for several centimeters. **C–E,** The rectal mucosa, rectal muscle, rectovaginal septum, and vaginal epithelium are closed, in succession, in this order. Success rates range from 84% to 100%.

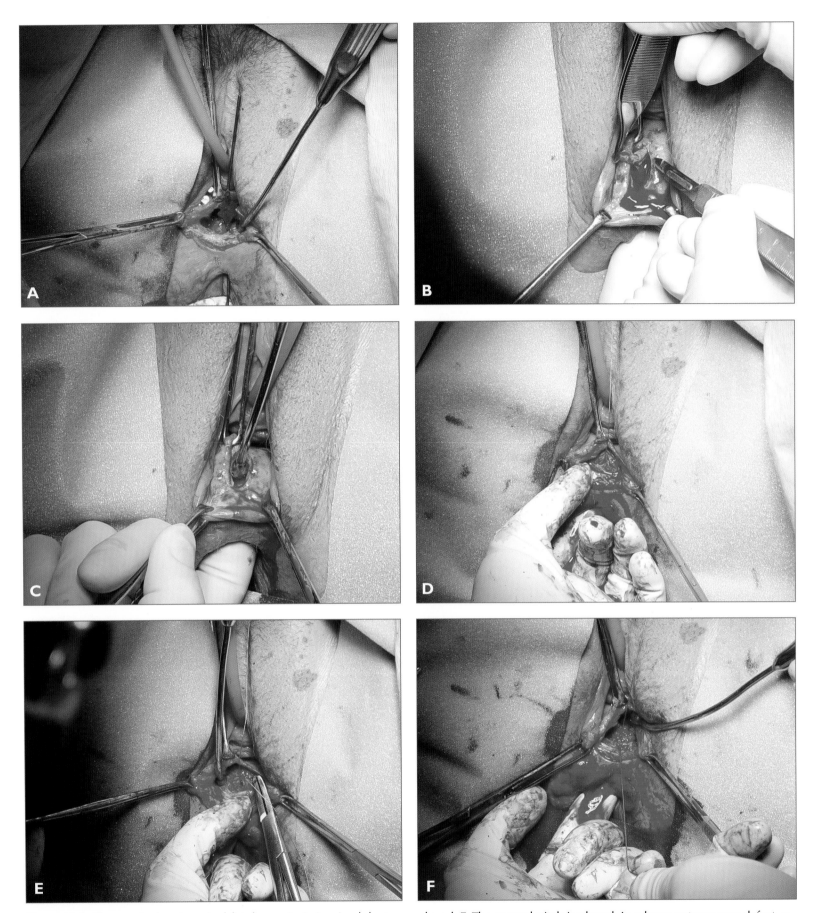

Figure 13-9. Transvaginal rectovaginal fistula repair. **A**, Lacrimal duct probe delineates the fistulous tract. **B**, The fistulous tract is circumscribed, then dissected out. **C**, With the tract excised, the surgeon's gloved finger can be seen. **D**, The apical stitch in the fistula defect is placed. **E**, The second stitch is placed. In a large or transverse defect, a transverse repair will help prevent constriction or stenosis of the rectum in this area. **F**, With the fistula closed, the vaginal epithelium should be closed in the opposite direction to prevent overlapping of suture lines.

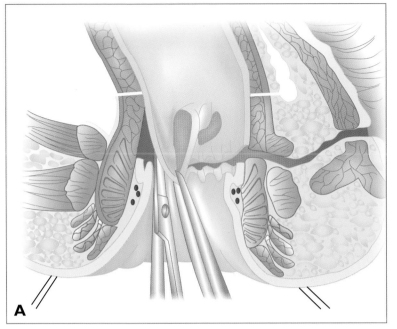

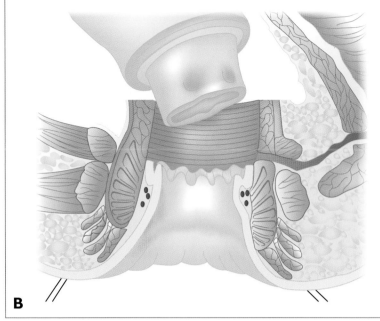

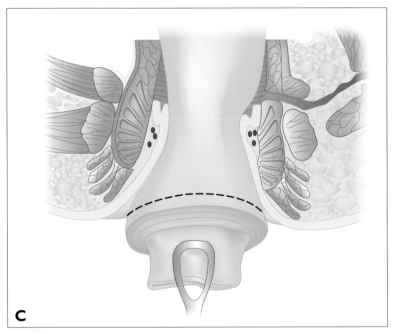

Figure 13-10. Advancement of the rectal sleeve. Distal rectovaginal fistulas (RVFs) can be closed in much the same way as transvaginal fistulas, with attention to the integrity of the anal sphincter musculature. **A,** Another option is the advancement of the rectal sleeve, which has been described for use in patients with Crohn disease, but with a disease-free rectum [9]. Material in a fistula flows downstream from an area of high pressure (the anorectum) to an area of relative low pressure (atmospheric pressure); therefore, full excision of the fistulous tract is not a necessity. **B,** The anal mucosa is circumcised just above the dentate line, then clamped to prevent any gross spillage. The mucosa is undermined for several centimeters and then the rectal muscularis is also circumcised. **C,** The now disease-free

rectum is drawn out through the anus, where the diseased segment can be excised and then re-attached to the healthy distal rectum segment just above the dentate line.

Novel closures have been attempted with varying success. Although some anecdotal reports of the closure of small RVFs with fibrin glue or sealant have been reported, large-scale good-quality studies have not been performed [16]. For patients who are poor surgical candidates but require symptomatic treatment, another physician group has developed an obturator or plug to temporarily deal with RVF symptoms [17].

Postoperative management includes optimization of stool consistency to avoid excessive straining at defecation. In the past, many physicians recommended a "low-residue" diet with little fiber, to keep the bowel at rest for as long as possible. However, the larger, softer stools afforded by fiber supplementation return the postoperative patient to normal defecation earlier with minimal straining required. Regularity may require any combination of twice- or thrice-daily stool softeners, fiber supplementation, lubricants (such as mineral oil), mild stimulants, or even careful enemas. Once a normal stooling routine is developed, treatment can be weaned to the least bothersome dose that still ensures stooling regularity.

The most common postoperative presenting symptom of an infectious complication is an increase in pain, followed by a foul discharge or fever. Excessive straining can lead to suture pull-through or dehiscence. Vaginal or anal intercourse should be discouraged until wound healing is complete. Perianal and ischioanal fossa ecchymosis are not uncommon. If hemostasis is not meticulous before closure, then a subcutaneous drain through a separate stab wound should be considered. Bowel stimulants should be avoided if a bowel obstruction has not been ruled out. Suspicion and anticipation are the keys to treating postoperative complications associated with rectovaginal fistula repair.

REFERENCES

1. Tsang CBS, Rothenberger DA: Rectovaginal fistulas: therapeutic options. *Surg Clin North Am* 1997, 77:95–114.

2. Venkatesh KS, Ramanujam PS, Larson DM, Haywood MA: Anorectal complications of vaginal delivery. *Dis Colon Rectum* 1989, 32:1039–1041.

3. Lescher TC, Pratt JH: Vaginal repair of the simple rectovaginal fistula. *Surg Gynecol Obstet* 1967, 124:1317–1321.

4. Bandy LC, Addison A, Parker RT: Surgical management of rectovaginal fistulas in Crohn's disease. *Am J Obstet Gynecol* 1983, 147:359–363.

5. Lowry AC, Thorson AG, Rothenberger DA, Goldberg SM: Repair of simple recto-vaginal fistulas: influence of previous repairs. *Dis Colon Rectum* 1988, 31:676–678.

6. Senagore A: Rectovaginal fistula. In *Surgery of the Colon, Rectum, and Anus*. Edited by Mazier WP, Levien DH, Luchtefeld MA, Senagore AJ. Philadelphia: WB Saunders; 1995:279–289.

7. Poen AC, Felt-Bersma RJF, Eijsbouts AJ, *et al.*: Hydrogen peroxide-enhanced transanal ultrasound in the assessment of fistula-in-ano. *Dis Colon Rectum* 1998, 41:1147–1152.

8. Fazio VW, Wu JS: Surgical therapy for Crohn's disease of the colon and rectum. *Surg Clin North Am* 1997, 77:197–209.

9. Brand MI, Saclarides TJ: Rectovaginal fistula. In *Atlas of Clinical Gynecology: Urogynecology and Reconstructive Surgery*. Edited by Stenchever MA, Benson JT. Philadelphia: Current Medicine; 2000:11.1–11.13.

10. Gilliland R, Wexner SD: Complicated anorectal sepsis. *Surg Clin North Am* 1997, 77:115–153.

11. Sands BE: New therapies for the treatment of inflammatory bowel disease. *Surg Clin North Am* 2006, 86:1045–1064.

12. Saclarides TJ: Radiation injuries of the gastrointestinal tract. *Surg Clin North Am* 1997, 77:261–268.

13. Rafferty JF: Rectovaginal fistula. In *Urogynecology and Reconstructive Pelvic Surgery*, edn 2. Edited by Walters MD, Karram MM. St. Louis: Mosby; 1999:277–283.

14. Turnbull RB, Cuthbertson A: Abdominorectal pull-through resection for cancer and for Hirshsprung's disease: delayed posterior colorectal anastamosis. *Cleve Clin Q* 1961, 28:109–115.

15. Lee BH, Choe DH, Le JH, *et al.*: Device for occlusion of rectovaginal fistula: clinical trials. *Radiology* 1997, 203:65–69.

16. Singer M, Cintron J: New techniques in the treatment of common perianal diseases: stapled hemorrhoidopexy, Botulinum toxin, and fibrin sealant. *Surg Clin North Am* 2006, 86:937–967.\

17. Tsang CB, Madoff RD, Wong WD, *et al.*: Anal sphincter integrity and function influences outcome in rectovaginal fistula repair. *Dis Colon Rectum* 1998, 41:1141–1146.

14

Injuries to the Genitourinary Tract: Prevention, Recognition, and Management

Walter S. von Pechmann and Sarah E. Camp

In women, the close embryologic and anatomic relationship between the reproductive and lower urinary tracts predisposes the lower urinary tract to involvement in gynecologic disease processes and places it at risk during pelvic surgery. Accordingly, the majority of surgical injuries to the lower urinary tract occur as a result of gynecologic surgery. The gynecologic procedures most commonly associated with lower urinary tract injury are abdominal and vaginal hysterectomies performed for the treatment of benign disease. The incidence of lower urinary tract injury at the time of major gynecologic surgery is 0.5% to 2.5%. Procedures performed for the treatment of incontinence or pelvic organ prolapse increase the risk of injury, as do hysterectomies performed for obstetric indications [1,2].

Of concern is the fact that the majority of these injuries are not recognized at the time of surgery. For instance, only 12.5% of ureteral injuries and 35.3% of bladder injuries are detected before cystoscopy. When these injuries are recognized and appropriately managed, postoperative morbidity is significantly reduced. Therefore, emphasis must be placed on the prevention, recognition, and management of lower urinary tract injuries that are associated with gynecologic surgery [3–6].

Preoperatively, the history and physical examination, urinalysis, urine culture, and blood chemistries may offer important information about the condition of the urinary tract and its involvement by pathologic conditions. Although routine preoperative urinary tract imaging has not been shown to reduce injury rates, intravenous or CT urograms are sometimes helpful in detecting congenital anomalies of the urinary tract and in documenting involvement by pelvic tumors, pelvic inflammatory disease, or invasive processes such as endometriosis or cancer [7]. Ureteral catheters may be used to assist in the identification and dissection of the ureters, but their need cannot always be predicted and their use can contribute to ureteral injury. For these reasons, many surgeons prefer to insert ureteral catheters when they are needed intraoperatively rather than preoperatively.

Intraoperatively, certain safety principles apply routinely. When surgery is performed within the peritoneal cavity, it is important that the anatomy be restored and the course of the ureters be identified. In dissecting retroperitoneally, the attachment of the ureters to the pelvic peritoneum should be preserved and the adventitial blood supply to the ureters should not be damaged. Most ureteral injuries that are the result of gynecologic surgery occur in the distal 4 to 5 cm; the types of injury vary and injuries are sometimes difficult to recognize. When ureteral injury is suspected, several procedures can be used to determine the location and extent of the injury. Bladder injuries are also more likely to occur in certain locations depending on the procedure type. For example, bladder injuries incurred during hysterectomy or anterior colporrhaphy are typically located in the bladder base whereas injuries that occur during incontinence surgery are usually located in the dome of the bladder. Cystoscopy should be performed immediately upon development of hematuria or pneumaturia and should be performed routinely during surgery for incontinence or pelvic organ prolapse [8].

Postoperatively, unrecognized lower urinary tract injuries or unsuccessful repairs should be considered when oliguria or anuria, fever, chills, or flank pain develops. Intraperitoneal or retroperitoneal leakage of urine may cause abdominal distention, ileus, and urinoma formation. Ultimately, a urinary fistula may develop or there may be ureteral obstruction with loss of renal function. Surgical injuries to the lower urinary tract that are recognized within days of surgery should be repaired immediately if the patient's condition permits. The timing of the repair of injuries that are diagnosed later in the postoperative period or are discovered in patients whose physical condition will not permit surgery must be individualized [9]. During the waiting period, urinary leakage may be managed with retrograde placement of ureteral catheters or by percutaneous nephrostomy catheter placement; bladder drainage, either transurethral or suprapubic; and, in the case of genitourinary fistulas, also by vaginal drainage devices.

PREVENTION

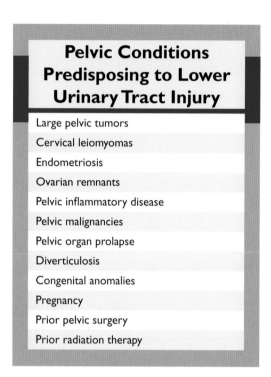

Pelvic Conditions Predisposing to Lower Urinary Tract Injury

Large pelvic tumors

Cervical leiomyomas

Endometriosis

Ovarian remnants

Pelvic inflammatory disease

Pelvic malignancies

Pelvic organ prolapse

Diverticulosis

Congenital anomalies

Pregnancy

Prior pelvic surgery

Prior radiation therapy

Figure 14-1. Pelvic conditions that predispose to lower urinary tract injury. Although these findings may predispose some patients to surgical injury of the lower urinary tract, most injuries occur at the time of hysterectomy performed for a benign condition in which none of them is a complicating factor. Injury is more likely to occur with abdominal hysterectomy than with vaginal hysterectomy. Most lower urinary tract injuries are not recognized at the time of surgery [3].

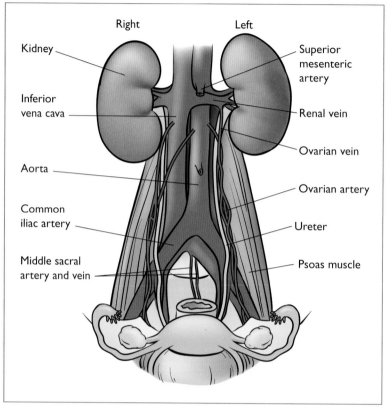

Figure 14-2. The upper pole of each kidney lies at the level of T12 and the lower pole at the level of L3; the right kidney is usually slightly lower than the left. The renal arteries arise from the aorta at right angles between L1 and L2.

The ureters originate from the renal pelvis at the level of L1 and descend 25 to 30 cm before entering the bladder. The abdominal ureters descend along the anterior surface of the psoas muscles, posterior to the ovarian vessels to the pelvic brim. The right ureter lies laterally to the inferior vena cava; the left ureter lies laterally to the aorta and passes beneath the inferior mesenteric artery, ovarian vessels, and colon. After passing over the bifurcations of the common iliac arteries, the pelvic ureters descend along the pelvic sidewalls, coursing laterally to the uterosacral ligaments. Each ureter then passes under the uterine arteries after which they pass through the cardinal ligaments, then medially and anteriorly over the lateral vaginal fornices to enter the bladder.

The ureters become more vulnerable to injury as they descend further into the pelvis due to their increasing proximity to the reproductive tract. For instance, the average distance from the ureter to uterosacral ligament is 2.3 cm at the level of the ischial spine but only 0.9 cm where the ligament meets the cervix [10]. Although the average distance between the ureter and the cervix is 2.3 cm, in 12% of women the distance is less than 0.5 cm [11].

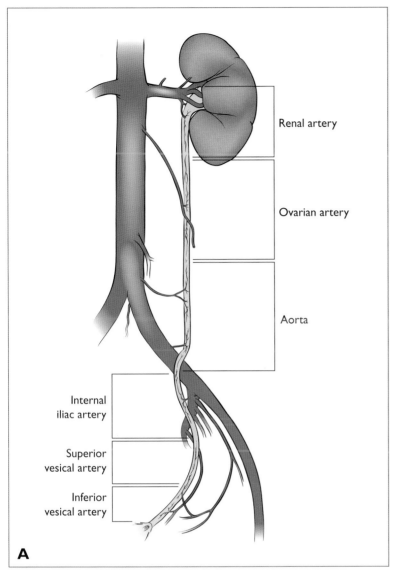

Renal artery

Ovarian artery

Aorta

Internal
iliac artery

Superior
vesical artery

Inferior
vesical artery

A

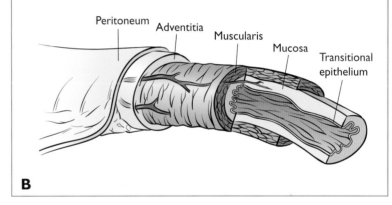

Peritoneum   Adventitia   Muscularis   Mucosa   Transitional epithelium

B

Figure 14-3. Blood supply to and anatomy of the ureter. **A,** The blood supply to the ureters is unpredictable. Normally, in their course from the kidneys to the bladder, the ureters receive ureteral branches from the renal arteries, ovarian arteries, aorta, internal iliac arteries, and the superior and inferior vesical arteries. The veins fol-low the correspondingly named arteries and terminate in the correspondingly named veins. **B,** The wall of each ureter is comprised of three layers: mucosa, muscularis, and adventitia. Their major blood supply forms a rich anastomotic network within the adventitia and gives small branches to the inner muscularis and mucosa.

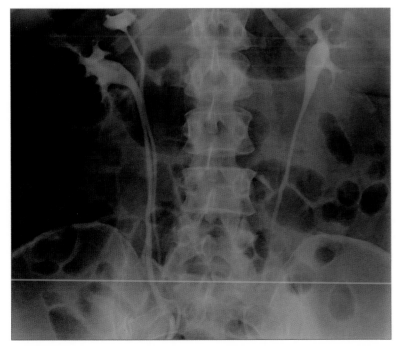

Figure 14-4. Preoperative imaging studies. In patients with genitourinary anomalies or prior urinary tract surgery, preoperative imaging studies can provide information that may help to prevent urinary tract injury during surgery. For example, this intravenous pyelogram was obtained from a patient who thought she had undergone a left nephrectomy as a child due to infectious complications. This study revealed that only the upper pole of the left kidney was removed and that bilateral kidney function was preserved. Additionally, there was the unexpected finding of complete right ureteral duplication.

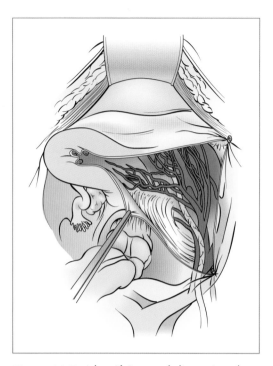

Figure 14-5. Identifying and dissecting the course of the ureters during abdominal procedures. The best method of preventing ureteral injury is to demonstrate the course of each ureter at the time of laparotomy or laparoscopy and then to keep them out of harm's way. The pelvic ureters are most easily identified as they enter the pelvis by passing over the bifurcations of the common iliac arteries. An alternative method of identification is to locate the external iliac arteries and to follow them toward their corresponding common iliac artery; the first structure crossing the external iliac artery will be the ureter [12]. The ureter is best identified by direct visualization of its characteristic peristalsis. During palpation, when the ureter is allowed to pass between the index finger and thumb, it will sometimes provide an audible "click" and impart a snapping sensation to the palpating fingers. On occasion, both of these findings may be rendered by palpating pelvic vessels or some other structure, making this a less reliable way of positively identifying the ureters. When dissecting the ureters, it is important to preserve their attachment to the overlying peritoneum and to perform the dissection outside of their adventitial sheaths to avoid injuring their blood supply. Routine dissections of each ureter usually do not go much below the level of the uterine arteries. Circumstances may require dissection of the distal ureter.

Surgical Principles for Protection of Pelvic Organs

Before surgical entry

Bowel preparation

Positioning in universal stirrups

Draping for abdominal and vaginal access

Bladder drainage

Examination under anesthesia

After surgical entry

Adequate exposure of surgical field

Adequate light within surgical field

Adequate suction for surgical field

Restoration of anatomic relationships

Traction and countertraction to exposure adjacent structures

Dissection of extraperitoneal "spaces"

Dissection along tissue planes

Maintaining hemostasis

Clamping, cutting, and suturing under direct vision

Avoidance of mass ligation of tissues

Restrictive use of electrocautery

Figure 14-6. Surgical principles for protection of pelvic organs. These principles are helpful in preventing injury to the lower urinary tract and bowel. When a difficult pelvic dissection is anticipated, the bowel should be prepared beginning 24 to 48 hours before surgery by prescribing a liquid diet, an oral bowel cleansing agent (eg, citrate of magnesia, electrolytes with polyethylene glycol), and enemas. Positioning the patient for surgery in universal stirrups; preparing her abdomen, vulva, vagina, inner thighs; and draping her with a drape that provides abdominal and vaginal access will simplify intraoperative vaginal manipulation and cystoscopy. For most major gynecologic surgery, it is best to provide continuous bladder drainage by inserting a balloon catheter and connecting it to a closed drainage system. This is usually done using a double-lumen catheter; however, if the need for bladder filling can be anticipated, it can be made easier by inserting a triple-lumen catheter and connecting it to a closed drainage system and to a bag containing a suitable sterile irrigating solution.

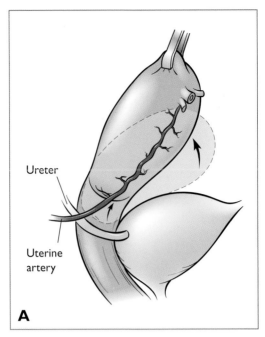

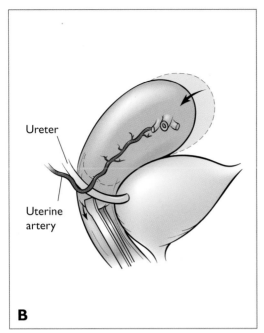

Figure 14-7. Effect of traction on the relationship of the uterus to the ureter. **A,** Upward countertraction on the uterine fundus during an abdominal hysterectomy normally increases the distance between the cervix and ureter at the level of the uterine vessels.

B, Downward traction on the cervix during a vaginal hysterectomy decreases the distance between the cervix and ureter at the level of the uterine vessels. Remembering this is important in preventing ureteral injury.

RECOGNITION OF LOWER URINARY TRACT INJURY

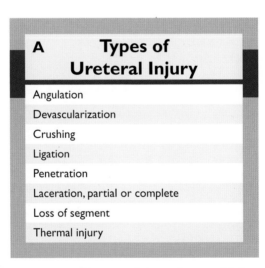

A	Types of Ureteral Injury
Angulation	
Devascularization	
Crushing	
Ligation	
Penetration	
Laceration, partial or complete	
Loss of segment	
Thermal injury	

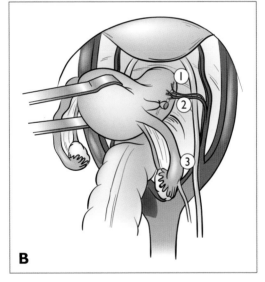

Figure 14-8. Types and sites of ureteral injury. **A,** Ureteral injuries may be direct or indirect. **B,** During gynecologic surgery, the most frequent sites of ureteral injury are at the level of 1) the cardinal ligaments, 2) the uterine vessels, and 3) the infundibulopelvic ligaments.

Methods of Detecting Intraoperative Ureteral Injury
Dissect the course of the ureter
Cystoscopy or cystotomy
Intravenous injection of indigo carmine
Ureteral catheterization
Intravenous urography
Retrograde pyelography

Figure 14-9. Methods of detecting intraoperative ureteral injury. If intraoperative ureteral injury is suspected, one or more of these procedures may be used to prove the condition and function of a ureter.

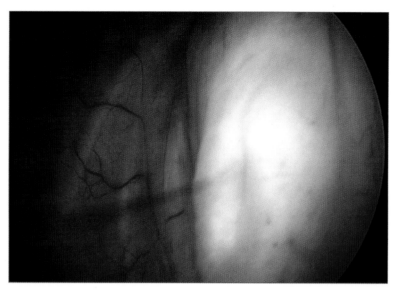

Figure 14-10. Use of cystoscopy to rule out ureteral obstruction. Transurethral cystoscopy is facilitated by placing the patient in low lithotomy using universal stirrups. If urine is not visibly effluxing from both ureteral orifices, intravenously administering 5 mL of indigo carmine renders efflux more readily apparent [13]. If ureteral patency is not confirmed, retrograde ureteral stenting should be attempted. Alternatively, suprapubic cystoscopy, sometimes referred to as telescopy, can be performed during laparotomy. Telescopy is performed by distending the bladder with sterile water or saline, placing a pursestring of absorbable suture around what is to be a puncture site in the extraperitoneal dome of the bladder, puncturing the bladder with a scalpel, and inserting the cystoscope through the bladder dome [14]. After removing the scope, a suprapubic catheter can be placed through the cystotomy if required. The pursestring suture is then tied down to close the cystotomy.

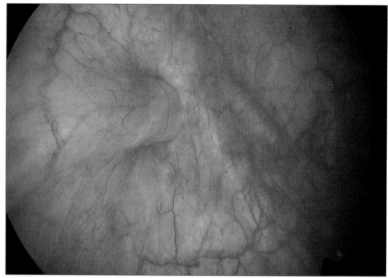

Figure 14-11. Use of cystoscopy to rule out bladder injury. In this case, routine intraoperative cystoscopy revealed an incidental cystotomy due to accidental passage of a trocar through the bladder dome during tension-free suburethral sling placement. Cystoscopy should be performed immediately if intraoperative hematuria develops and should be performed routinely during incontinence surgery. Retrograde filling of the bladder with methylene blue–stained sterile water can also be useful when looking for extravasation into the surgical field.

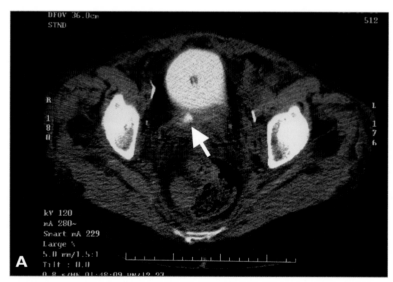

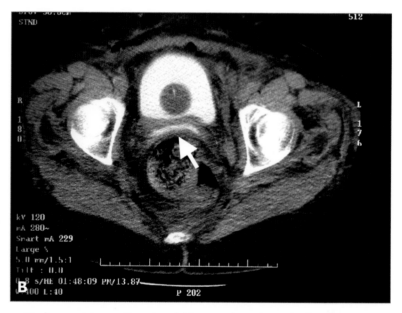

Figure 14-12. Postoperative diagnosis of urinary tract injury. When urinary tract injury is suspected postoperatively, investigative options include tampon testing, cystoscopy, and radiographic procedures such as intravenous pyelograms, cystograms, or CT urograms. Tampon testing is performed by placing a tampon in the vagina, followed by retrograde filling of the bladder with methylene blue–stained water. Staining of the innermost portion of the tampon confirms the presence of a vesicovaginal fistula. Alternatively, oral medications such as phenazopyridine or intravenous medications such as indigo carmine can be used to color the urine and will reveal fistulas from either the ureter or bladder. Staining of the tampon with oral or intravenous administration but not retrograde bladder filling is highly suggestive of a ureterovaginal fistula.

Radiographic studies should be employed routinely when urinary tract injury is suspected postoperatively. Imaging studies can be diagnostic in cases in which other measures are either not definitive or not feasible. Additionally, even when tampon testing or cystoscopy has confirmed a bladder injury such as a vesicovaginal fistula, upper tract imaging should be obtained to rule out ureteral involvement.

A, This CT urogram was obtained 3 days after total abdominal hysterectomy when the patient began complaining of leakage per vagina. Note the contrast-filled tract beneath the bladder base (*arrow*). **B,** This image from the same patient shows pooling of contrast within the vagina (*arrow*), confirming the presence of a vesicovaginal fistula.

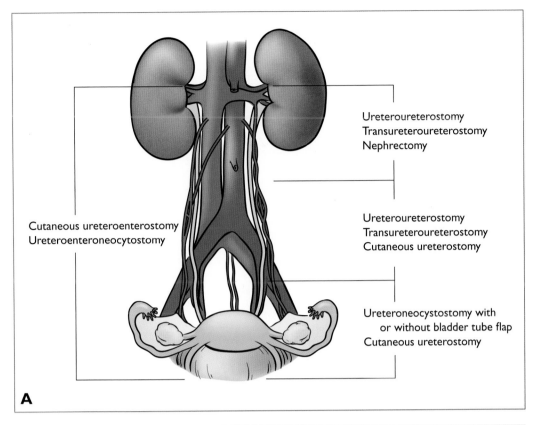

Ureteroureterostomy
Transureteroureterostomy
Nephrectomy

Cutaneous ureteroenterostomy
Ureteroenteroneocytostomy

Ureteroureterostomy
Transureteroureterostomy
Cutaneous ureterostomy

Ureteroneocystostomy with
or without bladder tube flap
Cutaneous ureterostomy

A

B   Principles for Successful Ureteral Repair

Perform meticulous ureteral dissection using atraumatic instruments.

Preserve ureteral blood supply by leaving peritoneal attachments and dissecting outside the adventitial sheath.

Perform a tension-free anastomosis.

Use a minimal amount of the smallest absorbable suture that is needed to obtain watertight anastomosis.

Surround anastomosis with retroperitoneal fat or omentum to assist healing.

Drain the retroperitoneal anastomotic site to prevent the accumulation of urine.

Consider proximal urinary diversion, with or without stenting.

Figure 14-13. Surgical procedures and principles for the repair of ureteral injuries. **A,** The selection of a reparative procedure depends on the location and extent of the injury [4]. Other factors that must be considered are the cause of injury, condition of the tissues, renal function, patient prognosis, and experience of the surgeon.

In cases of suspected ureteral obstruction, retrograde passage of ureteral stents should be attempted via cystoscopy or cystotomy. In the event of ureteral ligation, careful ureterolysis will sometimes allow relief from the obstruction. Ureteral stents can then be left in place temporarily to prevent edematous obstruction or fibrosis from developing in the early postoperative period. When ureterolysis does not relieve the obstruction or when more significant injuries such as ureteral transection occur within the distal 5 cm, ureteroneocystostomy is the preferred method of repair. Ureteroureterostomy is the preferred procedure for more proximal injuries. Procedures such as transureteroureterostomy, ureteroenteroneocystostomy, and cutaneous ureterostomy are rarely required for iatrogenic injuries. When the diagnosis of ureteral injury is made more than 72 hours postoperatively, urinary diversion with percutaneous nephrostomy will frequently be employed to allow edema to subside before returning for surgical repair. **B,** The principles for successful repair are listed [15].

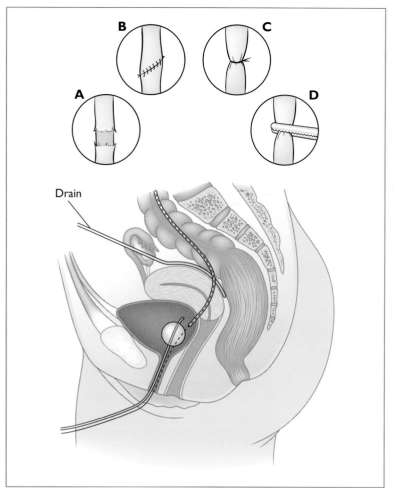

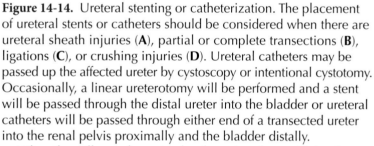

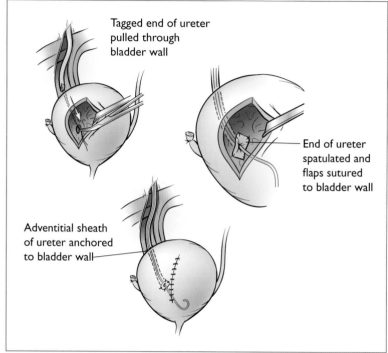

Figure 14-14. Ureteral stenting or catheterization. The placement of ureteral stents or catheters should be considered when there are ureteral sheath injuries (**A**), partial or complete transections (**B**), ligations (**C**), or crushing injuries (**D**). Ureteral catheters may be passed up the affected ureter by cystoscopy or intentional cystotomy. Occasionally, a linear ureterotomy will be performed and a stent will be passed through the distal ureter into the bladder or ureteral catheters will be passed through either end of a transected ureter into the renal pelvis proximally and the bladder distally.

When the stiffness of a ureteral catheter interferes with its placement, a small silicone pediatric feeding (5-F) tube may be substituted. If this is done, it is important to know the location of openings within the end of the tube and to confirm that it is placed at a location within the upper renal tract, which will ensure the drainage of urine.

When linear stents or catheters are left in place for urine drainage, they may be brought out of the body alongside a transurethral or suprapubic catheter. The urethral stent or catheter should be anchored to the transurethral or suprapubic catheter to maintain its position within the urinary tract. Urethral and bladder catheters will require separate closed-drainage urine collection systems. A ureteral catheter will rarely be brought out directly through the skin as a temporary method of urinary drainage.

Sometimes it is helpful to have ureteral catheters or stents placed to help identify the course of one or both ureters during surgery. This may be done preoperatively or intraoperatively by cystoscopy or cystotomy. Ureteral catheterization is not without hazard: the placement of ureteral stents or catheters may cause ureteral injury resulting in hematuria, edema, and perforation. Surgeons who dissect ureters containing stents or catheters should be aware that the catheters or stents may impart a stiffness to the ureter, which may predispose it to injury.

Figure 14-15. Abdominal ureteroneocystostomy. This procedure is recommended for injuries to the distal 5 cm of the ureter. The pelvic ureter is meticulously dissected to prevent damage to its adventitial sheath and blood supply. The distal end of the ureter is ligated with a permanent suture at the ureterovesical junction. Any damaged ureteral segment is excised. A 3-0 suture is used to tag the proximal ureter approximately 0.5 cm from its end.

An extraperitoneal cystotomy is created in the dome of the bladder and the ureteral orifices are identified. A finger is placed inside the fundus of the bladder, which is displaced toward the cut end of the ureter to determine the best site for a tension-free reimplantation. The entire thickness of the bladder wall is perforated with a right-angle clamp from within the bladder at the site selected for reimplantation and the perforation is opened approximately 1 cm in diameter to allow passage of the tagged end of the proximal ureter. The end of the ureter is drawn into the bladder for a distance of 1 cm and then the end of the ureter is spatulated approximately 0.5 cm on the opposite sides of its circumference. The tagging suture is removed and then four 3-0 absorbable sutures are placed to secure the distal ureteral flaps to the inside of the bladder wall. Several 3-0 delayed-absorbable sutures are used to anchor the adventitial sheath of the ureter to the outside of the bladder wall. A ureteral catheter is placed to prevent obstruction from edema and then the cystotomy is closed.

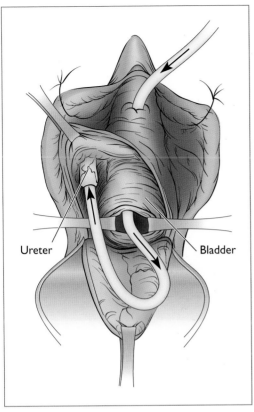

Figure 14-16. Vaginal ureteroneocystostomy. This technique may be used for injuries of the terminal 3 cm of either ureter [16]. The distal end of the ureter is identified and ligated with a permanent suture at the ureterovesical junction. The proximal end of the ureter is identified, trimmed, mobilized, spatulated bilaterally for a distance of approximately 0.5 cm, and catheterized. The catheter is passed through a cystotomy incision and brought out of the urethra. The spatulated end of the ureter is drawn into the bladder through a cystotomy and is sewn to the inside of the bladder with two 4-0 absorbable sutures. The adventitial sheath is anchored to the external surface of the base of the bladder with two or three 3-0 interrupted delayed-absorbable sutures.

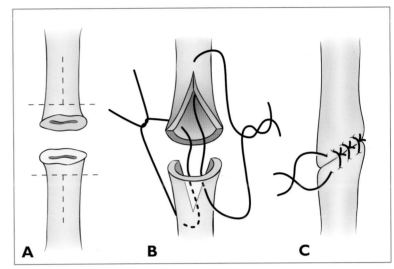

Figure 14-17. Ureteroureterostomy. This technique is recommended for significant ureteral injuries above and just below the pelvic brim. In performing an end-to-end anastomosis of a ureter, trim the cut ends to healthy tissue (**A**), spatulate both ends to allow an oblique anastomosis and reduce the incidence of stenosis (**B**), and approximate the ends over a properly placed ureteral catheter using interrupted 4-0 chromic catgut or delayed-absorbable suture (**C**). The anastomosis should be watertight, but not ischemic. The anastomotic site should be drained by an extraperitoneal suction drain. The end of the drain should be adjacent to but not in contact with the ureteral anastomosis.

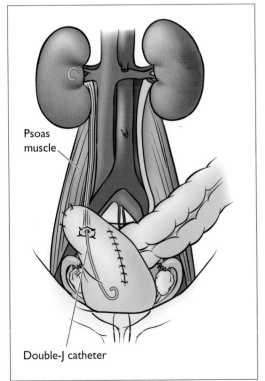

Figure 14-18. Vesicopsoas hitch. A vesicopsoas hitch is recommended when performing a ureteroneocystotomy or ureteroureterostomy to ensure a tension-free ureteral anastomosis. The upward mobility of the bladder may be increased by freeing the dome of the bladder from its loose attachments to the retrosymphysis. The vesicopsoas hitch is performed by placing one or two fingers through an anterior extraperitoneal cystotomy in the dome of the bladder and displacing the bladder toward the end of the damaged ureter. The leading point of the outer wall and muscular layer of the bladder is sutured to the psoas major fascia with several interrupted 2-0 or 1-0 delayed-absorbable sutures.

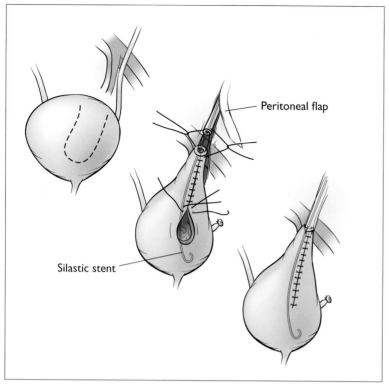

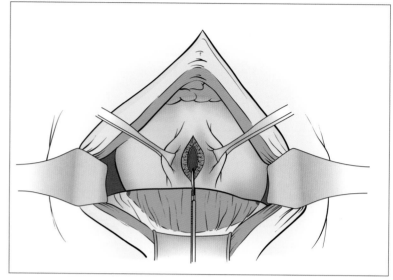

Figure 14-19. Boari–Ockerblad bladder flap. A Boari–Ockerblad bladder flap is used to extend the bladder a greater distance toward a shortened ureter than is possible by using a vesicopsoas hitch [17]. The bladder is mobilized by freeing its attachments to the retrosymphysis. A vesicopsoas hitch is performed on the side in which the ureter is to be reimplanted. A full-thickness, wide-based bladder flap is cut out of the anterior bladder wall. The distal ureter is reimplanted directly or by way of a submucosal tunnel into the upper end of the bladder flap with 4-0 interrupted absorbable or delayed-absorbable sutures. The cut edges of the flap are approximated with one layer of interrupted 4-0 or 3-0 absorbable or delayed-absorbable sutures.

Figure 14-20. Cystotomy. A cystotomy for inspection of the bladder, ureteral catheterization, or ureteroneocystostomy is best performed in the extraperitoneal portion of the dome of the bladder. A cystotomy for the repair of a genitourinary fistula may have to be placed through the portion of the bladder that is covered by peritoneum. Cystotomies should be closed in two layers with absorbable or delayed-absorbable suture. It is helpful to cover transperitoneal cystotomies and those in the base of the bladder with an intact layer of peritoneum or a flap of omentum. A suprapubic or transurethral catheter should be placed for postoperative bladder drainage.

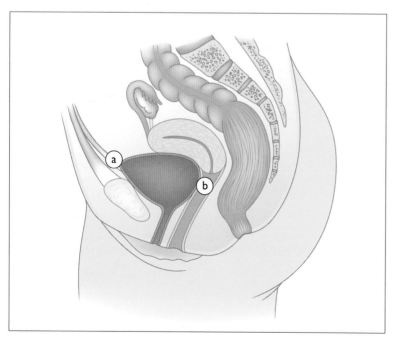

Figure 14-21. Frequent sites of bladder injury. The dome of the bladder (a) is the most frequent site of injury, usually at the time of entry into the abdomen or during incontinence operations. The base of the bladder (b) is subject to injury when separating the bladder from the cervix during abdominal or vaginal hysterectomy and when clamping and suturing the vaginal cuff.

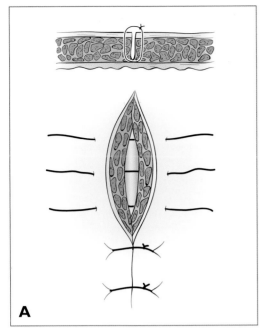
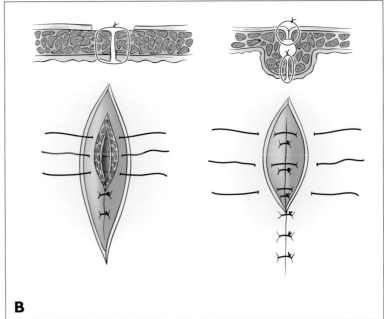

Figure 14-22. Management of bladder injuries. The need for surgical repair depends on the size, nature, and location of the injury. If recognized intraoperatively, injuries to the bladder dome incurred during tension-free suburethral sling placement are typically so small that they require nothing more than 24 to 48 hours of continuous bladder drainage once the sling arm has been removed and replaced outside the bladder. In general, repairs to the bladder dome are simpler and less prone to failure than injuries to the bladder base. After repairs to the bladder base, continuous drainage is typically performed for 7 to 14 days due to the risk of vesicovaginal fistula formation if catheters are removed prematurely. A cystogram can be obtained if necessary to confirm bladder integrity prior to catheter removal. In most cases, bladder injuries incurred during vaginal surgery are best repaired vaginally and those sustained during laparotomy or laparoscopy are best repaired abdominally.

A, Partial-thickness injuries are repaired by placing a single layer of 3-0 absorbable sutures through the muscular and serosal layers. **B,** Full-thickness injuries are repaired in two layers with the first layer incorporating the muscular and mucosal layers of the bladder wall and the second layer imbricating the deeper layer by the placement of Lembert sutures through the serosal and muscular layers of the bladder.

Postoperative Urinary Drainage

Ureteral catheter

Ureteral damage may require 5–7 d of urinary diversion with an excretory urogram and possible cystogram prior to catheter removal.

Ureteral transections or resections may require 6–8 wk of urinary diversion with an excretory urogram and possible cystogram before catheter removal.

Bladder catheter

Period of continuous catheter drainage must be individualized.

Consider transurethral catheters for < 24–48 h of continuous drainage.

Consider suprapubic catheters for > 24–48 h of continuous drainage or when there is risk of postoperative voiding dysfunction.

Intermittent clean self-catheterization may be used instead of continuous drainage as a means of bladder drainage.

Figure 14-23. Postoperative urinary drainage. Ureteral catheters should be positioned to drain urine from the renal pelvis into the bladder or out of the body. Double-J catheters will maintain their position as a result of their coiled tips. Straight catheters must be anchored to a bladder-drainage catheter or to the skin to prevent dislodgement.

The bladder can be drained with either transurethral or suprapubic catheters. Balloon transurethral catheters of 14 or 16 Fr are usually adequate. Percutaneously placed suprapubic catheters are typically 12 Fr except in rare instances where the catheter is placed for long-term use, in which case larger-caliber catheters should be selected. When hematuria is present, temporary dual drainage with both transurethral and suprapubic catheters can be performed to minimize the risk of blood clots obstructing catheter flow.

References

1. Vakili B, Chesson RR, Kyle BL, et al.: The incidence of urinary tract injury during hysterectomy: a prospective analysis based on universal cystoscopy. Am J Obstet Gynecol 2005, 192:1599–1604.

2. Carley ME, McIntire D, Carley JM, Schaffer J: Incidence, risk factors, and morbidity of unintended bladder or ureter injury during hysterectomy. Int Urogynecol J Pelvic Floor Dysfunct 2002, 13:18–21.

3. Symmonds RE: Ureteral injuries associated with gynecologic surgery: prevention and management. Clin Obstet Gynecol 1976, 19:623–643.

4. Hurt WG, Segreti EM: Intraoperative ureteral injuries and urinary diversion. In Gynecologic and Obstetric Surgery, edn 2. Edited by Nichols DH, Clarke-Pearson D. St. Louis: Mosby; 1999.

5. Goodno JA Jr, Powers TW, Harris VD: Ureteral injury in gynecology surgery: a ten-year review in a community hospital. Am J Obstet Gynecol 1995, 172:1817–1822.

6. Saidi MH, Sadler RK, Vancaillie TG, et al.: Diagnosis and management of serious urinary complications after major operative laparoscopy. Obstet Gynecol 1996, 87:272–276.

7. Piscitelli JT, Simel DL, Addison W: Who should have intravenous pyelograms before hysterectomy for benign disease? Obstet Gynecol 1987, 69:541–545.

8. Harris RL, Cundiff GW, Theofrastous JP, et al.: The value of intraoperative cystoscopy in urogynecology and reconstructive pelvic surgery. Am J Obstet Gynecol 1997, 177:1367–1371.

9. Witters S, Cornelissen M, Vereecken R: Iatrogenic ureteral injury: aggressive or conservative treatment. Am J Obstet Gynecol 1986, 155:582–584.=

10. Buller JL, Thompson JR, Cundiff JW, et al.: Uterosacral ligament: description of anatomic relationships to optimize surgical safety. Obstet Gynecol 2001, 97:873–879.

11. Hurd WW, Chee SS, Gallagher KL, et al.: Location of the ureters in relation to the uterine cervix by computed tomography. Am J Obstet Gynecol 2001, 184:336–339.

12. Manetta A: Surgical maneuver for the prevention of ureteral injuries. J Gynecol Surg 1989, 5:291–294.

13. Kwon CH, Goldberg RP, Koduri S, Sand PK: The use of intraoperative cystoscopy in major vaginal and urogynecologic surgeries. Am J Obstet Gynecol 2002, 187:1466–1472.

14. Timmons MC, Addison WA: Suprapubic teloscopy: extraperitoneal intraoperative technique to demonstrate ureteral patency. Obstet Gynecol 1990, 75:137–139.

15. Schlossberg SM: Ureteral healing. Semin Urol 1987, 5:197–199.

16. Thompson JD, Benigno BB: Vaginal repair of ureteral injuries. Am J Obstet Gynecol 1971, 3:601–610.

17. Boari A: Contributo sperimentale alla plastica dell uretere. Atti Acad Sci Med Nat Ferrara 1894, 68:149–157.

A

Acupuncture, 131
Ambiguous external genitalia
  in congenital adrenal hyperplasia, 17
  differential diagnosis of, 15
  in hermaphroditism, 16
  in pseudohermaphroditism, 18
Anal anatomy, 162
Anal incontinence, 67
Anal manometry, 155
Anal reflexes, 49
Anal sphincter
  anatomy of, 7
  artificial, 172
  innervation of, 38
  laceration of, 152
  repair of, 161–170
  ultrasound of, 153
Anatomy
  pelvic, 1–7
Androgen insensitivity syndrome, 18
Antidiarrheal medications, 161
Antimuscarinic drugs, 129–130
Artificial anal sphincter, 172
Autoaugmentation, 65
Autonomic neurons, 29–30
Autonomic testing, 50
Axon terminals
  urethral, 26

B

Behavioral therapy, 112
Bethanechol supersensitivity testing, 50
Bicornuate uterus, 23
Biofeedback, 113–114
Bladder. *See also* Bladder dysfunction
  diverticula of, 143
  neurogenic, 59, 63
  neurophysiology of, 30, 34–36, 54–55
  overactive. *See* Overactive bladder
  surgical injuries in, 260, 263–265
Bladder dysfunction. *See also* Overactive bladder
  autoaugmentation in, 65
  cystoplasty in, 65
  in diabetes, 76
  in multiple sclerosis, 76–78
  neuromodulation in, 63
  pathophysiology of, 53–59
  pharmacotherapy in, 63
  in spinal cord injury, 72–73
  urinary diversion in, 66
  urodynamic evaluation in, 64

Boari-Ockerblad bladder flap, 264
Botulinum toxin, 63, 132–133
Bowel training, 160
Bulking procedures, 120

C

Calculi
  urethral, 232
Catheterization, 61–62
Cauda equina syndrome, 73–74
Cerebrovascular accidents, 70
Cloaca embryology, 10
Colostomy, 172
Colpoperineopexy, 209–212
Colporrhaphy
  complications of, 183
  for pelvic organ prolapse, 204–216, 218–227
Computed tomography urography, 260
Congenital adrenal hyperplasia, 17
Congenital genitourinary anomalies, 9–24, 257
  See also specific anomalies
Constipation
  causes of, 150
  evaluation of, 156–157
  overview of, 149, 159
  treatment of, 159, 170–171
Continence tampons, 115
Conus medullaris syndrome, 73–74
Cough profile, 100
Crohn's disease, 152
Cube pessary, 198–199
Cystitis, 106
Cystocele, 206–207
Cystometry, 91, 93
Cystoplasty, 65
Cystoproctography, 184
Cystoscopy
  in possible surgical injury, 260
  in urinary incontinence, 103–106
Cystotomy, 264
Cystourethroscopy
  of fistulas, 240
  of urethral diverticula, 233
  in urinary incontinence, 102–103

D

Defecation
  normal, 157
Defecography, 156
Dermatomes, 43

Detrusor–sphincter dyssynergia
  pathophysiology of, 59, 70
  in spinal cord injury, 72–73
Diabetic neuropathy, 75–76
Dilation of vaginal agenesis, 20
Donut pessary, 193–194
Double-balloon catheterization, 108, 234
Duloxetine, 116, 119

E

Electrical stimulation therapy, 114, 129, 134–138
Electrodiagnostic testing, 44
Electromyography
  in fecal incontinence, 154
  in pelvic floor disorders, 44–45
  in urinary retention, 143
Endopelvic fascia anatomy, 3–5
Enteric nervous system, 37
Enterocele repair, 223–225
Episiotomy repair, 163
Estrogen replacement therapy
  in pelvic floor prolapse, 189
  in urinary incontinence, 116–119
Exercises
  pelvic floor, 113–114, 160, 187–188
External genitalia
  ambiguous, 15–18
  stages in development of, 13

F

Fascia
  pelvic, 3–5
Fecal continence, 25, 36–38
Fecal incontinence
  causes of, 150–151, 160
  evaluation of, 149–156
  nonsurgical treatment of, 159–161
  overview of, 149–150, 159
  pathophysiology of, 67
  surgery for, 161–170, 172
Female pseudohermaphroditism, 18
Fistulas
  diagnosis of, 240
  genitourinary, 237–245
  rectovaginal, 247–253
Functional electrical stimulation, 114

G

Gastrointestinal disorders
  functional, 150

Gehrung pessary, 194–195
Gellhorn pessary, 197–198
Genital duct embryology, 12
Genital hiatus, 180
Genital tract anomalies, 9, 14–24
Genital tract embryology, 9–13
Genitourinary anomalies, 9–24, 257
  See also specific anomalies
Genitourinary fistulas, 237–245
Genitourinary injuries, 255–265
  diagnosis of, 259–260
  management of, 261–265
  overview of, 255–256
  prevention of, 256–259
Gonadal dysgenesis, 18

H

Halban enterocele repair, 224
Hemivagina, 20
Hermaphroditism, 15
High-fiber diet, 160, 170
Hymen anomalies, 14

I

Imperforate hymen, 14
Incontinence
  fecal, 149–157, 159–172. See also Fecal incontinence
  urinary, 81–108, 111–145. See also Urinary incontinence
Indwelling catheters, 61–62
Injuries
  obstetric, 68–69, 163–164
  pelvic plexus, 74–75
  spinal cord, 71–74, 160
  surgical, 255–265
Intermittent catheterization, 62, 144
InterStim system, 134–138
Intravenous pyelogram, 108
Intussusception
  colonic, 153
Irritative voiding, 105–106

L

Laceration of external anal sphincter, 152
Leak point pressure, 94–95
Levator ani muscle anatomy, 2–5, 205
Lifestyle changes
  in pelvic floor prolapse, 189

M

Male pseudohermaphroditism, 18
Manometry
  anal, 155
  in pelvic organ prolapse, 184
Marland pessary, 196
McCall culdoplasty, 225
Micturition
  lesions affecting, 57
  neurophysiology of, 36
Micturition reflex, 58
Mixed urinary incontinence, 81, 111
Moschcowitz enterocele repair, 224
Motor neurons, 27, 32
Multiple sclerosis, 76–78
Myotomes, 41

N

Nerve conduction testing, 46
Nerve stimulation, 114, 129, 134–138
Neurogenic bladder, 59
Neurologic examination
  in urinary incontinence, 85–86
Neuromodulation, 63, 145
Neurons
  anatomy and physiology of, 25–33
  classification of, 32
  spinal, 32–33
Neurotransmitters, 25–26

O

Obliterative pelvic surgery, 216–218
Obstetric injuries, 68–69, 163–164
Ovarian embryology, 11
Overactive bladder
  behavioral therapy in, 128
  biofeedback in, 128
  cystoscopy in, 105
  electrical stimulation in, 129
  overview of, 111, 127
  pathophysiology of, 53–55
  pharmacotherapy of, 129
  urodynamic testing in, 96–97

P

Pad testing, 90
Paravaginal defect repair, 206–207

Parkinson's disease, 70
Patient incontinence questionnaires, 83–84
Pelvic anatomy, 1–7, 74
Pelvic examination, 88
Pelvic floor
  anatomy of, 2
  muscle exercises for, 113–114
  neurologic examination of, 40–50
  in renal failure, 60
  sequelae of disorders of, 60
Pelvic organ prolapse
  clinical features of, 176–180
  diagnosis of, 175–185
  estrogen therapy in, 189
  exercises and lifestyle changes in, 188–189
  overview of, 175, 187, 203
  pessaries in, 190–200
  presurgical evaluation of, 180
  recording and sites of, 181–182
  recurrent, 183
  repair kits for, 226–227
  surgical procedures for, 203–227
  treatment complications in, 183
  vaginal delivery and, 68–69
Pelvic plexus
  anatomy of, 74
  nerve damage in, 75
Pelvic visceral function
  neurophysiology of, 25–50
  pathophysiology of, 53–78
Perineal membrane anatomy, 7
Perineal tears, 68
Perineoproctotomy, 250–251
Perineorrhaphy, 225
Peripheral nerve anatomy and physiology, 31–32
Pessaries
  general considerations in, 190–192, 200
  in pelvic floor prolapse, 190–200
  in urinary incontinence, 115
Postvoid residual assessment, 89
Pressure voiding study
  in urinary incontinence, 101
  in urinary retention, 142
Prolapse
  pelvic organ, 175–185, 187–200, 203–227
    See also Pelvic organ prolapse
Pseudohermaphroditism, 16, 18
Pudendal nerve
  damage to, 75
  testing of, 46, 153–154
Pulley suture, 215–216

Q

Quality of life tools, 84

R

Radiofrequency incontinence procedure, 121
Rectal prolapse, 182
  in fecal incontinence evaluation, 152
  repair of, 223–225
Rectal wall imbrication repair, 221
Rectoceles, 171, 185, 222–223
Rectovaginal fistulas
  causes of, 248
  classification of, 247
  diagnosis of, 248–249
  in fecal incontinence, 152
  surgical repair of, 250–253
Rectovaginal prolapse, 182
Rectovaginal septal defect repair, 219–220
Reflexes
  micturition, 58
  in pelvic floor disorder evaluation, 41–42, 48–49
Renal failure, 60
Renessa radiofrequency procedure, 121
Resiniferatoxin, 133
Ring pessary, 192–193

S

Sacral neuromodulation, 145
Sacral reflexes, 48, 88
Sacrospinous ligament fixation, 215
Sector ultrasound imaging, 89
Self-catheterization, 62, 144
Sensory neurons, 28, 32
Septate uterus, 24
Sexual ambiguity, 15–19
Sexual function
  pelvic floor disorders and, 60
  vaginal innervation and, 39
Shy-Drager syndrome, 70
Sigmoidocele, 185
Skin breakdown, 60
Sling procedures, 123–126
Somatosensory evoked potentials, 47
Sphincter motoneurons, 33
Sphincteroplasty
  anal, 161–170
Spinal anatomy
  neural, 31–33
  vascular, 71
Spinal cord injury, 71–74, 160
Stenting
  ureteral, 262
Stress incontinence
  ambulatory procedures for, 120–121
  behavioral treatment of, 112
  cough profile in, 100

electrical stimulation for, 114
  exercises for, 113–114
  overview of, 81, 111
  pathophysiology of, 53–55
  pessaries and tampons for, 115
  pharmacotherapy of, 116–119
  surgery for, 121–126
Surgical injuries, 255–256
  conditions predisposing to, 256
  prevention of, 257–259
  ureteral, 58–59, 259–263
  vesical, 263–265

T

Transient urinary incontinence, 56, 82
Trauma. *See* Injuries
Turner syndrome, 19

U

Unicornuate uterus, 24
Ureteral stenting, 262
Ureteroneocystostomy, 262–263
Ureteroureterostomy, 263
Ureters
  anatomy of, 256–257
  surgical injuries of, 58–59, 260–263
Urethra
  anatomy of, 5–6, 230
  neurophysiology of, 26, 30
Urethral calculi, 232
Urethral diverticula, 229–236
  clinical features of, 229–230
  diagnosis of, 107–108, 232–234
  proposed causes of, 231
  surgery for, 235–236
Urethral dysfunction
  pharmacotherapy of, 63
  urinary diversion in, 66
Urethral instability, 98
Urethral pressure profilometry, 98–99, 234
Urethral reflexes, 49
Urethral sphincter neurophysiology, 35
Urethrography, 234
Urethropexy, 123
Urethroscopy, 102–103
Urethrovaginal fistulas, 237, 239–242
Urethrovesical junction mobility, 90
Urge incontinence, 81, 111, 112, 114, 128–139
  See also Overactive bladder
Urinary continence
  anatomic mechanism of, 5–6
  neurophysiology of, 25, 34–36

Urinary diary, 85–86
Urinary diversion therapy, 66
Urinary drainage
  postoperative, 265
Urinary incontinence. *See also* Specific types
  acupuncture for, 131
  behavioral therapy in, 112, 128
  causes of transient, 56, 82
  classification of, 112
  cystometry in, 91
  cystourethroscopy in, 102–106
  electrical stimulation in, 112, 114, 129, 134–138
  exercise therapy in, 113–114
  imaging techniques in, 107–108
  overview of, 81–82, 111
  pathophysiology of, 53–58
  patient history in, 82–86
  pessaries and tampons in, 115
  pharmacotherapy of, 116–119, 129–130, 132–133
  physical examination in, 86–90
  pressure-flow study in, 101
  Renessa radiofrequency device in, 121
  surgery for, 121–126
  treatment options in, 112
  urodynamic testing in, 91–100
Urinary retention
  causes of, 140
  definitions of, 139
  diagnosis of, 141–143
  management of, 143–145
  signs and symptoms of, 141
Urinary tract
  brain pathways to, 34
  dysfunction of. *See* Urinary tract dysfunction
  embryology of, 10
  neurophysiology of, 34–36
  spinal nerves and, 33
Urinary tract dysfunction. *See also* Specific disorders
  in diabetes, 76
  lesions affecting micturition in, 57
  in multiple sclerosis, 76–78
  pathophysiology of, 53–60
  spinal cord injury and, 72–74

Urine testing in incontinence, 89
Urodynamic testing
  in pelvic organ prolapse, 184
  in urinary incontinence, 91–100
  in urinary retention, 141–142
Uroflowmetry, 91–92
Urogenital ducts, 12
Urogenital fistulas. *See also* specific fistulas
  steroid pretreatment of, 240
Urogenital ridges, 9
Uterine anomalies, 22–24
Uterine didelphys, 23
Uterovaginal pelvic organ prolapse, 177–179

V

Vagina
  anatomy of, 1, 4, 204
  anomalies of, 20–21
  embryology of, 12
  neurophysiology of, 38–39
  in pelvic organ prolapse, 176–182, 204–227
Vaginal cones, 113
Vaginal delivery, 68–69, 176
Vaginoplasty
  for prolapse, 204–227
  for vaginal agenesis, 21
Vanilloids, 63, 133
Vesicopsoas hitch, 263
Vesicovaginal fistulas, 238–239, 243–245
Videourodynamics, 107
Viscerosomatic reflexes, 49
Voiding cystogram, 107
Voiding dysfunction
  causes of, 140
  diagnosis of, 50, 141–143
  treatment of, 143–145